GOD DOES HEAL TODAY

GOD DOES HEAL TODAY

Pastoral Principles and Practice of Faith-Healing

Robert Dickinson

Published for Rutherford House

by

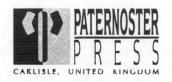

CARLISLE, UNITED KINGDOM

First published 1995
by The Paternoster Press, P.O. Box 300, Carlisle, Cumbria
CA3 0QS U.K., and Rutherford House, 17 Claremont Park
Edinburgh EH6 7PJ, Scotland

01 00 99 98 97 96 95   7 6 5 4 3 2 1

British Library Cataloguing in Publication Data

Dickinson, Robert
God Does Heal Today: Pastoral Principles
and Practice of Faith-Healing
I. Title
615.852

ISBN 0-946068-56-9

Typeset by Rutherford House, Edinburgh

Printed in Great Britain by BPC Wheatons Ltd, Exeter

CONTENTS

PART I • THE BIBLE TEACHING

PART II • THE CHURCHES HEALING

PART III • MODERN HEALING MINISTRIES

Individual Healers:

(i) Healing and evangelism
(ii) Healing and 'prophecy'
(iii) Other problems
(iv) Gunstone's questions

PART IV • PASTORAL PRINCIPLES AND PRACTICE

Acknowledgements

I should like to express my sincere thanks to Rev. Principal T. S. Reid, B.A., B.D., M.Th., Dip.Ed., of Union Theological College, Belfast whose advice and encouragement throughout made this project the more enjoyable. I should like also to acknowledge the helpful cooperation of the five practitioners of the ministry of healing who provided personal insight into the nature and methods of their work. My thanks are also due to Mrs. D. McDowell, the librarian at Union Theological College for her gracious and ready assistance in making available much of the resource material, and to my son, Rev. J. R. Dickinson, B.A., B.D., Minister of Seaview Presbyterian Church, Belfast, for his considerable help both with his computer and photocopier.

I am indebted beyond measure to my wife Pat whose loving devotion and care nursed me back to health from the 'valley of the shadow' many years ago, who has been my loyal and indispensable partner through all the years of my ministry in the Gospel, and who reared our four children each of whom is now engaged in the ministry of the church. Above all, I would humbly acknowledge the unchanging love of my heavenly father and the boundless grace of my saviour who, in his infinite mercy and goodness, saved me, called me, equipped me, healed me, guided me, chastened me, pardoned me, made me his, and has given me the inestimable privilege for more than forty years of ministering in word and prayer his power to heal and 'save to the uttermost all who come unto God by him'.

Author's Note

Since the publication of this book began, the author has suffered a grave illness and been healed of cancer, thus experiencing at first hand the principles of Divine healing which have been discerned in the Word of God and set forth in this study.

It is, therefore with deep conviction that 'God *Does* Heal Today' both through and far beyond the resources of human wisdom, skill, love and care which he provides and which have been extended to me in such abundant measure by my devoted wife and family, by doctors, nurses and Hospital staff, and by a host of colleagues and Christian friends throughout the length and breadth of the church and far beyond in their concern and continuing prayers, that this work goes forth with the desire and hope that in some small way it may be of help to others who may be wrestling with these deep and divine issues, and above all, that in everything Christ may have the pre-eminence and the glory.

Robert Dickinson

PREFACE

The problem with 'faith-healing' is not that it happens, or even that it doesn't happen when it is sought or expected. It is that so often the claims that are made for its availability, and the excuses that are made for its failure are based upon superficial understanding or interpretation of the Scriptures coupled with a deep Christian compassion for those who suffer and a genuine concern to glorify the Lord Jesus Christ by seeking to follow his example and to fulfil what is perceived to be his command not only to 'preach the word' but also to 'heal the sick'.

The 'healing' ministry is as inseparable from the calling of the Christian believer and of the church as it was from the life and work of Christ and of the Apostles. Through the grace of Christ the believer himself experiences forgiveness, reconciliation and peace with God which is able to resolve the guilt and inner conflict of mind and soul which can, and often do, give rise to all sorts of physical and psychological symptoms and disorders. And when the causes are removed, the effects too will disappear. But even when physical disease or disorder is not the result of inner guilt, conflict or failure on the part of the sufferer, saving faith in Christ creates a new relationship with God in which the power of prayer and the counsel of God's Word make available, according to the sovereign purposes of God's love, the possibility either of physical healing through the direct intervention of the divine power, or the healing of mind and heart which rests on the grace which is 'sufficient' and the infallible assurance that 'all things work together for good to them that love God' (Rom. 8:28).

But not only do believers themselves experience such healing. They also become dispensers of such healing through the ministry of prayer and intercession on behalf of others, and through the 'ministry of reconciliation' to which they are called and committed (2 Cor. 5:18). As members of the church of Christ they are individually and together engaged in a community of healing in which the love of Christ constrains them, either directly or indirectly to feed the hungry, care for the lonely, the sad, the oppressed, the afflicted and the dying without regard to race, class, age or circumstance. The proclamation of the Good News of salvation is reinforced, and the saving power of

Christ demonstrated, in the personal and practical ministry of love and self-sacrifice in order that others might believe. By the consecrated use both of 'natural' talents and of those special gifts which the Holy Spirit bestows to equip for any and every situation, it is the privilege and the responsibility of the believer and the church (the believers together) to be the harbingers of the divine grace and power which are able 'to do exceeding abundantly above all that we ask or think' (Eph. 3:20).

The doctor, by means of medicine, surgery or psychiatry seeks, through his God-given and divinely effective resources of wisdom and skill, to heal for the sake of restoring or preserving bodily or mental health and vigour to live an active and purposeful life. The Christian believer and the church seek through prayer, counsel and the spiritual resources of faith, hope and love to be the means of communicating the divine power and grace that can restore and preserve body, mind, *and spirit* in that 'newness of life' both in time and eternity which is made possible only through the redemption obtained for us sinners through the atoning death of Christ on Calvary and 'the power of his resurrection' (Phil. 3:10). The healing administered by the doctor is divine healing addressed primarily (though not necessarily exclusively) to the needs of body and mind. The healing communicated by the Christian believer and the church is divine healing addressed through body and mind to the needs of the soul—it is the 'wholeness' of the whole person both in time and eternity.

This ministry of wholeness is communicated by the church in many ways. In the New Testament times, and since the Protestant Reformation, it is offered primarily through the preaching of the Good News of the Gospel of Jesus Christ 'which is the power of God unto salvation to everyone that believeth' (Rom. 1:16). But the implementation of the Gospel involves worship, prayer, and demonstration in practical and material terms of the love of Christ within and through the fellowship of God's people. Thus all Services of Worship are, or ought to be, occasions of healing in so far as they provide opportunity for thanksgiving, praise, intercession, forgiveness, instruction in the Word of God, counsel, admonition and mutual encouragement in word or sacrament. The church also provides the ministry of healing through the particular ministries of pastors, elders, teachers and leaders of the young, and of the various departments of congregational life and witness, and through the ministry of those members who exercise special gifts of wisdom, counsel, sympathy and service both within and beyond the fellowship of believers. All of this is truly the ministry of divine healing without which any congregation or Christian fellowship would simply not be the church of Christ as revealed and constituted in the New Testament. So let it be understood that 'divine healing' is alone the work of God which all Christians have experienced and therefore in which all devoutly believe. And the ministry of 'divine healing' is an essential aspect of the life and witness of the Christian church.

In more recent times the ministry of healing has also been developed by Christian agencies without any relationship to particular Churches, congregations or fellowships, who claim to exercise the 'gift of healing' endowed by the Holy Spirit. Such ministries are carried on by means of radio, television, telephone, correspondence or mass rallies, and because of their form and nature they are open to particular dangers. For example, there is the tendency to create personality cults of those whose 'star' performances make the normal pattern of pastoral ministry seem unimpressive; a sensational overemphasis or concentration on one particular form of healing to the exclusion of the others; and the temptation to play-up, or even invent, 'success' where it is not in evidence. But, to be fair, the same might be said, perhaps to a lesser degree, of the 'private' practice of faith-healing by any individual whose help may be sought on the basis of his 'reputation for success' rather than on any response to the Word of God.

Within the ministry of 'divine healing' which takes many forms and uses a variety of means, there is one particular application. It is the healing of physical or psychological disease or disorder by means of God's power apart from the use of medical or psychiatric knowledge or techniques.

That is the subject of the following pages.

SUMMARY

The thesis is in four parts and seeks from the pastoral principles and practice of faith-healing set forth in the Scriptures to establish an appropriate pattern for such a ministry today.

PART I, having set parameters for the scope of the enquiry, examines the Bible teaching and practice as illustrated in both the Old and New Testaments, and especially in the work of Christ and the Apostles which is normally regarded as the basis for the practice of faith-healing in modern times. The nature and purpose of 'miracles' and the phenomenon of 'demons' are also examined. The nature of 'spiritual gifts' and the debate concerning their continuance beyond the Apostolic era is discussed. The implications of the James 5 passage are dealt with as are the nature and relevance of the 'faith' element in healing, the failure of faith-healing, and the ultimate fact and significance of death in relation to the question of healing whether for the believer or the unbeliever.

PART II gives a brief account of faith-healing as taught and practised in various Churches since the Apostolic period with particular reference to the Church of the Fathers, the Roman Catholic Church and the Reformed Churches as represented by the Anglican, Methodist, Pentecostal Churches and the Presbyterian Church in Ireland.

PART III deals with the teaching and practice of faith-healing in modern times. The results of interviews with five local practitioners are tabulated and compared. The work of a medical consultant who is also involved in the faith-healing ministry is reviewed. And three healing movements; an Anglican, a Roman Catholic and a Charismatic are examined in some detail.

PART IV seeks to draw together the principles discerned and the conclusions arrived at in the preceding sections, and from these to formulate pastoral principles and practice for today.

1

SETTING LIMITS

I. A SUITABLE NAME

That people are healed apart from the use of medical or psychiatric means is not in question. Whether in the physical or mental sphere, there are those who claim to have been healed or cured through prayer, faith, Christian Science, transcendental meditation, the occult, the veneration of saints or relics, the ministry of healers exercising particular 'gifts' or charms, *etc*. In these pages it is proposed to examine the phenomenon of non-medical healing which is to be found in both the Old and New Testament Scriptures, in the teaching and practice of the early days of the Christian church, and in various forms within the Christian community ever since.

There is, however, an immediate problem—to find a satisfactory designation for the practice. To call it 'Divine Healing' is not satisfactory because Christians regard all healing, by every legitimate means, as part of the sovereign Providence and activity of God in the world. Christian doctors, moreover, regard themselves and their skills as but the instruments of the Divine Physician.

'In the healing of every disease of whatever kind', writes Dr Henry E. Goddard, 'we cannot be too deeply impressed with the Lord's part of the work. He is the operator. We are the co-operators. More and more I am impressed that every patient of mine who has ever risen up from his sick bed on to his feet again has done so by the divine power. Not I, but the Lord, has cured him. And it is this fact that the Lord does so much, that gives to different systems of healing their apparent cures.'[1]

To call it 'Miracle Healing' presents similar difficulty with the added complication that the 'miracle' may refer either to the nature of the healing itself or to the mere fact of it. The Lord may use perfectly 'natural' means to accomplish his ends, but, of course, he may sovereignly dispose them at his divine discretion in an unnatural or supernatural way.

To call it 'Faith-Healing' is also difficult because it appears to lay the efficacy of the event upon 'faith', or at least to place the emphasis upon 'faith' in the accomplishment of the healing or cure when, as will later be made evident, 'faith', whether in the sense of theological faith in God as the divine Creator and Redeemer or simply confidence in his power to heal, may or may not be seen to be involved on the part of the sufferer. Nor may the effectiveness of the healing be determined by the degree of faith exhibited. Nevertheless, in so far as the healing is effected through prayer, and all effective or 'believing' prayer requires the exercise of faith on the part of the one who prays, whether on his own behalf or on behalf of others, 'faith' must in fact be a necessary element in the healing process.

To call it 'Spiritual Healing' is not appropriate either because what we are dealing with is really physical or psychological healing by spiritual means. Moreover, 'spiritual healing' may more properly refer to the healing of conditions which relate to specifically spiritual or religious rather than physical causes, or even be thought to refer to 'spiritualist' healing.

So, since some identification is necessary, for the purpose of this study the term 'faith-healing' will be used in spite of its limitations, simply because of its widespread acceptance as a convenient, if to some a somewhat disconcerting, term of reference to the teaching and practice of healing based not upon the use of medical or psychiatric skills and resources, but upon the divine intervention of God directly in response to the human cry for help.

II. BODY, MIND AND SOUL

The phenomenon which we propose to examine in some detail is not the question of health, physical, mental and spiritual, in general terms. It is accepted that the spiritual condition of any person has direct relation to and effect upon every aspect of personality, character, physical, mental and total wellbeing. Both the Old Testament and the New insist upon such a relationship.

> The significance of the virtual absence of the word 'body' from the pages of the Old Testament is that health is not presented there in primarily physical terms. This is in contrast to the

modern popular concept of health which is mainly physical in character.[2]

In the Old Testament health is 'wholeness', 'completeness', 'shalom', whether in the sphere of the physical, mental, spiritual, individual, social or national (Ps. 29:11; Isa. 54:13; Mal. 2:5, 6). Such health is procured by obedience to God's law (Deut. 30:15, 16), and by the establishment and maintenance of a right relationship to God (Isa. 26:3), whereas disobedience may result in disease and affliction (Isa. 48:22; Ezek. 7:25). Here is the very essence of the doctrine of the 'fall' in Genesis. All sickness, disease and death is the consequence of the fall of our first parents from 'the estate in which they were created'.[3] In this sense, and in this sense only, it can be said that all sickness is the consequence of sin. In this sense too it may be said that it was not God's initial design or purpose that mankind, or any part of the creation, should be the victim of pain, weakness, disease, destruction, decay, despair or death. All of these are revealed to be the direct and inevitable consequence of man's estrangement from God by sin (Gen. 2:17). Health is the restoration of all that has been forfeited by man's revolt against God's sovereign decrees, not only in terms of human restoration, but also of the restoration of creation itself (Rom. 8:19–24).

> It is only when man's being is whole and his relationships right that he can be truly described as healthy. The basic relationship of all is man's relationship to God and when this is disturbed all human relationships are disturbed whether they are of man to himself, to his fellows, or to his environment.[4]

The New Testament concept of health is precisely the same as that of the Old Testament. But the concern of the New Testament is more immediately to reveal how man's health, shattered by the 'fall', can be restored in Christ. It might best be summed up in the words of Christ himself, 'I am come that they might have life and that they might have it more abundantly' (John 10:10). The apostle Paul may be said to define health in 1 Thessalonians 5:23 thus: 'I pray God your whole spirit and soul and body be preserved blameless unto the coming of our Lord Jesus Christ'. The possibility of such health was personified in the earthly life of Jesus who although 'touched with the feeling of our infirmities' and 'in all points tempted like as we are' yet was 'without sin' (Heb. 4:15). And the actuality of it was secured by his death and resurrection. Thus as Matthew says he fulfilled the prophecy of Isaiah 53:4, 'Himself took our infirmities and bare our sicknesses' (Matt. 8:17). It is also asserted in the use of the verb *sozo* in reference both to healing and to the work of redemption:

> it is clear that its wide application in the Gospels indicates that the Christian concept of healing and the Christian concept of

salvation overlap to a degree which varies in different situations, but are never completely separable. Healing of the body is never purely physical, and the salvation of the soul is never purely spiritual, but both are combined in the total deliverance of the whole man, a deliverance which is foreshadowed and illustrated in the healing miracles of Jesus in the gospels.[5]

It is also accepted that the church's ministry of healing has, of necessity, the widest possible application to the suffering of individuals and of human society, both in terms of the support and promotion of medical, social and welfare services, either directly or as provided by national or local government, and in terms of its fulfilment of its biblical charter as the agent of 'reconciliation'—'all things are of God, who hath reconciled us to himself by Jesus Christ, and hath given to us the ministry of reconciliation; to wit that God was in Christ, reconciling the world unto himself...and hath committed unto us the word of reconciliation' (2 Cor. 5:18, 19).

So we see the church as a family of those who love the Lord Jesus Christ. We are his agents in this twentieth century world, through whom he can care for the vagrant; stand by the alcoholic; mend broken marriages, broken minds or broken bodies. Each local church must take up the work to which it is called in its locality, and adapt the pattern of its life accordingly.[6]

Indeed, it is strongly argued by some that failure to deal with the question of healing in this context is a fundamental mistake:

Part of our difficulty in the Christian healing ministry in the past has been our tendency to subordinate health to healing. This has led to an emphasis on the individual at the expense of the community, an emphasis on the sacramental at the expense of the social, an emphasis upon signs and wonders at the expense of a responsible theology of suffering and death. Fortunately we are now beginning to recognise the dangers implicit in this lack of balance. The continuing challenge...is how we hold these different perspectives in a fruitful and creative tension.[7]

There is, of course, truth in this assertion of the need for such a 'balance' in the church's ministry of healing. But in our present study we shall be concerned with the particular phenomenon of the healing of physical or psychological disorder in the individual by the power of God apart from medical or psychiatric treatment, which we call 'faith-healing', rather than the wider issues of the social and political implications of the healing of divisions, memories, conflicts, injustices and cruelties which also is, or ought to be, rightfully the concern and ministry of the church in the world.

III. THE ULTIMATE 'GUIDEBOOK'

All this being assumed then, it is our purpose primarily to examine what the Bible teaches in regard to the doctrine and practice of 'faith-healing' and that from a 'Reformed' position which holds that

> The Word of God set forth in the Scriptures of the Old and New Testaments is the only infallible rule of faith and practice and the supreme standard of the church.[8]

Inevitably elements of the discussion in regard to 'faith-healing' will involve the silence of Scripture. But no doctrine or practice can be promulgated on the basis of the silence of Scripture, nor can any doctrine or practice be accepted on such a basis either. Two matters arise from this position: (1) it is accepted that not every healing ever performed by Jesus or the Apostles is recorded. Indeed, at the close of the Gospel of St John this is forthrightly stated, 'there are also many other things which Jesus did, which, if they should be written every one, I suppose that even the world itself could not contain the books that should be written' (John 21:25). Obviously the Scriptural historians had to be selective in their writing, just as Jesus and the Apostles had to be selective in their healing. This means that we must be the more careful in our assessment of what is recorded. It does not give warrant for assuming or supposing what is not there. And (2) it is an accepted principle in Reformed interpretation of the Scriptures, as stated in the Scriptures themselves, that 'no prophecy of the Scripture is of any private (*i.e.* individual) interpretation' (2 Pet. 1:20), but that

> the infallible rule of interpretation of scripture is the scripture itself; and therefore, when there is a question about the true and full sense of any scripture, (which is not manifold but one), it must be searched and known by other places that speak more clearly.[9]

This means that, for example, the unique instance of the blind man who received his full sight as the result of being touched twice by Jesus, cannot alone be made the basis of a theory that divine healing is to be effected by a gradual process, unless such a process can be confirmed by other Scriptures.

This is not to say that the experience of the church after the New Testament period is not of interest or value. But it is evident that, after the passing of the Apostles, the church quickly began to depart from the teaching and example of the Scriptures and became subject to all kinds of heresy and superstitious practices which, in many instances, were contrary to or beside the Word of God.

> Some have been unable to see in the later developments anything but what was bad—corruption of primitive truth and degen-

eration from a purer type. The simplicity of scriptural teaching has been, it is argued, from the apostolical age onwards, ever more and more contaminated. Men were not content with the divine revelation and sought to improve upon it by all kinds of human additions and superstitions. Above all, the church and the priests, the guardians of the revelation, perverted it in every way they could to preserve their own selfish interests, and so was built up the great system of ecclesiastical doctrines and ordinances under which the simplicity and purity of apostolic Christianity was altogether obscured and lost.[10]

Whatever interest therefore may be found in extra-biblical records or experience, they can have no place in the formulation of church doctrine or practice, except in so far as they conform to the teaching and example of Scripture.

Similarly, evidence derived from the experience of faith-healers may be of interest or value in comment on, or illustration of, biblical doctrine or practice, but it cannot formulate or establish doctrine or practice apart from the authority or precedence of Scripture. This, of course, is not to call in question the truth of claims that may be made, although it must be acknowledged that unsubstantiated evidence or claims which cannot be, or have not been, submitted to medical or other reliable and competent investigation, do present real problems of assessment. Nor is there any predisposition to dispute that, in his sovereign love and power, God may and does intervene in miraculous ways in human and personal experience. But only such opinion or experience as conforms to the requirements or example of the Scriptures can determine how the life and work of the church is to be ordered.

Whatever conclusions may be drawn, therefore, must be based upon the teaching of Scripture or must be open to correction or amendment in the light of evidence produced from or sustained by Scripture.

NOTES

1 As quoted in *Counterfeit Miracles*, B. B. Warfield, Banner of Truth Trust, 1972, p. 172 from *The New Church Review*, Vol. XV, 1908, pp. 415ff.

2 J. Wilkinson, *Health and Healing,* Handsel Press, Edinburgh, 1980, p. 4.

3 *Shorter Catechism,* J. G. Eccles, Edinburgh, 1981, Q. 13.

4 J. Wilkinson, *Health and Healing,* Handsel Press, Edinburgh, 1980, p. 1.

5 J. Wilkinson, *Health and Healing,* Handsel Press, Edinburgh,

1980, p. 33.
6 M. Wilson, *The Church is Healing,* London, SCM Press, 1966, p. 15.
7 D. Dale, *Health and Healing*, No.1, Churches' Council for Health and Healing, London, 1989, p. 1.
8 *Constitution and Government of the Presbyterian church in Ireland,* Belfast, 1980, p. 10.
9 *Westminster Confession of Faith*, J. G. Eccles, Edinburgh, 1981, chap. 1:9.
10 J. F. Bethune-Baker, *An Introduction to the Early History of Christian Doctrine,* Methuen, London, 1949, p. 33.

2

THE MASTER HEALING

I. THE BASIC PATTERN

Since the primary justification of the doctrine and practice of faith-healing is said to be the fact that Jesus healed and that he commanded or commissioned his disciples to do so, we begin by examining what Jesus himself did.

The accompanying Tables I–III catalogue the healings wrought by Jesus. In them we are immediately made aware of the limitation of the data that is available to us. There are, in fact, only twenty-six individual incidents covered by the four Gospels, and only twelve incidents of multiple healings. These must surely constitute only a small but representative proportion of Jesus' 'mighty works'. And they present us with a number of problems.

For example, it is not always possible to be sure that the Gospel references are to the same incident (*e.g.* Matt. 8:28–34 refers to two men while Mark and Luke refer to only one. Again, Matt. 20:29–34 refers to two blind men whereas Mark and Luke refer to one whom Mark names as Bartimaeus. Or again, in the case of duplicate accounts there are differences of detail which do not affect the nature of the evidence).

Equally, it is not always possible, especially in the records of multiple healings, to distinguish positively between cases of physical healing and those of exorcism of demons. With regard to the reasons or motives for healing, the question of compassion arises. While it must be assumed that Jesus did have compassion for all who suffered, there are only three individual instances and two multiple healings where compassion is stated to have been the motive. It would be unsafe, therefore, to rule out compassion in those cases where it is not specifically mentioned. But, on the other hand, it is unwarranted to claim, as some do, that compassion was the motive in every case (for example, William Barclay, *And He had Compassion on Them*).

The question of 'touch' is also somewhat complicated. Some would make much of the fact that Jesus touched his patients and find in this a weighty justification of the practice of 'laying on of hands'.

> Why do we lay on hands? Chiefly because it was Jesus' usual method, so much so that when people asked for healing their words of request very often were: 'Come and lay your hands on him or her'.... It is evident therefore that while Jesus could heal by his mere word, he seems to have resorted chiefly to the laying on of hands. The reason probably was that while the Divine Healing Grace could be communicated by means of speech and thought, it was more effective on direct contact...it is clear from the Bible record that he healed many more by his touch than by his word to judge from the cases of which details are given.[1]

But the fact is (Tables I and II) that in only three individual incidents out of the twenty-six is Jesus specifically said to have healed by touch while in eight he is said to have used both word and touch, and in twelve word only. In the remaining two we are not specifically told but since they were exorcisms it most probably was by word alone (see pp. 11ff.).

Of particular interest to us is the factor of faith in the healings of Jesus. In the records of general or multiple healings the question of faith nowhere is mentioned. In the individual incidents, out of the twenty-six recorded, faith is not mentioned in fourteen of them. Again, caution must be exercised in drawing conclusions. The absence of a specific reference to the exercise of faith by the patient may not always mean that it was totally absent or irrelevant. But it must surely make any claim that healing was dependent upon the exercise of faith by the patient at least precarious.

Again there is the problem as to whether Jesus healed all who were sick and came to him. We are told, for example, that in Nazareth 'He could there do no mighty work, save that he laid his hands upon a few sick folk, and healed them' (Mark 6:5). Does this mean that none, or only a few sought and received healing or that while many sought only a few actually received it? In six instances we are told he healed 'many', and in three that he healed 'some'. This leaves open the question as to whether or not all who came were healed. Since there is not a single reference to anyone having been refused healing or turned away by Jesus, it would appear reasonable to conclude that all who came were in fact healed, and certainly, as we might expect, there is no recorded instance of Jesus' word or touch ever having failed. Such an event, we may be sure, could not possibly have failed to be noted by the enemies of Jesus if not by his friends.

It would be wrong to conclude from the fact that in total only thirty-eight instances of healing, whether individual or multiple, are specifically recorded in the three years of Jesus' public ministry, healing was therefore a rare or insignificant aspect of his earthly ministry. But equally, it must be wrong to conclude that it constituted the most persistent or important aspect of his work.

Two facts are inescapable. First, in only four of the twenty-six individual incidents, and possibly six of the twelve multiple incidents, is Jesus said to have taken the initiative. It might also be noted that in five cases, Jesus having healed gave specific instructions to the patients not to reveal what had happened. The reasons for this procedure will be looked at later, but at least it seems *prima facie* to indicate that his activity in healing was not intended to be the primary purpose of his ministry or the supreme evidence of the nature of his person and work. Second, the incident at the Pool of Bethesda in John 5:1–16 seems to indicate the very selective nature of Jesus' healings. We are told that in the five porches 'lay a great multitude of impotent folk, of blind, halt, withered, waiting for the moving of the water' (John 5:3). Doubtless the Master had a particular reason for choosing to heal only one, but the fact that he left all the others, whom he might have healed, to their unhappy plight would seem to reinforce the view that he did not regard healing as the primary purpose of his mission in the world.

In general, therefore, it appears that healing is carried out in the context of preaching and teaching in the gospels rather than the other way round. In other words, healing as an activity of Jesus is practised in illustration of his preaching and teaching rather than as their text and occasion.[2]

II. ONCE AND FOR ALL

The incidents recorded present important and instructive principles of which we may take note. When Jesus healed the effect was immediate and obvious. This was so in every individual case except two: (1) the blind man (Mark 8:22–26) who was not completely healed at once but whose cure was effected in two stages, and (2) the other blind man who having been touched by Jesus was sent to the Pool of Siloam to wash the clay from his eyes and obtain his sight (John 9:7). Since no explanation of Jesus' procedure on these occasions is given it is idle to speculate. But this much can be said. There was no question of a prolonged course of treatment, or of a second visit to the healer. Nor were the blind men told that their sight would gradually improve and eventually be restored. Whatever the reason for the method used by Jesus, it is clear that the healing was totally effected in the one operation and was not the result either of the normal processes of healing or of repetitive visits to the healer. Furthermore, in both cases the healing was immediately obvious to others, as is evidenced in the case of the man blind from birth by the reaction of the 'neighbours', and in the case of the other by the command of the Lord that he should go home directly and not disclose it to those 'in the town' of Bethsaida.

This matter of the immediacy of healing upon the word of Christ is strikingly demonstrated in three particular cases in each of which the person healed was not in the presence of Christ at the time. The healing nevertheless took place, at a distance, though precisely at the moment when the word of divine power was spoken. The centurion's servant was 'healed in the very same hour' (Matt. 9:13) so that when those who were sent by the centurion to ask for the help of Jesus returned they 'found the servant well that had been sick' (Luke 7:10). And in the case of the daughter of the Syrophoenician woman, it is reported that when Jesus spoke the word of healing 'her daughter was made well from that very hour' (Matt. 15:28). Another report states, 'when she was come to her house, she found the demon gone out and her daughter lying upon the bed' (Mark 7:30). The nobleman's son at Capernaum was healed while his father was still talking to Jesus at a day's journey distant from the home. When the father returned home to find the son, who had been 'at the point of death', already well, it is explicitly reported that 'Then inquired he of them the hour when he began to improve. And they said unto him, Yesterday, at the seventh hour, the fever left him. So the father knew that it was at the same hour in which Jesus said unto him, Thy son liveth' (John 4:52, 53). In each case, then, the healing was not the result of a prolonged or repetitive process, but rather, instant upon the word spoken by Christ.

In modern practice instant healing usually does not take place. Indeed it would appear that so far as some faith-healers are concerned, it is almost unfair to expect it to do so. For example, J. C. Peddie writes,

> Some sufferers come expecting us to perform instantaneous cures as Jesus did, and many lose patience and give up hope when cure is delayed. But with faith and patience, especially patience, every rheumatic condition yields.[3]

He explains the difference between the immediate effectiveness of Jesus' healing and that of modern-day practitioners thus,

> We require more time to impart and maintain benefit, not to speak of effecting a complete cure, because we are inferior to Jesus

Christ in surrender, purity, sanctification, and in our sense of unity with God. A consequence of our inferiority is that God has to make up in time what we lack in spiritual qualifications. If Jesus Christ were here, every case, even the most difficult, would be instantaneously and completely cured, as we learn from the Bible. We do however have occasional instantaneous results.[4]

Michael Wilson goes further suggesting that the whole concern and enquiry with regard to the practice of healing in the New Testament may be, and often is, a spurious business seeking to apply or impose upon present-day situations conditions which are no longer relevant. He says,

At present there is emphasis in the church's ministry of healing, on the New Testament miracles of Christ and on trying to reproduce them. Much of this work is fantasy, concerned with imposing principles on life, rather than examining the reality of life as it is. In the church we must take medicine seriously as the work of God which he is entrusting to men.[5]

But few even of those who most diligently pursue the practice of faith-healing deny for a moment the God-given nature and value of medicine and medical practice, or would regard faith-healing methods as a general substitute for normal medical procedures. For example, George Jeffreys, founder and leader of the Elim Foursquare Gospel Alliance, who had a remarkable ministry of evangelism and healing throughout the British Isles between the two world wars when many thousands were converted and vast numbers healed through prayer, says,

When we come to consider the human creation, we find that God in his love and mercy has provided the means of healing for all mankind, saints and sinner alike, by the operation of the natural law which is inherent in the human organism. Physicians and nurses through much study have become acquainted with this natural law of healing: consequently they can intelligently assist nature to heal or re-assert itself. They minister in the realm of the natural, and it is the duty and privilege of every Christian to pray for them in their work.[6]

Commenting on Psalm 115; 121:2; 124:8; 134:3; 146:6; Genesis 14:9; Acts 7:49, where God is declared to be the 'Maker of heaven and earth', Brooks says,

He is Creator and Sustainer alike of the miracle processes of heaven and of the natural processes of earth. The miraculous may transcend the natural. But there is no antagonism. This is so in respect of healing and health.... But there are two channels by which health may flow to man: (a) the miraculous channel; (b) the natural channel (in which are to be included medicine, surgery, herbs, *etc.*, and various psychological techniques, such

as the 'power of mind over matter'). Along whichever channel
we receive healing, we ought humbly to recognise God as its
source and glorify Him as the giver.[7]
It may be that there are those in the more extreme Christian sects who
press their belief and practice of faith-healing to foolish and sometimes
dangerous extremes, but then there are many medical practitioners who
are so prejudiced as to be unable to consider the possibility of the
efficacy of faith-healing or to countenance even the factual evidence
of those who actually have been so healed.

Michael Wilson's statement that,

> The New Testament images of the church are fluid, adaptable and
> dynamic. There is no reason whatever why she should not
> penetrate the new healing world of science—indeed she must.
> But the Church's official 'healing ministry' as it exists today is
> too frozen in ecclesiastical moulds, or busy trying to prepare the
> way for the wind of the Spirit by a literal imitation of the biblical
> methods of long ago, and is diverting thought and energy very
> badly needed for this new task[8]

needs careful qualification. It would appear that in his view not only
should we not be expecting healing to happen as it did in the ministry
of Jesus, but that we should rather be turning away from biblical
patterns of healing activity to dependence solely on modern medical
techniques.

In both of these positions, therefore, there is a fundamental flaw.
Peddie's explanation for the modern failure to produce instantaneous
effect founders on the fact that he appears to believe that the ability
of God to heal is in some way determined by the condition of the
healer. But, as even the Christian doctor will acknowledge, the power
to heal lies in the sovereign power of the Divine Physician, not in the
qualifications of the healer or the perseverance of the patient.
Moreover, it is the same power as that manifested by Christ. Since the
healing claims to be done in the name of Christ (*i.e.* by his authority
and power) there is no reason why the same result should not be
obtained. But the truth sadly is that, in spite of the most strenuous
denials on the part of faith-healers, there is a tendency sometimes to
link the expectation of success to the expertise of the healer or the
'faith and patience' of the patient. Wilson's position would appear to
be a straightforward distrust of the efficacy of faith-healing methods
and a preference for traditional, if updated, medical or psychiatric
resources.

In the experience of those healed by Jesus there was never any
confusion between the physical effects and the spiritual. This is made
particularly plain in the case of the man sick of the palsy when Jesus
dealt first with his spiritual condition and afterwards with his physical.

There is no suggestion whatever that psychological or spiritual benefits derived from his visit to Jesus should have been regarded as a substitute for physical healing. In fact, the Lord expressly used the physical healing as a proof of the spiritual rather than the other way round—'that ye may know that the Son of Man hath power on earth to forgive sins, then saith he to the sick of the palsy, Arise, take up thy bed, and go unto thine house' (Matt. 9:6). Yet how often when sick folk have failed to experience physical healing as the result of the ministrations of a faith-healer, are they not comforted by being given the hope or assurance that at least they may enjoy psychological or spiritual benefit instead.

> What, they may say, of those who get no benefit and are left to suffer in discomfort, pain and mental agony till the end? The answer is that in this ministry there are no complete failures. Everyone who is sincere in his seeking and is prepared patiently to wait upon God, receives a blessing mental and spiritual, if not physical, to an exceptional degree and doctors admit this is so.[9]

The point being made is not that any or all of the three forms of healing or help may not be experienced simultaneously, they often are, but that the one should not be confused with, substituted for, or used to explain away the failure of the other. Jesus is never recorded as having said to anyone, 'I can't guarantee a physical cure, but I am sure you will experience some other kind of blessing'.

Later we shall examine in more detail the 'faith' factor in faith-healing, but we note at once that while it is said that Jesus 'could do no mighty work' in at least one place 'because of their unbelief', nowhere is anyone's failure to be healed upon the word of Christ attributed to a failure of faith either in nature or degree on the part of the individual sufferer. How cruel and unwarranted it can be for the faith-healer to explain or justify the failure to effect a cure by laying the responsibility on the want of faith of the sufferer. It is clear that in some instances Jesus called for faith on the part of the sufferer (Matt. 9:29), or on the part of those seeking his help, while in others faith was neither asked for nor expressed.

Clearly then the matter before us is not a simple one—to heal or not to heal. Any claim to be obeying the command or following the example of Jesus Christ can only be substantiated by a strict conformity to the nature and circumstances of his healing activity. If we claim his authority and power for such activity, then we cannot restrict such authority or power to certain diseases or certain applications. If the exercise of the ministry of healing is to be undertaken by the command, and according to the pattern, of Christ, then it must include, for example, the ability to restore parts of the body that have been, by one means or another, amputated (*cf.* Malchus' ear, Luke 22:51); or the renewal of limbs that have atrophied (*cf.* Matt. 12:13); or the straightening of bones that have become deformed (*cf.* the woman doubled in two, Luke 13:13); and, of course, it would include the raising again to life of the dead (*cf.* Luke 7:15; Mark 5:42; John 11:44). These particular forms of healing are important because they provide no loophole for deception or doubt. Like the restoration of sight, hearing, speech or reason, they can be tested and proved or disproved. Yet, significantly, it is often these very needs which leave the faith-healer impotent to help.

We note also that there is no use by Jesus of any kind of symbolic procedure. We read that often 'He laid hands on' folk or 'touched' them. Much is made by modern faith-healers of the 'laying on of hands' and we shall deal with this phenomenon more fully later. For example, as we have already noted, J. C. Peddie writes,

> It is evident therefore that while Jesus could heal by his mere word, he seems to have resorted chiefly to the laying on of hands. The reason probably was that while the Divine Healing Grace could be communicated by means of speech and thought, it was the more effective on direct contact.[10]

This, of course is clearly quite wrong as is demonstrated decisively by the fact that some of the most dramatically effective instances of healing on Jesus' part took place at his word spoken 'a day's journey' from the place where the patient was (John 4:52, 53). He was equally wrong when speaking of a case where another prayed for a patient but did not lay on hands,

> Had he had sufficient faith in himself to lay on hands, as an instrument of God, the result would have been the same as in my case, perhaps better.[11]

In many cases Jesus' touch or contact would appear to have been strictly functional rather than symbolic. For example, it would be natural for him to touch blind people or deaf people since they might not otherwise have been able to discern his immediate presence or attention to them. It is noteworthy that he did not need to touch blind Bartimaeus because he had told his friends to bring him forward, and thus Bartimaeus was well aware of what was happening. He touched others for the purpose of assisting them to fulfil his instructions. For example, to help Jairus' daughter to sit up in bed (Mark 5:41, 42); to help the deformed woman to straighten herself (Luke 13:13); to help Peter's mother-in-law to get up out of bed (Matt. 8:15); to help the convulsed boy get up from the ground where he had been lying in a fit (Mark 9:27); to help the man with dropsy to stand (Luke 14:4); and, of necessity, to replace the ear of Malchus which had been severed (Luke 22:51).

In many instances Jesus did not touch the sufferer at all, for example, the paralytic man (Matt. 9:6); the Gadarene demoniac (Matt. 5:13); the woman with the issue of blood who rather touched him (Luke 18:44); the man with the withered hand (Matt. 12:13); blind Bartimaeus (Luke 18:42); the man at the Pool of Bethesda who evidently was able to move albeit with difficulty (John 5:7, 8). Of note too is the fact that in the case of the son of the widow at Nain, Jesus touched not the boy but 'the bier' on which he lay evidently to indicate that the funeral procession should stop (Luke 7:14).

This survey of the practice of the Lord in healing would not be complete without reference to the fact that the only substances ever used by him were saliva—on a number of occasions when dealing with blindness, deafness or dumbness (Mark 8:23; John 9:6; Mark 7:33)—and clay—only once in dealing with blindness (John 9:6). There is never any reference to the use of oil by the Lord either medicinally or symbolically. And finally, it is important to notice that in his healing no period of convalescence was required, no rehabilitation necessary, and no relapse recorded.

III. THE PURPOSE OF MIRACLES

One further consideration requires closer examination. Were the healing miracles of Jesus intended to be 'proofs' of his divinity or were they rather demonstrations of the nature and power of the Kingdom which he came to establish on earth?

(i) 'Proof'

Percy Dearmer is categorical in his view:

> it is clear that these miracles were not wrought in order to convince men of Christ's Divinity. They were not arguments; they were acts of kindness. They were in fact not primarily evidential.[12]

Indeed he reacts with startling vehemence to the idea of the miracles as proof or even evidence which he apparently regarded as being unnecessary or even unworthy, to judge by the following strange outburst:

> In the seventeenth and eighteenth centuries (when the Deists worshipped a Sultan and the Calvinists worshipped a devil) miracles were put forward as the evidence of Christianity; the whole burden of proof was laid on them because, as Archbishop Trench said, the deeper mysteries of our faith were thrust greatly out of sight by a cold, unspiritual theology which required external evidence and mathematical 'proofs'.[13]

His conclusion on the matter is:

> We may, therefore, safely say that our Lord did not heal men in

order to prove his own Divinity, though his healing them 'by the finger of God' (Luke 11:20) or 'by the Spirit of God' did indeed show that the Kingdom of God was come upon them (Matt. 12:28).[14]

The truth is, of course, that we may 'safely say' nothing of the kind. Alfred Plummer takes the view that while

He worked miracles for the good of mankind, and he was willing to use them as credentials of his authority…this was a secondary use; primarily they were acts of beneficence. He wrought nothing that was a mere wonder, a mere exhibition of power; and this was what the Scribes and Pharisees wanted…they ask to be miraculously convinced, and this he refuses.[15]

It is also claimed that Jesus' demand that some of those healed should on no account make it known, was evidence that he did not intend that his miracles should be used as 'proof' of his divine authority and power.

It was, perhaps, to show that our Lord in his great love could heal just for the sake of healing that the Evangelists have recorded certain cases in which he enjoined secrecy…. These instances prove that it could not have been only for his own glory that he healed the sick, and therefore that another reason must be found—that other reason being that he healed the sick because he was 'doing good'.[16]

But the two purposes are in no way in conflict. Both are thoroughly valid. Besides, A. E. J. Rawlinson, rejecting the theory of W. Wrede that,

the Messiahship of Jesus is a secret, and is meant to be kept as a secret, during his life on earth: no one except the Lord's chosen disciples is to know about it: only after the resurrection is the veil removed[17]

concludes that,

Taken as an historical picture this entire representation of the life of Jesus is beset with contradictions, and is unintelligible…. It is, indeed, part of the witness to Jesus that the mighty acts in which his power was manifested could not and did not remain concealed; and therefore Mark represents the injunctions of secrecy as being disobeyed (Mark 7:36, 37).[18]

(ii) 'Signs'

The question of the purpose of Christ's healing miracles centres around the meaning of *semeion* or 'sign' which is the word which John used to refer to the miracles which Jesus did and which were recorded 'that ye might believe that Jesus is the Christ, the Son of God; and that believing ye might have life through his name' (John 20:30, 31). John also believed that the miracle of turning the water into wine was 'the beginning of miracles (which) Jesus did in Cana of Galilee, and manifested forth his glory' (John 2:11). By his 'glory' (*doxa*) John meant,

> the presence and power of God in the person and work of Jesus. This can be seen in such verses as John 9:3; 11:4, 40 as well as 4:54 with which should be compared 2:11 since this verse makes clear that the function of a sign (*semeion*) was to manifest the glory of Jesus. The healing miracles are therefore a revelation of the deity of Jesus Christ, an indication that his presence and power is the presence and power of God.... It cannot be denied that there is an evidential aspect to the healing miracles in the gospels for they do witness to the fact that Jesus is the Christ, the Son of the living God. Their occurrence caused men to acknowledge that Jesus manifested the glory of God as he lived and walked amongst them on earth.[19]

'Signs' were important to the Jews (1 Cor. 1:22). Yet repeatedly Jesus regards the demand for a 'sign' as the mark of an 'evil generation' (Matt. 12:38; 16:4; Luke 11:29), or as the evidence not of the desire to believe on Him, but rather as an excuse for unbelief by its absence (Mark 8:12; Luke 11:16; John 4:48). On the other hand, even while rejecting the demand for an immediate 'sign' he did say 'There shall be no sign given unto it (the wicked and adulterous generation) but the sign of the prophet Jonas' (Matt. 16:4) by which he evidently meant that the ultimate and only sign of his divine power and authority would be seen in his resurrection on the third day prefigured in the experience of Jonah.[20]

'But', says A. E. J. Rawlinson, 'the demand for a "sign" was not confined to the Pharisees, or to the period of Jesus' life on earth. Men wanted evidence in Apostolic days that Christianity was true; and a "sign" was needed, not indeed for the "evil and adulterous generation" of those whom no "sign" could convince, but for the reassurance of those who were disposed to believe, but whose faith was weak.'[21]

Again, Leslie Weatherhead asserts,

> although no modern theologian uses the healing miracles as evidence of divinity, to the early Christian they formed part of his credentials. The view that the early Christians first recognised Christ as Lord by a divine intuition, and then came to interpret his miracles as 'signs' of the Rule of God cannot be sustained.[22]

A. H. McNeile takes *semeion* clearly in the sense of 'proof', thus,

> The *semeion* which they wanted was something more than a 'miracle' of healing, in which sense the word, though characteristic of the 4th Gospel (*cf.* also Mark 16:17, 20) is not used by the Synoptists. They asked for something which would

substantiate his unique claims to authority.[23]

G. H. C. Macgregor sees a difference between the reasons given for Jesus' performing of miracles in the Synoptic Gospels and that of John.

> According to the Synoptists it is because he is 'moved with compassion' (Mark 1:41; 8:2), according to John Jesus' signs are evidence of his divine power (and the more miraculous the more convincing the proof) and therefore 'display his glory' (2:11). Whereas for the Synoptists faith is a condition of miracle (Matt. 13:58), John regards miracle as the supreme inducement to faith (14:11).[24]

(iii) 'Mighty works'

The final word must rest with the Lord himself. On the occasion when John the Baptist sent from prison to inquire whether Jesus was indeed the Messiah of whom at the beginning he had proclaimed 'Behold the Lamb of God' (John 1:36), the reply sent back by the Master was unmistakable. 'Go and show John again those things which ye do hear and see; the blind receive their sight, and the lame walk, the lepers are cleansed, and the deaf hear, the dead are raised up, and the poor have the gospel preached to them' (Matt. 11:5). In other words the ultimate 'proof' of the power and authority of Christ, as presented by himself, was indeed the evidence of his 'mighty works'. As William Barclay put it,

> In the time of John's doubts, Jesus is depicted as pointing to his acts as the things which would accredit Him to John.[25]

We have dealt with this matter at some length because it seems to have important implications regarding the future ministry of the church in respect of the exercise of divine power especially in healing, as we shall later consider.

IV. THE PROBLEM OF DEMONS

There are six recorded cases of the casting out of demons by the Lord (see Tables I and II). Wilkinson classifies them thus: two of major epilepsy (the Synagogue demoniac Mark 1:26; Luke 4:35; and the epileptic boy Matt. 17:15 *etc.*); one of acute mania (the Gadarene demoniac Matt. 8:28 *etc.*); one of inability to speak (the dumb demoniac Matt. 9:32, 33); one of mutism and blindness (Matt. 12:22; Luke 11:14); and one in which no manifestations are described (the Syrophoenician girl Matt. 15:22; Mark 7:25). One further case is reported in the Acts of the Apostles (the girl in Philippi Acts 16:16–18). The subject of demon-possession, or 'demonisation' as it has been termed in more recent times, raises issues some of which are relevant to our present purpose. For example, Wilkinson says,

Demon possession is often regarded as a concept which has been
rendered unnecessary by modern psychiatry. What ancient
writers called demon-possession is said to be mental disorder of
the various types which are familiar to psychiatrists today. It is
then argued that since modern psychiatry can explain the
phenomena formerly attributed to demon possession we no
longer need to believe in the existence or activity of demons...
However, the matter is not as simple as this view would suggest,
for the introduction of psychiatry by no means excludes the
possibility of demon possession.[26]

And indeed, a clear distinction between demon-possession and disease
physical or mental is indicated in the New Testament (Matt. 4:24; 8:16;
Mark 1:32). Psychiatry may indeed describe the symptoms in
psychiatric terms, but this is not to identify or explain the cause. While
'epilepsy' or 'manic-depressive psychosis' or 'acute mania' may
describe the effects of demon-possession they do not account for the
cause.

Conversely, for example, in the case of the 'bent woman' (Luke
13:11–17), her condition may be identified in medical terms as
'spondylitis ankylopoietica'

the only case of a rheumatic disease which is identifiable in the
Bible[27]

as Wilkinson says. But Jesus described her as 'a daughter of Abraham
whom Satan hath bound, lo, these eighteen years' (Luke 13:16) and he
'loosed' her 'from her bond'. She is not referred to in Scripture as a
case of demon-possession, nor is exorcism said to have taken place,
yet Jesus attributes her physical condition to the malignant activity of
Satan. And Wilkinson concludes,

The main contribution which this account of the healing of the
bent woman makes to the Biblical view of health and disease is
its clear implication that disease is due to the activity of Satan',
and 'The cure of disease is therefore an illustration of the power
of God over evil and over Satan which is revealed and expressed
in the Life, Death and Resurrection of Jesus Christ.[28]

The Greek verb *exorchizo* ('exorcise') occurs only once in the New
Testament in Matthew 26:63 where in the trial of Jesus before
Caiaphas, the High Priest says, 'I adjure (*exorchizo*) thee by the living
God, that thou tell us whether thou be the Christ, the Son of God'. The
verb *orchizo* occurs twice: Mark 5:7 where the Gadarene demoniac
addressing Jesus says, 'I adjure (*orchizo*) thee by God, that thou
torment me not', and Acts 19:13 where the 'wandering Jews', who are
described by the noun (*exorchistes*) as 'exorcists', and who were using
the name of Jesus 'over them who had evil spirits', said, 'We adjure
(*orchizo*) you by Jesus whom Paul preacheth'. Thus the concept of

'exorcism' is never used with reference to the casting out of demons by Jesus. In fact, Wilkinson, with reference to the commission of Jesus to the Twelve in Matthew 10:8, 'cast out demons', says,

> Demon possession is clearly distinguished from sickness and from leprosy, and its treatment is to be of different character from theirs. Jesus does not call this exorcism, for this word by derivation means the casting out of demons by oaths, incantations and magic, and is not used in the New Testament of the casting out of evil spirits by Jesus or by the Apostles. The disciples cast out demons in the name and by the power of Jesus Christ.[29]

Kurt Koch notes the present day dangers amongst Christians either too readily to attribute physical or mental malady to demon-possession or to deny the existence of demonic activity entirely.

> On the theological front liberal and neorationalistic theologians continue to deny the existence of not only Satan, but of the angels and demons as well. As they see it the demonic is merely the reflection of either the sub- or superconscious within man.... To such people the stories in the New Testament concerning those who were demon possessed, simply mean that Jesus was a child of his own times, holding the primitive concepts of those around him. Possession is therefore a form of mental illness—at least that is what they say.

On the other hand, he says,

> Some primitive Christian groups are prone to read the demonic into almost everything they cannot understand, organically-based depressions and headaches included.... One continually needs to warn people to avoid hastily labelling someone as being possessed.... The opposite extreme of denying the existence of the demonic, is usually based on either ignorance, arrogance or both.[30]

Koch identifies important differences between mental illness and demon-possession. For example, the use of sedatives is effective in the treatment of mental illness but is quite ineffective in dealing with possession; there is no behavioural reaction on the part of the mentally ill while being prayed for, whereas the possessed usually reacts immediately with screams or curses when the name or power of Christ is applied. In fact, in the story of the Gadarene demoniac he finds eight symptoms which he says,

> distinguish demon possession from mental and nervous diseases.[31]

They are: (1) the demons are resident in the person concerned as the counterpart of the indwelling of the Holy Spirit in the believer; (2) unusual physical strength; (3) visible conflict within the possessed person similar to what psychiatrists diagnose as schizophrenia; (4)

resistance to the name and presence of God; (5) clairvoyance, for
example in regard to the sins of others; (6) the ability to speak with
voices other than their own or languages they have not learned; (7) the
possibility of immediate deliverance as distinct from the process of
medical or psychiatric treatment; (8) the possibility of transference of
the possession to other persons or creatures. Some of these, however,
may be evident in mental illness or even in alcoholic or drug
intoxication.

It would appear that for Koch the most prevalent reason for demon-
possession is involvement, directly or indirectly (by transference from
a relative or other person), with occultism, parapsychology, or
spiritism.

> Hundreds of thousands of people are suffering oppression either
> directly or indirectly as a result of occult influences. The tools of
> medicine and psychology are inadequate for the task of dealing
> with this problem. Rationalism has blocked the door to a true
> understanding of the nature of the effect that the demonic can
> have upon people.[32]

He classifies 'occultism' under four forms—superstition, fortune-
telling, magic and spiritism which in its religious form becomes
'spiritualism'.

'In England', he says, 'this is manifested in the numerous
spiritualistic churches and healers who claim to be working in the name
of God, yet who in fact further the work of Satan. The Bible itself often
suffers the abuse of being used and quoted in magic spells and
formulae'.[33]

His verdict on occultism and its consequences is clear:

> Occultism is not a hobby in which people may dabble. It is rather
> a problem and task which faces every minister and counsellor of
> Christ. It is the duty of the disciples of the Lord Jesus to give aid
> to those who have fallen prey to, and become ensnared by, the
> powers of darkness, whether through ignorance, through
> curiosity, or with a knowledge of the consequences involved. The
> only help and deliverance available is that which comes through
> Christ. Without him we would not be able to stand against the
> forces which occultism conceals.[34]

A Dictionary definition of 'exorcism' is,

> act of exorcising or expelling evil spirits by certain ceremonies:
> a formula for exorcising.[35]

As we have already noted, the concept is never used of the casting out
of demons by Christ. He, of course, needed no 'formula' to do so. It
was a simple word of command which spoken by the Son of God could
not be resisted (as the demons themselves acknowledged). It is true that
the Apostles cast out demons 'in the name of Jesus Christ', but there

is no 'formula' or 'ceremony' prescribed in the New Testament other than a simple command given in the name and by the authority of the Lord Jesus Christ. Moreover, this command was only effective when spoken by those who themselves were possessed by the Holy Spirit, that is, Christian believers (Acts 19:13–16). And unlike the healing of disease by Jesus there evidently was the possibility of relapse in the case of demon-possession (Matt. 12:43–45). The whole paraphernalia, therefore, of a ritual of exorcism relating to persons or places is foreign to the Scriptures.

Nevertheless, John Richards recounts how

> The Bishop of Exeter...appointed a commission in the early sixties which reported to each diocesan bishop in 1964.[36]

This Report contained, amongst other things, Liturgical Forms for 'The Exorcism and blessing of a place' and 'The Exorcism and blessing of a person' said to be possessed. These 'Forms' included certain safeguards, for example,

> No exorcism of a person may take place...without the explicit permission of the diocesan bishop of the place...given for every individual case concerned.... An exorcism may be performed only by a trained exorcist who holds a current licence to practice....[37]

Following the 'occult explosion' especially amongst young people in the 1960s, further episcopal guidance was sought in May 1970, and Richards reports,

> It was not forthcoming, so those who were discovering deliverance as part of the healing ministry, if they were not strongly within the sacramental tradition, tended to base their ministry on the American 'pentecostalist' writing which was spreading to this country. Thus there grew up a second approach to exorcism, one which was less formal, less ritualistic, less priestly, and almost exclusively concerned with the healing of disturbed personalities rather than places.[38]

Richards goes on to present 'Guidelines' in which he deals at length with such matters as diagnosis, discernment and directives, before providing Orders of Service for the practice of exorcism.

Let Kurt Koch have the final word:

> Jesus is the only one able to free people from occult oppression. Psychiatrists, psychologists and theologians at most are only a poor substitute. Satan is a powerful enemy. He has only been defeated once: at the cross on Golgotha where the archenemy was dethroned. If an oppressed person is unwilling to come to Jesus he can hold out no hope of being delivered.[39]

V. SUMMARY

We may therefore summarise the characteristics of the Lord's healing technique thus:

1. It constituted an essential part of his ministry.

2. His healing miracles were an important evidence of his divine person and power.

3. His healing work was a demonstration of the nature of the Kingdom he had come to establish, especially in his dealing with demons.

4. Healing was immediate and complete without convalescence or relapse.

5. There was no necessity or occasion for a second or more treatments.

6. The effect of the healing was immediately evident to others.

7. The sufferer did not always require to be in the presence of Christ at the time of healing.

8. There was no confusion between physical healing and other psychological or spiritual benefits.

9. In some instances Jesus touched the sufferer but usually this was functional rather than symbolic.

10. Jesus used no material substances or symbolism except saliva or clay.

11. Faith on the part of the sufferer or those seeking Jesus' help on his or her behalf was required in some instances but not in others.

12. No individual sufferer is ever said not to have been healed because of want or weakness of faith.

13. No instance is ever recorded of Jesus having refused or failed to heal any who came to him.

14. The power to heal included the complete restoration of diseased or mutilated physical organs, and the restoration to life of the dead.

NOTES

1 J. C. Peddie, *The Forgotten Talent,* London, Fontana Books,1966, pp. 77f.

2 J. Wilkinson, *Health and Healing,* Handsel Press, Edinburgh, 1980, p. 39.

3 J. C. Peddie, *The Forgotten Talent,* London, Fontana Books, 1966, p. 55.

4 *Ibid.,* p. 58.

5 M. Wilson, *The Church is Healing,* London, SCM Press,1966, p. 101.

6 G. Jeffreys, *Healing Rays,* Victory Press, 1932, pp. 5, 6.

7   N. Brooks, *Sickness, Health and God,* Advocate Press, USA., 1965, p. 50.
8   M. Wilson, *The Church is Healing,* London, SCM Press, 1966 p. 103.
9   J. C. Peddie, *The Forgotten Talent,* London, Fontana Books, 1966, p. 116.
10 *Ibid.,* p. 77.
11 *Ibid.,* p. 78.
12 P. Dearmer, *Body and Soul,* Dutton, New York, 1923, p. 169.
13 *Ibid.,* p. 169.
14 *Ibid.,* p. 172.
15 A. Plummer, *An Exegetical Commentary on the Gospel according to St Matthew,* Robert Scott, London, 1928, p. 182.
16 P. Dearmer, *Body and Soul,* Dutton, New York, 1923, p. 170.
17 A. E. J. Rawlinson, *The Gospel according to St Mark,* Methuen, London, 1947, p. 259.
18 *Ibid.,* pp. 260ff.
19 J. Wilkinson, *Health and Healing,* Handsel Press, Edinburgh, 1980, pp. 43f.
20 *cf.* A. Plummer, *An Exegetical Commentary on the Gospel according to St Matthew,* Robert Scott, London, 1928, p. 183.
21 A. E. J. Rawlinson, *The Gospel according to St Mark,* Methuen, London, 1947, p. 257.
22 L. D. Weatherhead, *Psychology, Religion and Healing,* Hodder and Stoughton, London, 1951, p. 40.
23 A. H. McNeile, *The Gospel according to St Matthew,* Macmillan, London, 1949, p. 181.
24 G. H. C. Macgregor, *The Gospel of John,* Hodder and Stoughton, London, 1928, pp. xvf.
25 W. Barclay, *And He had Compassion on Them,* Church of Scotland, Edinburgh, 1966, p. 31.
26 J. Wilkinson, *Health and Healing,* Handsel Press, Edinburgh, 1980, pp. 25, 26.
27 *Ibid.,* p. 74.
28 *Ibid.,* p. 79.
29 *Ibid.,* p. 163.
30 K. Koch, *Demonology, Past and Present,* Kregel Publications, Grand Rapids, USA, 1981, pp. 47, 48.
31 *Ibid.,* p. 136.
32 *Ibid.,* p. 94.
33 *Ibid.,* p. 96.
34 *Ibid.,* pp. 100,101.
35 *Chambers' Twentieth Century Dictionary,* W. R. Chambers, London, 1959, p. 373.

36   J. Richards, *Exorcism, Deliverance and Healing: Some Pastoral Guidelines,* Grove Books, Notts. 1979, p. 9.
37   *Ibid.,* p. 10.
38   *Ibid.,* p. 11.
39   K. Koch, *Demonology, Past and Present,* Kregel Publications, Grand Rapids, USA, 1981, p. 148.

3

THE APOSTLES HEALING

We have examined in some detail the extensive evidence of healing in the work of Christ. When we turn to the experience of the twelve original disciples, and the Apostles in the early days of the church, the situation is somewhat different. Although much is made by some of the Lord's commission to his disciples to heal the sick and cast out demons, there is, in fact, very little record of such activity on their part.

I. THE 'TWELVE' AND THE 'SEVENTY'

The Twelve would seem to have had a particular commission to 'Go not into the way of the Gentiles.... But go rather to the lost sheep of the house of Israel. And as ye go, preach, saying "The kingdom of heaven is at hand." Heal the sick, cleanse the lepers, raise the dead, cast out devils' (Matt. 10:5, 6). Their primary mission evidently was to preach, and the special powers given to them were to demonstrate the divine authority of their ministry and message. That ministry was also strictly limited in its scope and effective only in the fulfilment of this particular assignment rather than any general commission.

The 'Seventy' seem also to have been similarly commissioned for a particular operation (Luke 10:9), and having completed their mission they reported back to the Lord and were apparently discharged from their assignment (Luke 10:17–20) since there is no further reference to the existence of the group or the continuance of their mission. We need not here go into the whole question of the fact or the nature of the mission of the Seventy. As J. M. Creed notes,

> The appointment of the seventy (-two) disciples is unknown to the other Gospels and the rest of the N.T..

What is of interest for our purpose is that,

> The main content of the charge (vv. 2–11, 16) is in Matthew 9:37f. conflated with Mark 6:7–13 and forms part of the charge to the Twelve.[1]

Creed goes on to point to a number of problems regarding the record of the event, but for us it is the command to 'heal the sick' (Luke 19:9) and the fact that on their return they reported that 'even the devils are subject unto us through thy name' (Luke 10:17) which is of consequence. Whatever the reason for sending out the Seventy, as distinct from the Twelve, it would not appear that their mission was a general commission to all disciples, but a particular dispensation of God's power for the purpose of demonstrating that the same power which was made available to the Jews through the ministry of the Twelve, also extended to the Gentiles as symbolised by the Seventy:

> The number 'seventy' probably has a symbolic value as corresponding with the number of the nations of the earth in Genesis 10 (70 in Heb., 72 in LXX), as the Twelve correspond to the number of the twelve tribes.[2]

At any rate, it would seem clear that they provide no enlightenment regarding the exercise of the power to heal or exorcise beyond that of the Twelve whose original mission accomplished the same degree of surprise and success (Mark 6:30).

Even in the case of the Twelve, apart from the occasion of their first commission and sending out only to the Jews, there is only one instance recorded of their being involved in a healing situation, and that was on the tragic occasion of the demon-possessed boy whose father sought the help of the nine who were not on the Mount of Transfiguration with Jesus only to find they were unable to fulfil his request.

We are not told how the disciples went about trying to heal the boy. It would appear that they may have done so without prayerful preparation of themselves or perhaps without adequate dependence on, or acknowledgement of, the fact that it was only in the name or power of Jesus that the miracle could be effected. Thus, it would appear that even the commission of the Twelve was for specific occasions rather than for general practice, and that only on such occasions was it effective. When they went out on the specific instructions of the Master there is no report of any instance of failure due to lack of faith on their part. On the contrary, their success exceeded their expectations. Why then did they fail on this occasion?

Plummer sees their failure as simply, in the words of Matthew, 'Because of your unbelief' (Matt. 17:20), thus,

The fault lay in themselves. His power to heal was with them as before, but they had lost the power of making use of it. Unconsciously they had fallen away into a condition of mind in which they trusted either too much in themselves, as if the power were their own; or too little in Christ, as if in this difficult case he might fail them.... It was not their faith in Jesus as the Messiah that had failed them, but their faith in the commission to heal which he had given them.[3]

Rawlinson comments on Mark 9:28, 29 thus,

Matthew 17:20 gives a different answer to the disciples' question, to which in some texts a version of Mark 9:29 is added as a further comment. It seems likely that here, as elsewhere, the esoteric conversation with the disciples reflects the experience of the early church; in which case the words 'and fasting' are probably a genuine part of the Marcan text. The church, it would seem, ascribed cases of failure to exorcise demons successfully to spiritual deficiencies on the part of the exorcist; and there were certain types of demon who would yield only to an exorcist who was conspicuously an ascetic and a man of prayer.[4]

There is only one other instance in the New Testament of an attempted miracle-working which failed and which, though different in circumstance, may not be without relevance here. In Acts 19:13–18 we read of certain Jews, including the seven sons of Sceva, the chief priest, who attempted to exorcise evil spirits by using the name of Jesus, but without success. In one spectacular case 'the man in whom the evil spirit was leaped on them, and overcame them, and prevailed against them, so that they fled out of that house naked and wounded' (Acts 19:16). Here, it would appear, the name of Jesus was being used as a kind of charm or magic by those who presumably professed no faith in or commitment to him, rather than as an exercise of personal faith in Christ and devotion to his purpose and glory. They were acting not on the basis of Christ's authority or commission but simply attempting to do what they had seen others do by the use of the name of Jesus.

We remember too that Simon Magus (Acts 8:13–24), who had also formerly practised magic, but had professed faith in Christ and had been baptised by Philip, thought, in his spiritual ignorance, that he might purchase the ability to bestow the power of the Holy Spirit on others, only to receive the stern rebuke of Peter and the judgment of God.

Now this is not to suggest that in the case of the epileptic boy the disciples had acted out of superstition or selfishness. But from the extended form of the answer which Jesus gave privately to their question 'Why could not we cast him out?', it might appear that they had taken upon themselves to perform a miracle in the name of Jesus,

(1) without due recognition that the right to do so rested not in themselves, even as his disciples, but in his express commission—may this have been the real significance of Jesus' reference to 'prayer and fasting' which were the normal procedure in the church for commissioning people for particular work, for example Luke 6:12, 13; Acts 13:2, 3; 14:23?; (2) without adequate recognition that the power to do so lay not in themselves or in the mere use of his name, but in the total commitment of themselves to him and reliance upon the working of his Spirit in them—faith; and (3) without that depth of spiritual oneness with him which would ensure that the motivation of their action was singleness of purpose to glorify not themselves but him—prayer. W. M. Taylor explaining Jesus' reply to their question says,

> He wished them to understand that the power which wrought miracles, even through their instrumentality, was his power, and that therefore it was equal to every emergency. They were able to work miracles only in so far forth as they were in living union with him; and as the bond of union between them and him was faith, they could be powerful in his service only when they really believed in him. But when their faith was real, then, though it were little, it would enable them to do what to others was impossible. One with him, they were one with omnipotence, and on that they could always draw for all things that are right and necessary for them to do. Or, as Paul put it afterwards, 'they could do all things through Christ which strengthened them'.[5]

Their failure evidently was the result of a foolish presumption rather than a wilful neglect or disobedience. But it serves to show that even the best intentions can be no substitute for want of spiritual knowledge and discipline, nor justification for action which does not have his express authority.

There can be no doubt, however, that in the earliest days of the newly-established Christian church, and principally before the conversion and ministry of the Apostle Paul, multiple healings did take place, some on a large scale. These are said to have been effected by the 'Apostles' without any indication as to whether the whole twelve were involved or whether Peter and John acted on behalf of the others. This phenomenon has also been evident from time to time, and in various parts of the world, down to the present day when the Spirit of God has visited the church in a special work of 'revival'. Such periods have often been characterised by remarkable events including multiple healings. But it has always been a temporary phenomenon which ceased after the period of special outpouring of God's Spirit and grace had passed. It would probably be fair to say also that except in the case of the extensive healing activity which was associated with the spiritual revival which took place in Samaria as the result of the evangelising ministry of Philip, the work of healing was restricted to the Jews, as indeed was the commission of Christ to the Twelve when he sent them out on their evangelistic tour (Matt. 10:5, 6). But whereas in our Lord's ministry multiple healings were fairly frequent, in Apostolic times they were more rare and would seem to have occurred only in the very early days of the church.

II. POST-PENTECOST

When we examine the situation after the ascension of the Lord and the outpouring of the Holy Spirit at Pentecost, the results are equally surprising. True, we have in Mark's record of the general commission to the disciples, when Christ was about to leave them and return to the Father, the words, 'they shall lay hands on the sick and they shall recover' (Mark 16:18). Moreover it is said not just of the eleven who were present, but of 'those who believe' (Mark 16:17).

Unlike the charge given by Jesus to the Twelve and the Seventy, however, while all mention preaching and teaching there is no reference to healing in the accounts of Jesus' final commission to the disciples (Matt. 28:19, 20; Acts 1:8) except in the Marcan version. Even here it is not a command to heal, but a prophecy of what will happen. Wilkinson comments,

> If this longer ending belongs to a later time than the rest of the Gospel of Mark the omission of a command to heal is even more significant than if it belonged to the original text of the Gospel. According to the original gospel tradition Jesus had not included a command to heal in his final commission to his disciples. If the longer ending of Mark was added to the gospel at a later time this was an opportunity to add such a command if Jesus had ever given it, and for the church to record it, if the church felt the need to have his authority for its healing activity. The fact that such a command was not included indicates that Jesus never gave it in explicit terms, but only commanded his disciples to preach and to witness as Peter said in Acts 10:42.[6]

Moreover, when we turn to the record of the early years of the Christian church, we find no fulfilment of such a general commission to heal, nor any general programme of healing.

(i) Changing pattern

In both number and magnitude the healings in the Acts of the Apostles are less than in the time of Jesus' ministry. But there can be no doubt that in the early church healing was expected and practised. Morris Maddocks puts it this way,

They knew they would be given the power and grace to heal if they responded with obedience to what their Master had taught them. They were therefore gladly obedient. Obedience led to expectancy. It is obvious from the record of Acts that the early Christians invariably expected that the power to heal would be present. They knew that if they obeyed Jesus' commission he would be true to his promise to be with them and would 'confirm the word with signs following'.[7]

But the pattern of healing in the New Testament church exhibited important similarities to, and differences from that which took place in the days of Jesus' healing. There are eight instances of individual healings recorded in the Acts of the Apostles (see Table IV). We note that of the Apostles only three are mentioned by name—Peter, John and Paul—as having engaged in healings. In addition Philip the Evangelist, Stephen the Martyr, and Ananias are credited with healings, and Barnabas is associated with Paul in the multiple healings in Iconium.

Amongst the individual healings there is only one case of exorcism recorded in the Acts of the Apostles (16:16–18)—the demon-possessed girl in Philippi who followed Paul and became an embarrassment to his work. It is also interesting to note that here the reaction of the demon was similar to that in the Gospels when Jesus dealt with them. It is worthy of note too that healing was not designed to be a part of the evangelistic strategy of the Apostles, though, as in the case of the healing of the lame man at the gate of the Temple (Acts 3:1–10), it could be made the occasion of evangelistic witness by Peter and John. And again, it would appear that the Apostles took the initiative more frequently in their cases of healing (seven out of eight) than did Jesus (four out of twenty-six). We notice, moreover, that the question of 'faith' on the part of the patient is scarcely mentioned in the Acts of the Apostles. As before, of course, this does not necessarily mean that 'faith' or 'expectant trust' as Weatherhead prefers to call it, was not involved, but it underlines the need for caution in assessing the necessity or importance of it. Nor in the Acts of the Apostles is there any mention of the practice of anointing with oil, but the 'laying on of hands' is reported in the case of the restoration of Paul's sight by Ananias (9:17) although this can hardly be regarded as a normal case of healing since it was also apparently an act of 'commissioning'. It is also mentioned in the case of the healing of the father of Publius (28:8).

Weatherhead gives a useful summary of the changing pattern of healing as time passed,

as we get farther from the experience of Pentecost, there seems:
(i) a less powerful energy at work;

(ii) a uniform method of treatment and one which made a much smaller demand on the healer;

(iii) a treatment becoming more and more similar to those practised by contemporary non-Christian exorcists.

When we pass on in the history of the early church and leave behind us the Gospels and the Acts of the Apostles, we find these three factors are more and more obvious.[8]

We shall later discuss the implications of this analysis of the changing pattern (see Section 2 'The church of the Fathers'), but for now it is sufficient to note that in the days of the Apostles the pattern of our Lord's healing work was not rigidly maintained even though the purpose remained the same.

(ii) 'Exceptional powers'

There are only seven instances of multiple healings recorded in the Book of Acts (see Table IV). Amongst these the most extraordinary and difficult cases are those in (a) 5:15, and (b) 19:12.

(a) What are we to make of the statement, 'they brought forth the sick into the streets, and laid them on beds and couches, that at the least the shadow of Peter passing by might overshadow some of them'? Are we to conclude that it was actually believed that the 'shadow' of Peter falling on someone could affect healing, and, if so, could such a presumption be justified?

Wilkinson makes the point that Luke does not specifically say that Peter's shadow was the means of healing. But if not, what was the purpose in mentioning it? He suggests two reasons,

First, to show how near to Peter the people brought their sick. They were near enough for his shadow to fall on some of them as he passed by. Second, to reflect the people's superstition that healing was to be found in the shadow of an apostle. But the shadow fell only on some of them and we are told that all were healed (5:16).[9]

His first point, however, is not very convincing. If that were all that Luke intended, the suggestion that healing was somehow expected is removed. His second reason has greater substance—that it was 'to reflect the people's superstition'. But his argument, that while Peter's shadow only fell on some, all were actually healed, proves little since we are not told that it actually fell on any, but rather that it was the intention that it should do so. And again, it is not absolutely clear that the references in verses 15 and 16 are to the same groups of people.

F. F. Bruce neatly evades any problem or explanation by simply referring the one passage to the other without comment.[10] R. B. Rackham is more positive:

The people (who) thronged the apostles, sought to derive benefit

even from St Peter's *shadow*. This savours of superstition. But
miracles are 'signs', and the best signs for the instruction of the
simple-minded; and by this, and similar instances in the case of
the Lord (*the hem of his garment*) and S. Paul (*cloths from his
skin*), the lesson is taught that spiritual influence can be conveyed
through material things. The instances however are few and the
appeal has the least permanent effect.[11]

Dearmer is more positive still:

Here we have that atmosphere of enthusiastic faith in some
particular saint which to our minds is very mediaeval. Some
writers have therefore condemned it. But there is no con-
demnation in the text: on the contrary, it is given as the result of
the increase of believers...and we can hardly doubt that the
passage in the next sentence is added to tell us that, in addition
to the sick of Jerusalem, multitudes were brought from the towns
in the neighbourhood, and it concludes by telling us that all were
healed.[12]

Weatherhead adds another perspective:

This may have been the origin of cure by sacred relics so far as
Christian healing is concerned.[13]

and he goes on to recall the practices in the catacombs of Rome.

(b) In Acts 19:12 there is another development. Nothing in the
earlier case suggests that Peter personally was party to or approved the
expectation of healing from his shadow. But in the case of Paul and
the 'sweat-cloths and aprons', it would seem that the Apostle must
have at least co-operated in supplying the articles in question. Here it
is acknowledged that the miracles were 'special' or extraordinary
which were wrought 'by the hands of Paul'. Wilkinson says,

As the result of the extraordinary miracles performed by his
hands, the people came to regard anything which had been in
contact with his skin as potentially able to heal the sick.[14]

And as in the case of Peter's shadow, he refers the actual healing not
to the cloths and aprons but to the hands of the Apostle:

The fact that he would not have had a great number of these
items suggests that they were not in fact the means of healing the
sick. The first clause of verse twelve describes not the method by
which the sick were healed, but the result of the healing by which
the people took away cloths which had been worn by Paul in the
superstitious belief that they would convey healing to the sick
equally with his hands. Luke does not in fact tell us what effect
they had on the sick.[15]

No. But surely it is clearly implied that the healing was effected in the
absence of the Apostle himself through the cloths.

Dearmer has no doubts in the matter:

How scornful would a Protestant writer have been if he had come upon this account in some story of the thirteenth century. For here is something hardly to be distinguished from the use of relics; and so far from reprehending it, the writer of the Acts declares that God worked in this way and that the cures were successful.[16] The Ephesians were particularly impressed by the miracles ('exceptional powers') which God wrought by the hands of Paul. Thus Rackham says,

> This idea gave rise to superstitious practices.... In each case, both at Jerusalem and Ephesus, we have an instance of the divine condescension or accommodation: to a superstitious people a superstitious appeal is allowed. But there is a further explanation, of special application to Ephesus. The manifestation of divine power was needed to convict the false power—'the power and signs and lying wonders with all the deceit of unrighteousness' (2 Thes. 2:9, 10)—which had kept the Ephesians in bondage.[17]

So what are we to make of the commentators? Are we to believe that the Scripture actually supports or endorses a superstitious understanding of the exercise of the healing power displayed by the foremost of the Apostles in the early church? Are we to accept that Paul, the champion of the sovereignty of divine power, and the relentless exposer of heathen ignorance and Satanic deception should actually have been involved in the encouragement of the human propensity for the magical and the superstitious? Are we to give credence to the suggestion that he whose Word is truth actually was prepared to compromise that truth and integrity in order to 'accommodate' or even use the spiritual ignorance of those whom he purposed to redeem and heal? Are we to believe that the Holy Spirit whose specific mission in the world is to 'guide into all the truth' (John 16:13) actually led these early believers into ignorance and superstition?

Surely not! Besides, we have already noted that whenever any element of superstition did creep into the exercise of healing power, the result was embarrassment and failure (Matt. 17:14–21; Acts 19:13–16). Indeed, one of them actually occurred directly as the result of the very case with which we are dealing. Evidently it was when the Jewish exorcists saw what had happened as the result of the healings which had taken place apparently through the receiving by some of sweat-cloths or aprons from Paul that they attempted to use the name of Jesus as a similar kind of 'charm' with disastrous results.

How then are we to understand or explain what happened in Acts 5:15 and 19:12? In the first case it is clear from the record that whatever the expectations of those who brought their friends into the streets in the hope that even if they could not touch or be touched by Peter, his shadow falling upon them might perhaps bring them healing and relief, Luke does not attribute the healing to Peter's shadow. Nor is there anything to suggest that their quite understandable eagerness to obtain help, and their readiness to attribute such power not only to the Apostle but even to his shadow, actually was fulfilled in this way. It is true we are told in verse 16 of those who came 'they were healed every one'. But there is nothing whatever to indicate that the healing was the result of the shadow of Peter having fallen upon them.

In the second instance (Acts 19:12) we note that Luke specifically points to the fact that in Ephesus (and nowhere else or ever again!) did God work 'miracles of no ordinary kind' through Paul. Henry Alford comments thus:

> The rationalists, and semi-rationalists, are much troubled to reconcile the fact related, that such handkerchiefs and aprons *were instrumental in working the cures* with what they are pleased to call a popular notion founded in superstition and error. But in this and similar narratives Christian faith finds no difficulty whatever. All miraculous working is an exertion of the direct power of the All-powerful; a suspension *by him* of his ordinary laws.... In the present case, as before in chap. 5:15, it was his purpose to exalt his Apostle as the Herald of his gospel, and to lay in Ephesus the strong foundation of his church. And he therefore endues him with this extraordinary power—But to argue by analogy from such a case—to suppose that because our Lord was able, and Peter, and Paul, and in O.T. times Elisha, were enabled to exert this peculiar power, therefore the same will be possessed by the body or relics of every real or supposed saint, is the height of folly and fanaticism. The true analogy tends directly the other way. In *no cases but these* we find the power, even in the apostolic days.[18]

Our conclusion regarding this particular instance of healing must be that it was a unique occurrence, unparalleled and unrepeated in the history of the New Testament church, and was not an accommodation to superstitiousness, but rather a special providence evidently deemed by the divine physician to be appropriate to the particular circumstances of Paul's ministry in Ephesus at the time. It could not therefore conceivably provide a precedent or justifiable basis for the use of 'prayer-cloths' or other objects as the conveyancers of the divine power for healing.

By contrast, there are a number of important instances recorded in which either the exercise of miraculous healing did not arise, or, if it were attempted, failed. For example, Timothy suffered from a gastric complaint for which Paul could only prescribe 'a little wine' as medicine (1 Tim. 5:23). Why, we may ask, didn't he heal him? Again, Trophimus was so ill that he had to be left behind by Paul at Miletus

(2 Tim. 4:20). Epaphroditus, who at the time was indispensable to Paul, was almost at the point of death and Paul evidently could do nothing but leave him to the mercy of God (Phil. 2:27). But why didn't he heal them? And, of course, there is the case of the Apostle himself and his 'thorn in the flesh'. Now whatever the nature of the 'thorn' may have been, neither could he heal it himself, nor would God do so even though he prayed for relief on three specific occasions and was specifically told that he must learn to live with it (2 Cor. 12:7–9). It is also worthy of note that the Apostle Paul who claimed to have the gift of 'tongues' and to have used it more fully and frequently than any other member of the church (1 Cor. 14:18), at no time claimed to have the 'gift of healing' though he actually healed on a number of occasions.

(iii) 'Signs following'

The purpose of the healing practice was the same both for the Lord and for the Apostles. He healed in order to add to the authority of his word the visible sign of the power it possessed; but also in order to give assurance that he was indeed the One 'who should come' (Matt. 11:4, 5). His dealings with evil spirits were intended to demonstrate the power of the Holy Spirit over all other spirits, and his sovereignty over the realm and activity of Satan. The Pharisees realised this and tried to misrepresent what Jesus was doing, so that he declared, 'If I cast out demons by the Spirit of God, then the kingdom of God is come unto you' (Matt. 12:28).

Here was one of the 'signs'. His healing of those afflicted with leprosy proclaimed the end of separation between clean and unclean; they were seen no longer to be excluded from God's covenant of grace. His healings were not intended merely to be spectacular means of drawing attention to himself or arousing the curiosity of others for its own sake—hence his command, 'Tell no man but go unto thine own house'. Nor were they carried out merely as acts of compassion and concern for the sufferers (though, of course, they did indeed reflect such compassion and concern). They were 'signs' of the presence of the Son of Man and of the nearness of his reign.

So also in Apostolic times the healings were an important part of the vindication of the words and witness of the Apostles who by the commission of Christ 'went forth and preached everywhere, the Lord working with them, and confirming the word with signs following' (Mark 16:20). The fact that the members of the church in the early days realised this is evidenced by the terms in which they prayed—'And now, Lord, behold their threatenings; and grant unto thy servants, that with all boldness they may speak thy word, by stretching forth thine hand to heal; and that signs and wonders may be done by the name of thy holy child, Jesus (Acts 4:29, 30).

Dearmer goes to some length to dispute this assertion. He speaks of a holy 'reticence' on the part of the Apostles (pp. 205–209). For example, he says,

> we may say it reverently and truly of our Lord and his Apostles that they were gentlemen, and therefore could not blazon their powers abroad.... It would then have been most rash and unwise had the Apostles taught that they were to be believed because they had strange powers, and thus have led men to think that all who can heal should be believed.[19]

But has he forgotten that Jesus once said, 'Believe me that I am in the Father, and the Father in me: or else believe me for the very works' sake' (John 14:11); and that in seeking to prohibit Peter and John from witnessing as they had been doing in Jerusalem, the Council privately conceded, 'What shall we do to these men? For that indeed a notable miracle hath been done by them is manifest to all them that dwell in Jerusalem; and we cannot deny it' (Acts 4:16), in response to the claim of Peter and John. Besides, Dearmer has in the end to acknowledge,

> The witness of healing, then, is and was invaluable. And perhaps for this reason more than any other—that it shows people who are always apt to believe only in ponderable materialities, how real and great are the spiritual forces: 'That ye may know that the Son of Man hath power on earth to forgive sins, he saith to the sick of the palsy, I say unto thee, Arise, take up thy bed'. [20]

As in the healing activity of the Lord, so too in the Apostolic practice, there was no period of convalescence or rehabilitation required for those who were healed. The effect was immediate and there was no relapse. Moreover, the power to heal included for the Apostles, as it did for the Lord, the power to give back life to the dead. But the Lord's miracles of healing were not indiscriminate or universal. Nor could Paul heal in certain cases which we have already noted, and in others could only recommend the use of medicine. This is in itself an evidence of the fact that the gift of healing was not exercised indiscriminately or for its own sake, but the normal medical procedures were used except on specific occasions under the sovereign direction of the Holy Spirit.

(iv) 'Greater works'

One particular reference by the Lord himself to the 'works' of his followers requires consideration. 'He that believeth on me, the works that I do shall he do also; and greater works than these shall he do; because I go unto my Father' (John 14:12). These words evidently referred specifically to those to whom they were addressed. The disciples were alarmed and despondent at the prospect of being left in the world when the Lord returned to heaven. He was therefore at pains to show them that his own relationship with the Father while he was on earth would be maintained with them after he left them, and, as he had lived and worked in fellowship with the Father's power and purpose, so too they would do so through the indwelling presence of the Holy Spirit (John 14:16–18). This, of course, has been the privilege of all believers since the outpouring of the Holy Spirit at Pentecost.

The words 'greater works than these shall he do' have been taken by some to mean that believers working through the power of the Holy Spirit would do greater and more numerous miracles than Christ did. But what could be a greater miracle than raising the dead to life, or feeding 5,000 people from five small loaves and two fishes, or causing a storm to cease in a moment? Certainly, as we have seen, there is no evidence whatever that the miracles performed by the Apostles were more numerous or more impressive than those performed by Christ.

We must conclude, therefore, as the biblical commentators do, that the Lord was not speaking of more numerous or more spectacular achievements in the field of miracle-working than his own, to be accomplished by the believers who followed him. It is certainly not such incidents as those in Acts 5:15 or 19:12 that are here in mind. The contrast is rather between the few disciples of Jesus and the vast numbers of those to be converted by the preaching of the Apostles; between the mission of Jesus restricted to the Jews, and the mission of the Apostles extended to the world. These are the 'greater works'.

Macgregor comments thus:

> They will perform 'still greater deeds than these', than Christ's own—because with Christ's departure the full power of the Holy Spirit will be liberated into the world. These 'greater deeds' (*cf.* 1:50; 5:20) include all the missionary triumphs of the church which will be achieved in the power of the Spirit of the departed Christ (*cf.* Luke 24:29; Acts 1:8; Eph. 4:8ff.; Phil. 4:13). This comes out in the next clause: 'For I am going to the Father'; and, as in 16:23f., the power of prayer is made contingent upon the diffusion of the Spirit following upon that return to the Father.[21]

Jesus is not speaking of a surfeit of miracle-working as the hallmark of the church, as the later record of the Acts of the Apostles clearly proves, but rather of the extension of means and resources, of vision and opportunity, of blessing and fruitfulness which would be evident both in the Spirit-filled believer, and in the Spirit-filled church. William Temple comments:

> In scale, if not in quality, the 'works' of Christ wrought through his disciples are greater than those wrought by him in his earthly ministry. It is a greater thing to have founded hospitals all over Europe and in many parts of Asia and Africa than to have healed

some scores or some hundreds of sick folk in Palestine; and it is
to the Spirit of Christ at work in the hearts of men that we owe
the establishment of hospitals.[22]

Such is the generally accepted understanding of Jesus' words to Philip.
But it leaves a number of issues unclear. First, we must ask, to whom
does the statement relate—to the disciples to whom Jesus was talking,
or to all who would become believers? We shall discuss the question
more fully later, but for now we note that Jesus' answer is in the
singular number. He is not speaking evidently of the combined
activities of believers in the work and witness of the church, but of the
experience of the individual believer in his own relationship to the
Father, and his discharge of his personal responsibility with the further
assurance that 'Whatsoever ye shall ask in my name, that will I do, that
the Father may be glorified in the Son' (John 14:13). The prophecy or
promise therefore relates to the work and witness of the individual
believer.

Second, we must ask, to what is Jesus referring when he speaks of
'the works that I do'? The word used is *erga* and there can be no doubt
that in the New Testament it had reference to all kinds of activity including what we commonly call 'miracles'. W. M. Taylor commenting
on the word *erga* says,

Taken in connection with the emphatic assertion of the deity of
Jesus Christ, in the opening section of John's gospel, this
description of the miracles is most suggestive, as indicating that
what by men were regarded with wonder as indicating mighty
power, were in the estimation of the Lord himself simply works
requiring no more exertion at his hands than that which was
common or ordinary with him as divine.[23]

It is not sufficient therefore to explain (or perhaps attempt to explain
away) the meaning of Jesus' promise to Philip in terms of normal
human activity alone, such as building or equipping hospitals. The
'works' of Jesus did include the natural as well as his supernatural
doings. But, of course, his greatest 'work' was his work of redemption
by his death and resurrection to which all the others ultimately pointed.

Third, we must ask, what then could his reference to 'greater works
than these' refer? If we are to judge by the experience of the early days
of the church, it is clear that some of the Apostles and others preached
the Word, healed diseases and raised the dead to life as Jesus did. They
did so individually through the working of the Holy Spirit but with
wider scope and often greater response in terms of those who became
believers than the Gospel narratives record. We read of 'thousands' and
'multitudes' responding to the Word of God and being added to the
church. But, as we have seen, we do not read of miracles being
performed on anything like the same scale as in Jesus' ministry.

We must conclude, therefore, that when Jesus promised his disciples that 'greater works' would follow his return to the Father and his sending of the Holy Spirit to dwell and empower those who would constitute his 'Body' in the world, he was referring not to an increase in miracle-working, but to a vast extension of opportunity and fruitfulness of Gospel witness in speech and action, beginning in Jerusalem and spreading to 'Judea, Samaria and unto the uttermost part of the earth' (Acts 1:8), as indeed there was.

III. SUMMARY

We may summarise the characteristics of the Apostles' healing thus:

1. It was an important part of their ministry though less evident than in the ministry of Jesus.

2. Its purpose was the same as in the ministry of the Lord—to give added authority and authenticity to their witness.

3. Before Pentecost it was successfully effected only by special commission of the Master and not by any general commission.

4. Any attempt to use the name of Jesus superstitiously or wrongly resulted in failure to heal or exorcise.

5. It was immediate and complete without convalescence or relapse.

6. With one exception it took place in the presence of the Apostles (not at a distance as in the work of Jesus).

7. It was done mainly by word or touch with only two references to the 'laying on of hands', one by Ananias and the other by Paul.

8. It was usually done on the initiative of the healer rather than of the patient or friends.

9. The issue of 'faith' on the part either of the healer or the patient is not mentioned.

10. It included the power to raise from the dead.

11. It was not always used as a substitute for the normal use of medicine.

12. It was not part of the evangelistic strategy of the Apostles but it could be associated with an outbreak of 'spiritual revival'.

NOTES

1 J. M. Creed, *The Gospel according to St Luke,* Macmillan, London, 1950, p. 143.

2 *Ibid.,* p. 144.

3 A. Plummer, *An Exegetical Commentary on the Gospel according to St Matthew,* Robert Scott, London, 1928, p. 242.

4 A. E. J. Rawlinson, *The Gospel according to St. Mark,* Methuen, London, 1947, p. 125.

5   W. M. Taylor, *The Miracles of our Saviour,* Hodder and Stoughton, London, 1906, p. 326.
6   J. Wilkinson, *Health and Healing,* Handsel Press, Edinburgh, 1980, p. 84.
7   M. Maddocks, *The Christian Healing Ministry,* SPCK, London, 1981, p. 85.
8   L. D. Weatherhead, *Psychology, Religion and Healing,* Hodder and Stoughton, London, 1951, p. 85.
9   J. Wilkinson, *Health and Healing,* Handsel Press, Edinburgh, 1980, p. 100.
10 *cf.* F. F. Bruce, *The Acts of the Apostles,* Tyndale Press, London, 1951, p. 138.
11 R. B. Rackham, *The Acts of the Apostles,* Methuen, London, 1947, p. 69.
12 P. Dearmer, *Body and Soul,* Dutton, New York, 1923, p. 199.
13 L. D. Weatherhead, *Psychology, Religion and Healing,* Hodder and Stoughton, London, 1951, p. 81.
14 J. Wilkinson, *Health and Healing,* Handsel Press, Edinburgh, 1980, p. 100.
15 *Ibid.,* p.100.
16 P. Dearmer, *Body and Soul,* Dutton, New York, 1923, p. 200.
17 R. B. Rackham, *The Acts of the Apostles,* Methuen, London, 1947, p. 353.
18 H. Alford, *The Greek Testament,* Vol.II, Rivingtons, London, 1857, p. 196.
19 P. Dearmer, *Body and Soul,* Dutton, New York, 1923, pp. 206, 207.
20 *Ibid.,* pp. 208f.
21 G. H. C. Macgregor, *The Gospel of John,* Hodder and Stoughton, London, 1928, p. 308.
22 W. Temple, *Readings in St. John's Gospel,* Macmillan, London, 1945, p. 235.
23 W. M. Taylor, *The Miracles of our Saviour,* Hodder and Stoughton, London, 1906, p. 4.

4

HEALING IN THE OLD TESTAMENT

There is comparatively little material to be found in the Old Testament in terms of incidents of healing. And, as might be expected, the Old Testament has nothing to add to what we have already found in the New Testament. But it does provide interesting and important confirmation of many of the principles and patterns of New Testament healing. There are twenty-one incidents in all (see Table V) only one of which relates to a mental condition, three of which are actually cases where healing was explicitly refused, and three in which individual healing is not mentioned but sickness and death were prevented by the exercise of miraculous power.

One other phenomenon is found in the Old Testament which does not occur in the New Testament, namely, instances of sickness or suffering which are explicitly stated to have been inflicted by God as a judgment upon particular failure and later healed in response to penitence (Nos 5–9 Table V). This does not conflict with what we have already seen in the New Testament, however, since it was acknowledged that while, according to Jesus (John 9:3), it would be wrong to conclude that personal sickness or suffering must of necessity be the consequence of particular sin, nevertheless in the sovereign providence of God, or the normal processes of physical nature, it could be so.

I. INDIVIDUAL HEALINGS

The individual healings in the Old Testament may be classified as follows:

(i) The cure of childlessness

There are four cases of miraculous deliverance from this affliction.

1. Sarah (Gen. 18:14);
2. Abimelech's wife and maidservants (Gen. 20:17, 18). A. S. Peake (*Commentary on the Bible* p. 153) attempts to explain away the miracle by attributing the barrenness of the women to 'Abimelech's malady' (20:17). He suggests that Sarah's honour was preserved by the same fact. But this is in direct contradiction to the statement in verse 4 that 'Abimelech had not come near her', and to the word of the Lord in verse 6 'I also withheld thee from sinning against me: therefore allowed I thee not to touch her';
3. Rebekah (Gen. 25:21);
4. Rachel (Gen. 30:22–24). Again A. S. Peake (*Commentary on the Bible* p. 158) strains to call in question the miracle by the unlikely suggestion that

> In its original form the story of the mandrakes presumably explained the fruitfulness of Rachel.... The mandrakes, the earlier form of the story probably went on to say, removed the disability from which Rachel, like Sarah (Gen. 16:1f.) and Rebekah (25:21) suffered so that Joseph was born[1]

whereas the Word of God explains the miracle as a direct answer to prayer.

In three of these instances the healing was a direct answer to prayer either on the part of the sufferer (Rachel, Gen. 30:22); the sufferer's husband (Isaac, Gen. 25:21); or someone else (Abraham, Gen. 20:17). In the remaining case God acted sovereignly and revealed his intentions beforehand to his faithful servant (Abraham, Gen. 18).

(ii) Association with judgment

There are six cases of God's healing of his people after he had inflicted sickness upon them as a judgment upon sin.

1. Miriam's leprosy which was a punishment for her part in the conspiracy with Aaron against Moses was removed after one week (Num. 12:14) in answer to the prayer of Moses.
2. After those who had taken part in the rebellion led by Korah had been swallowed up by the ground which opened under their feet by the command of God, the people of Israel rebelled against Moses and, as a result, God sent a plague upon them through which 14,700 lost their lives before Aaron made atonement and thus the plague was halted (Num. 16:47, 48).
3. When the people of Israel again murmured against Moses and God in the wilderness, as a judgment God caused them to be attacked

and bitten by poisonous snakes, but on instruction from God they were healed when they looked at a bronze snake mounted on a pole by Moses (Num. 21:9). G. W. Wade appears at first to regard the story as an example of ancient magic,

> The means whereby the injury they (the serpents) inflicted was remedial was perhaps originally an instance of sympathetic magic inverted (like the cure of a dog's bite by a hair of the dog), though in antiquity serpents were widely credited with healing virtues in general.... The writer of Numbers naturally assigns the cure of the snake-bite not to magic but to Yahweh. It is held by several scholars that the present story is mainly an aetiological legend to explain the practice of the serpent-worship recorded in 2 Kings 18:4.[2]

But he finally acknowledges,

> By our Lord the uplifting of the brazen serpent was regarded as a symbol of his crucifixion (John 3:14)

4. King Jeroboam's hand with which he pointed for the prophet to be arrested, who had spoken against his unlawful altar, was healed of paralysis in answer to the prayer of the prophet (1 Kgs 13:1–6). Here at least Foakes-Jackson has to acknowledge,

> The story throughout is intentionally miraculous; the withering of the king's hand, the death of the prophet by a lion who refused to touch the corpse or to injure the ass, cannot be explained by any attempt to rationalise the story.[3]

5. King Hezekiah who was suffering from a terminal illness but who was healed and had fifteen years added to his life. He himself prayed for healing and Isaiah the prophet was sent to inform him that his prayer was to be answered in the affirmative, and to instruct him to use certain medicinal procedures (2 Kgs 20:1–11). His faith was also sustained by a further miracle in answer to a request for a 'sign'. But strangely, in spite of his merciful deliverance, Hezekiah's spiritual condition continued to deteriorate with serious consequences both for himself and for his people (2 Chron. 32:25).

6. Nebuchadnezzar who was stricken with mental derangement for an unspecified period and then restored to normal health with great spiritual benefit (Dan. 4:33, 36). H. T. Andrews finds several difficulties with this story. He says,

> The form differs in the Hebrew and the LXX. But there is a much greater difficulty with regard to the subject matter. The king's madness takes the form of lycanthropy, *i.e.* the sufferer imagines himself to be an animal. We have considerable evidence that such a disease was known in ancient time (*Century Bible*, p. 58), but there is not a shred of testimony to show that Nebuchadnezzar ever suffered in this way.... Probably the author is embodying

a floating tradition.... Many scholars think that our author has transferred to Nebuchadnezzar the doom with which he threatened Cyrus, but the evidence is obscure.[4]

How far some commentators will go to evade the plain truth of the biblical record! The healing in this case was obviously a sovereign act of God with no one else involved.

We note that in each of these instances the healing is granted by God in direct relief of the consequences of his earlier judgment and the repentance of the offenders. Wheeler Robinson notes:

If the individual Israelite were really in right terms with Israel's God, he would know it by his well-being in material things. That Psalm which describes most fervently the happiness of the forgiven man (Ps. 32) sees the evidence that the transgression is forgiven, the sin is covered, in the fact that the illness under which the poet groaned was removed after his penitent confession; this attitude is characteristic of Old Testament religion.[5]

(iii) Various healings

There are five such instances.

1. The son of the widow of Zarephath who was restored to life through the prayer of Elijah (1 Kgs 17:21, 22).

2. The son of the Shunamite woman killed by sunstroke who was restored through Elisha's prayer (2 Kgs 4:33, 35).

3. Naaman the Syrian (2 Kgs 5:14) who is referred to by Christ (Luke 4:27) in a comparison between the readiness of strangers and foreigners to accept the word of the prophet, and the unbelief and unreadiness of those who were specially privileged to hear his message to do so.

4. The story of Job deals at length with the problem of undeserved suffering and has important lessons to teach. For the moment our particular interest is in the fact that after much suffering and distress he was healed by divine power (Job 42:10).

Commenting on the phenomenon of 'undeserved' suffering Wheeler Robinson says,

If we exclude disciplinary suffering as being simply a natural extension of penal or retributive (an extension ultimately based on the gracious purpose of Yahweh), then we may say that the Old Testament offers five different attitudes to this problem of the suffering of the innocent (with the related fact of experience, the prosperity of the wicked). These five attitudes, in logical, though not chronological order, are (1) Wait! (2) There may be life beyond death for the righteous; (3) Life is a dark mystery; (4) Life is a bright mystery of a divine purpose higher than our grasp;

(5) The suffering of the innocent may avail for the guilty.[6]
The first suggests that either circumstances or a divine judgment will
in time remove the apparent contradiction (Hab. 1:13; 2:3, 4; Mal.
2:17; 3:14, 15, 18; Ps. 37). The second looks forward to resurrection
and immortality for the righteous (Ps. 73:24, 25; Job 19:25–27). The
third takes the view that there is no meaning or explanation but that
life is full of hopelessness and despair (Eccl. 9:2, 3). The fourth is the
answer which is arrived at in the experience of Job. The conclusion of
his three friends that his suffering was retributive is rejected; the
suggestion by Eliphaz and Elihu that it was disciplinary is also rejected.
While Job ultimately acknowledges his inability fully to comprehend
God's purposes, he is completely satisfied that they are good (Job
42:1–6). And the fifth reaches to the very concept of vicarious suffering
personified in the Suffering Servant of Isaiah 53:1–5 and the work of
atonement as set forth in the doctrine of the Apostle Paul and of the
New Testament.

> The most valuable thing the Old Testament has to offer is not a
> speculative solution. It is the inner certainty of God, which
> springs out of fellowship with him, and defying all the crushing
> proofs that the government of the world is unrighteous, holds its
> faith in him fast.[7]

5. The incident in 2 Kings 13:21 is particularly bizarre. It recounts how
when a corpse was hurriedly cast into the sepulchre of the dead prophet
Elisha and touched his bones it was revived. Peake remarks,

> The bones of the dead Elisha have more life-giving virtue than
> the prophet's staff in the hand of the living Gehazi.[8]

The purpose of the miracle would appear to be the authentication of
Elisha's divine authority in rebuking the king for his lethargy of faith
and in declaring the purpose of God to give deliverance to Israel. This
parallels the New Testament concept of miracles as 'signs' demonstrating the divine power and authority of Christ and of the Apostles acting
in his name and by his commission.

(iv) Healing refused

Three other cases are of special interest because they each culminate
in a refusal by God of healing.

1. King Jeroboam's son Abijah fell sick (1 Kgs 14:1–13). His father
sent his mother in disguise to Ahijah the prophet at Shiloh to ask
whether the child should recover or not. (This we take to mean that he
was, in fact, asking for healing.) Under the instruction of God, Ahijah
informed Jeroboam's wife that, because of his father's unfaithfulness
as king, the child would die, and a precise time was stated for it to
happen. But, strikingly, it is implied that the child's death would be an
act of God's mercy because, if he were to recover from this illness, he

would suffer a more terrible fate at the hands of those appointed to carry out God's judgment upon his father.

2. Ahaziah, King of Israel, who fell from an upper window and was seriously injured. He sent servants to inquire from a heathen deity as to whether he should recover (by which, we take it, he was asking for healing). But Elijah the prophet was sent by God to inform him that he would not recover (2 Kgs 1:4) and in fact that his illness would be fatal (2 Kgs 1:17).

3. Gehazi the servant of the prophet Elisha, who was unable to effect the miracle of God's power in the absence of Elisha himself, was stricken with leprosy (2 Kgs 5:27) as God's judgment upon his dishonesty and deceit, and apparently he was not only to die himself as a result, but the fatal disease was to become hereditary in his family.

These are not, of course, cases of healing, but, on the contrary, examples of the use by God of disease and death as a judgment upon sin. This is the one distinctive pattern in the Old Testament which is not seen in the New Testament, and obviously his chosen people the Jews took this solemn aspect of God's dealings with men very seriously, as is shown by the question of the disciples to Jesus on the occasion of the healing of the man born blind (John 9:2). There is nothing in the New Testament to correspond to this idea, and, as we have noted elsewhere, Jesus refuted the suggestion that this was a general principle. Even in the Old Testament there are only three recorded instances where healing was totally refused, and, while they stand as a solemn warning to us all against any presumption on God's patience and mercy, there is great comfort in the reaction of the Lord to the question of his disciples.

For the sake of completeness we should add three instances where individual healing did not occur, but where sickness and death were stopped or prevented by miracles performed by divine power through Moses and Elisha.

1. In Exodus 15:23–25 by casting a particular tree into the bitter or poisoned waters of Marah, Moses turned them to sweetness and purity.

2. In 2 Kings 2:21, 22 by casting salt into the poisoned spring Elisha purified it and prevented death and pollution.

3. In 2 Kings 4:38–41 by casting meal into the pottage which had been affected by poisonous herbs Elisha purified the food and enabled it to be eaten without harm or danger.

II. COVENANT HEALTH?

There are a number of general references to health and healing which call for consideration. Some would claim to find in the Old Testament a special kind of covenant relationship between God and Israel by which they were to be preserved from many of the natural afflictions and diseases to which other humans are prone. Some would even seek to give such a covenant a New Testament dimension and would make similar claims for God's people in Christ. But this is the result of faulty exegesis of Scripture.

Tony Dale writes,

> One of these marvellous names by which God has chosen to show himself is 'I am the Lord, your healer' (Exod. 15:26). To my mind, this ties up with statements of the Lord Jesus, such as 'I have come that they may have life, and have it to the full' (John 10:10), or 'In him was life, and that life was the light of men' (John 1:4).[9]

And having further considered such verses as Exodus 15:25, 26; Deuteronomy 34:7; 1 Thessalonians 5:23; he says,

> It seems to me that God holds out as a genuine possibility that the sanctifying work of his Holy Spirit can work in us so completely that we are brought in increasing measure into wholeness whether spiritually, in the realm of our soul, or in relation to our physical body.[10]

Now the conclusion may indeed be true but the premises on which it is based are not.

Or again, Gardner quotes from one of Kenneth Hagin's booklets in which he refers to a woman dying of tuberculosis who was instructed to repeat to herself every waking moment, 'According to Deuteronomy 28:22 consumption is a curse of the law. But according to Galatians 3:13 Christ has redeemed us from the curse of the law. Therefore I no longer have tuberculosis'. She got better and Hagin goes on

> You can Scripturally claim healing from any sickness, because Deuteronomy 28:61 says every sickness is a curse of the law. It will work for you too.[11]

While Herbert Carson, attempting to set things in their proper perspective writes,

> Some may point to the title that God revealed in Exodus 15:25, 26. He is Jahweh Rophecha, 'the Lord who heals you'. The assurance that none of the diseases of Egypt would affect them is cited as further evidence of God's concern with their bodily health. It must however be remembered that this was in the context of God's dealings with his people in the period of what Paul described as their infancy (Gal. 4:1–7).... Hence, when in the New Testament the emphasis is on the inward and the spiritual, the ceremonial law is abrogated and the health of the soul is seen as being of far greater importance.[12]

(a) In Exodus 15 we have the story of how the Israelites set out upon their wanderings in the wilderness of Shur and came to Marah

exceedingly thirsty after three days without water, only to find that the
water there was undrinkable. Moses heard their complaints, sought
God's face in prayer, and was instructed to cast a particular tree into
the waters of Marah in order to make them safe and palatable. In
addition, God made a covenant with his people there to the effect that
'If thou wilt diligently hearken to the voice of the Lord thy God, and
wilt do that which is right in his sight, and wilt give ear to his
commandments, and keep all his statutes, I will put none of these
diseases upon thee, which I have brought upon the Egyptians; for I am
the Lord that healeth thee' (Exod. 15:26).

This passage seems to be pivotal for Pentecostalists. Dr A. B.
Simpson, an American Presbyterian who was also a noted exponent of
Pentecostal doctrine, writes:

> The earliest promise of healing is in Exodus 15:25, 26.... The
> place of this promise is most marked. It is at the very outset of
> their journey, like Christ's healing of disease at the opening of
> his ministry.... This promise therefore becomes ours, as the
> redeemed people of God. And God meets us at the very threshold
> of our pilgrimage with the *covenant of healing*, declaring that as
> we walk in holy and loving obedience we shall be kept free from
> sickness, which belongs to the old life of bondage we have left
> behind us for ever. Sickness belongs to the Egyptians, not to the
> people of God. And only as we return spiritually to Egypt do we
> return to its malarias and perils.[13]

What a strange and incredible assertion in view of the facts both of
experience and of the teaching of Scripture. One of the most evident
and perplexing dilemmas facing us in the divine Word is the fact that
so often the wicked seem to be almost untouched by the pains and
tragedies of life, while those who walk most closely and serve most
diligently in the fellowship and witness of God's people are subject to
the deepest and most persistent distresses of body and mind. Indeed,
if such suffering is evidence of the 'bondage of Egypt' then the Apostle
Paul must never have crossed the river of redemption at all, for it is
evident that, under God's good hand, much of his life and experience
was moulded, if not determined, by physical weakness and suffering,
and he 'gloried' in his infirmities (1 Cor. 2:3; 2 Cor. 12:9, *etc.*). The
real meaning of Exodus 15:26 is different.

In the context of their situation it would appear that God was testing
the readiness of the Israelites to accept his promises through Moses to
provide for their physical and spiritual needs. God makes the covenant
that upon condition of obedience to his word, and trust in his loving
purposes, he will not inflict upon them the kind of plagues which he
had sent upon the Egyptians. The covenant does not relate to diseases
to which human beings are normally exposed, but rather to those

extraordinary afflictions to which the Egyptians were subjected as the result of the stubborn sinfulness of Pharaoh's refusal to allow the Israelites to leave his country.

The promise therefore in Exodus 15:26 is not a guarantee to the Israelites of immunity from natural diseases, nor even from God's particular judgments upon their failure to trust and obey him, but simply a promise that by obedience to his word they need not fear the terrors of his judgment as so recently experienced by the Egyptians. In fact, of course, the people of Israel were repeatedly subject to suffering as the result of their sin, as, for example, when they were bitten by the poisonous snakes (Num. 21:6), or when 14,700 of them died as the result of a plague (Num. 16:49).

As a 'sign' or seal of the covenant on this occasion God healed their immediate thirst by turning the bitter waters of Marah into the sweet waters of Elim. He did not thus establish a principle by which his people either under the Old Covenant or the New should expect any immunity from the natural diseases and disasters of life.

As Roux puts it,

> Thus not only health, prosperity and fertility, but also sickness, sorrow, and sterility are equally in God's hands the signs of blessing or of cursing, for the Lord 'kills and brings to life' and it is at his hand that we receive both good and evil (1 Sam. 2:6, 7; Job 2:10; Isa. 45:6, 7; Lam. 3:37–39).[14]

This surely was the great lesson which Job and Paul were to share in their bitterest experiences and in the ultimate conviction that 'all things work together for good to them that love God'.

The truth of the preceding point is demonstrated by the fact that in Deuteronomy 28:15–68 we have a terrifying catalogue of the consequences likely to befall these same people of God in the event of their disobedience and rebellion. We may note in particular the threat of disease and plague with specific reference to Egypt (vv. 27, 28). In fact, of course, the catalogue of punishment for disobedience far outreaches the terms of blessing in return for obedience and trust. So that if the one is to be applied as a covenant of special privilege, the other must equally be accepted as a covenant of special judgment. And, logically, if the one is to be applied to the children of God under the New Covenant, so must the other!

(b) There is an interesting statement in Deuteronomy 34:7, 'And Moses was an hundred and twenty years old when he died, his eye was not dim, nor his natural force abated'. Jeffreys sees the experience of Moses as an explicit demonstration of the fulfilment of the promise in Exodus 15:26. He writes,

> This blessing of healing was given to a people whose leader was undoubtedly a fully qualified physician. He was trained in all the

wisdom of a country that was noted for its medical knowledge (Acts 7:22). Moses miraculously enjoyed the full blessing of health until he was called home to higher service.[15]
The intended inference seems to be that such should also be the experience of all God's faithful servants. There is no doubt that having called Moses to the incredible task of leading the people of Israel from Egypt to the borders of Canaan with all the exhausting problems involved, God did sustain him in a special way beyond the natural limits of strength and endurance. But over against this, many distinguished servants of God have been sustained and remarkably used by God through weakness, pain, sickness or need (*e.g.* 1 Cor. 1:27, 28) according to his sovereign providences. So that while we glorify God for the evidence of his power and faithfulness in the life and vigour of his servant Moses, we cannot build any theory or principle upon it other than that God 'doeth all things well'.

(c) We come then to David the Psalmist. In Psalm 30:2 we read, 'O Lord I cried unto thee and thou hast healed me'. Here is a clear testimony to the Psalmist's experience of the effectiveness of 'the effectual fervent prayer of a righteous man' which 'availeth much' (Jas 5:16). Again, in Psalm 103:3–5 we read 'Who forgiveth all thine iniquities, who healeth all thy diseases; Who redeemeth thy life from destruction, who crowneth thee with lovingkindness and tender mercies, Who satisfieth thy mouth with good things, so that thy youth is renewed like the eagle's'. Some would see here again a place of special privilege for the believer in regard to physical health and healing.

But surely the Psalmist is simply pouring out his heart in thanksgiving as he calls to mind the extent and variety of God's blessings. It is right that he should specifically include the special blessing of healing and health since too often these are taken for granted even by God's people, until they are temporarily or permanently withdrawn. Only then are their value and preciousness realised and appreciated. The Apostle Paul could honestly recount the other side of God's providences when he wrote in 2 Corinthians 4:8–10, 'We are troubled on every side, yet not distressed; we are perplexed, but not in despair; persecuted, but not forsaken; cast down, but not destroyed; always bearing about in the body the dying of the Lord Jesus, that the life also of Jesus might be made manifest in our body'. There is a loving Providence that watches over us all and preserves us from harm and danger of all kinds often without our notice or gratitude.

(d) In Isaiah 35:5–7 the prophet looks forward to the work of redemption to be perfected by the coming of Messiah—the Suffering Servant. At that time, and in consequence of his coming, Isaiah says, 'Then the eyes of the blind shall be opened, and the ears of the deaf shall be unstopped. Then shall the lame man leap as an hart, and the tongue of the dumb sing'. These words, like those in 61:1–3, had a literal fulfilment in the coming and ministry of the Lord Jesus Christ, and he applied them specifically to himself (Luke 4:18, 19). That they also had a more eternal significance we shall see later.

(e) Finally we have an interesting reference in Malachi 4:2 to the coming of Messiah—'But unto you that fear my name shall the Sun of Righteousness arise with healing in his wings'. Here again the prophet's words found literal fulfilment both in the physical and spiritual sense in the coming and ministry of Jesus Christ.

In all of these references it is clear that physical healing is intended, and that the believing servant of God is given ground for hope and confidence in regard to faith and prayer concerning the needs of life including the problems of physical health or weakness. But there is no evidence that the Christian is in any respect different from others in being protected *from* the natural hazards of life in this 'present evil world'. He does, however, have the assurance of special protection and assistance *in* such circumstances. And, like others, he is protected by the divine Providence in many circumstances of harm or danger, either with or without his realisation of the fact. With God there are no 'accidents', and whether 'in sickness or in health, in joy or in sorrow, in prosperity or adversity' the believer is subject to the tests and trials of human life. But with this difference, he knows through faith in a living Saviour that 'all things work together for good to them that love God' (Rom. 8:28). And that knowledge sustains him and transforms every situation into an opportunity to prove God's power to heal and save according to his will. This is the secret of the New Covenant in Christ Jesus.

III. HEALING AND THE 'ATONEMENT'

A final word must be said with reference to the Old Testament relationship of healing and atonement. In Isaiah 53:4 we read, 'Surely he hath borne our griefs and carried our sorrows; yet we did esteem him stricken, smitten of God, and afflicted', and in Matthew 8:16, 17 'He healed all that were sick, that it might be fulfilled which was spoken by Isaiah the prophet, saying, he himself took our infirmities, and bore our sicknesses'. In 1 Peter 2:24 the prophet is also quoted in the words 'By whose stripes ye were healed'.

The Pentecostal interpretation of these verses is ambiguous. Simpson writes in comment on Isaiah 53:4,

> Therefore, as he has borne our sins, Jesus Christ has also borne away and carried off our sicknesses; yes, and even our pains, so that abiding in him, we may be fully delivered from both

sicknesses and pain. Thus 'by his stripes we are healed'.[16]
And in a further comment on Matthew 8:16, 17 he says,

> This is quoted as the reason why he healed all that were sick. It
> was not that he might give his enemies a vindication of his
> Divinity, but that he might fulfil the character presented of him
> in ancient prophecy.... Now this was the work of his life; and
> God would not have us forget that he spent more than three years
> in deeds of power and love before he went up to the Cross to die.
> And we need that living Christ quite as much as Christ Crucified.
> The Levitical types included the meal offering quite as much as
> the sin offering; and suffering human hearts need to feed upon
> the Great Loving Heart of Galilee and Bethany, as much as on
> the Lamb of Calvary.[17]

Here it would seem quite clear that the bearing and healing of our
sicknesses was to be identified with the incarnation of Christ rather
than his atonement. It relates to the life rather than the death of Christ.
If so, of course, it would have no application to any period of time
outside that of the earthly ministry of our Lord, and could not
constitute a promise of deliverance from all sickness on the ground of
faith in Christ's work of redemption.

But later in the chapter he says,

> But redemption finds its centre in the Cross of our Lord Jesus
> Christ, and there we must look for the fundamental principle of
> Divine healing, which rests on the atoning sacrifice.... If sickness
> be the result of the Fall, it must be *included in the atonement* of
> Christ, which reaches as 'far as the curse is found'. Again, this
> fundamental principle is most distinctly stated in the 53rd chapter
> of Isaiah, as we have seen.... Peter also states that 'His own self
> bare our sins in his own body on the tree...by whose stripes ye
> were healed'. In his own body he has borne *all our bodily
> liabilities* for sin, and our bodies are set free.... Thus our healing
> becomes a great redemption right, which we simply claim as our
> purchased inheritance through the blood of the Cross.[18]

Noel Brooks takes a different view. Having summarised the
foregoing theory of 'healing in the atonement', he writes,

> Tremendous emphasis has been placed on these texts and upon
> the theology of healing through the Atonement amongst
> Pentecostals.... Frequently...all restraint is thrown to the winds,
> and the most extravagant promises of physical healing through
> the atonement are made on the sole condition of 'faith'.... We
> must now point out, however, that not all, even amongst
> Pentecostals, consent to this popular presentation of healing
> through the atonement!...Dr Paul F. Beacham...an acknowl-
> edged Pentecostal teacher and leader, does not draw the same

conclusions from the concept of healing through the atonement.... According to his view there are physical benefits through
the atonement but until the second coming of Christ we may
expect only a limited realisation of them. I believe it is safe to
say that most Pentecostals who have given serious thought to it
have been driven to the same conclusion.[19]

Moreover, Mr. F. W. Woodford, a British Pentecostal leader, presented
a scholarly paper in 1956 to the Victoria Institute in London in which
he challenged the whole concept of 'healing through the atonement'.
Having considered in some detail the three texts in question he writes,

Perhaps the major defect in the popular presentation of 'healing
through the atonement' is that it puts the responsibility for being
healed almost entirely upon the sufferer himself. If Christ bore
all sickness and disease on the Cross, just as he bore all sin, why
am I not healed? The logical answer would seem to be, Because
I do not believe! But such a conclusion—one which many boldly
and uncompromisingly proclaim—has such terrible and
ridiculous implications and brings such torturing doubts and fears
into the minds of the unhealed, that it is small wonder that sober-
minded men feel the need to think again on the subject.[20]

Brooks himself comments,

Through the power of the Holy Spirit we may have an 'earnest'
and 'first fruits' of that deliverance, in which we may include
both these occasional miracles of healing which are witnessed in
the church, and these more frequent enablings of grace by which
the people of God transcend their bodily weaknesses to the praise
and glory of God. But full deliverance from all the workings of
death in the human body is not promised us, and cannot be
expected by us, until the return of Christ in glory, who at that
time 'will fashion anew the body of our humiliation, that it may
be conformed to the body of his glory' (Phil. 3:2).[21]

Hebrews 4:14–16 says, 'Seeing then, that we have a great high priest,
that is passed into the heavens, Jesus, the Son of God, let us hold fast
our profession. For we have not an high priest who cannot be touched
with the feeling of our infirmities, but was in all points tempted (*i.e.*
tested) like as we are, yet without sin, let us therefore, come boldly
unto the throne of grace, that we may obtain mercy, and find grace to
help in time of need'.

Three points are being made clear by the writer to the Hebrews:

1. That Jesus Christ in his redemption of us was our substitute in
the most specific sense. As Paul puts it in the *kenosis* passage, 'He
made himself of no reputation, and took upon him the form of a
servant, and was made in the likeness of men; and being found in
fashion as a man, he humbled himself and became obedient unto death,

even the death of the cross' (Phil. 2:7, 8). He not only took upon himself our human nature, but he lived in our world under our conditions in order to be identified not only with our nature but with our needs. In that sense 'He himself took our infirmities and bore our sicknesses' as Matthew, quoting Isaiah, says. His atoning work involved not only his being made like us, but also his actual submission to our needs and circumstances. Thus, and only thus, could he become the 'great high priest' who can be 'touched by the feeling of our infirmities' as the writer to the Hebrews says.

2. That our bodies and their afflictions were involved in his atoning work as were our souls and their sinfulness. Of course all our human sufferings and trials are the result of the fall of our first parents. Not only are our physical natures and their needs involved, but the whole of the created world is involved so that Paul could write to the Romans, 'Because the creation itself shall be delivered from the bondage of corruption into the glorious liberty of the children of God. For we know that the whole creation groaneth and travaileth in pain together until now...waiting for the adoption, that is, the redemption of the body' (Rom. 8:22). The work of Christ's atonement will only finally be consummated when, as the result of his coming again, and the great day of resurrection, all pain, disease, corruption and death itself will be past, body and soul will be reunited, and the new heaven and new earth will be ushered in. This is the great hope of the Christian. This is the moment of final triumph when 'death is swallowed up in victory'.

The 'resurrection of the body and the life everlasting' are the ultimate fulfilment of the work of the atonement. To suggest, as some do, that because Christ bore our sicknesses as well as our sin 'in his own body to the tree', believers have therefore the right to expect here and now deliverance from bodily sickness and distress is plainly contrary to the teaching and example of Scripture. No more can we expect the perfect re-creation of the body here in time than we can expect the sinless perfection of the soul. The Scripture teaches neither, but looks forward to their eternal realisation 'in that day', referring to the day of the Lord's return and the final resurrection.

3. But while neither physical nor spiritual perfection is promised to those who are believers in Christ, the writer to the Hebrews, explaining Isaiah and Matthew, assures us that Christ's substitution on our behalf enables him from personal experience as well as divine omniscience to understand, sympathise (or 'empathise' as the modern sociologist would say) with and sustain us in coping with the circumstances of life in this fallen world. So that while we await the ultimate and perfect fulfilment of our redemption we can 'come boldly unto the throne of grace, that we may obtain mercy and find grace to help in time of

need', the grace that is 'sufficient' (2 Cor. 12:9).

No, there is no promise to the Christian believer of deliverance in time from the hazards either physical or spiritual of life in this fallen world. But there is the blessed assurance of a glorious entrance, through the blood of Christ, into that kingdom where pain and suffering, sorrow and tears, weakness and despair can never come (Rev. 21:3, 4). In this confidence both the Old Testament and the New Testament are completely at one.

IV. SUMMARY

The following principles in regard to healing may be discerned in the Old Testament which have their counterparts and fulfilments in the teaching and example of the New Testament:

1. The sovereign power and authority of God in determining to heal or not to heal according to his righteous and loving purposes.

2. The effectiveness of believing prayer (the 'prayer of faith') as exercised by the person concerned or by someone else on his or her behalf.

3. The application of healing both to physical and mental illness.

4. The possibility of failure on the part of the healer (the case of the Shunamite's son).

5. The fact of death as an evidence of God's love and mercy and not the worst thing that can happen to a person (Abijah).

6. The possibility, though not necessity, of suffering as the consequence of personal sinfulness.

To these must be added the following 'negative' conclusions:

7. There is no promise of immunity for the people of God from the natural diseases and disasters of life in this present world.

8. There is no ground for believing in 'healing through the atonement' except in the sense of the ultimate restoration of all things at the Second Advent of the Lord and the Day of Resurrection.

NOTES

1   A. S. Peake, *Commentary on the Bible,* Nelson and Sons, London, 1919, p. 158.

2   G. W. Wade, *Peake's Commentary on the Bible,* Nelson and Sons, London, 1919, p. 223.

3   F. J. Foakes-Jackson, *Peake's Commentary on the Bible,* Nelson and Sons, London, 1919, p. 301.

4   H. T. Andrews, *Peake's Commentary on the Bible,* Nelson and Sons, London 1919, p. 527.

5   H. Wheeler Robinson, *Religious Ideas of the Old Testament,* Duckworth, London, 1947, p. 169.
6   *Ibid.,* p. 171.
7   A. S. Peake, *The Problem of Suffering in the Old Testament,* p. 144.
8   A. S. Peake, *Commentary on the Bible,* Nelson and Sons, London, 1919, p. 306.
9   O. R. Barclay, *Signs, Wonders and Healing,* IVP, Leicester, 1989, p. 58.
10 *Ibid.,* pp. 60, 61.
11 R. Gardner, *Healing Miracles,* Darton, Longman and Todd, London, 1958, p. 156.
12 H. Carson, *Spiritual Gifts for Today?,* Kingsway Publications, Eastbourne, 1987, pp. 97, 98.
13 A. B. Simpson, *The Gospel of Healing,* Morgan and Scott, London, 1915, pp. 7f.
14 H. Roux, *Vocabulary of the Bible,* Ed. J-J Von Allmen, Lutterworth Press, London 1958, p. 403.
15 G. Jeffreys, *The Miraculous Foursquare Gospel—Doctrinal,* Elim Publishing Co., London, 1929, p. 36.
16 A. B. Simpson, *The Gospel of Healing,* Morgan and Scott, London, 1915, p. 12.
17 *Ibid.,* pp. 13f.
18 *Ibid.,* pp. 31f.
19 N. Brooks, *Sickness, Health and God,* Advocate Press, USA, 1965, p. 54.
20 F. W. Woodward, cited in *Sickness, Health and God,* Advocate Press, USA, 1965, p. 56.
21 N. Brooks, *Sickness, Health and God,* Advocate Press, USA, 1965, p. 59.

5

THE GIFT OF HEALING

I. GIFTS AND CHARMS

Human 'gifts' take a variety of forms. We talk about 'natural' gifts by which we mean the development to a particularly high degree of natural talents and abilities. But the very fact that we recognise these as 'gifts' at least suggests that they are in some sense un-natural. For example, we have at least heard of, if we have not known, child prodigies who at an amazing early age have displayed extraordinary faculties of mind and body. We think of musicians like Beethoven or Mozart, people whose mathematical skills can match the computer, those who have the capacity to learn and speak fluently a great many different languages, those who display remarkable potentiality of genius or personality which sets them apart from and far ahead of others. All of these we call 'gifted' people.

There are those too who appear to possess healing gifts with or without reference to religion or the spiritual realm. Often their activities are frowned upon or discredited by the medical profession out of ignorance, arrogance, or professional prejudice. But they nevertheless practise their healing arts with remarkable success, and often with an even greater degree of success in dealing with particular maladies than orthodox medical practitioners, as, for example, those whose sensitive fingers can locate and restore displaced bones, sinews, muscles, discs, etc.

Or, as Leslie Weatherhead says,

After much consideration, it is my view that there are certain people with strange psychic gifts who, without doubt, have brought healing to some. As far as I know, there is no satisfactory explanation of this gift. The power of suggestion plays a part in such cures, but does not wholly explain them. The gift is often quite separated from any profession of Christianity, or from any adequate knowledge or understanding of medicine or psychology. Yet, to be quite fair, this so-called gift of healing is not always a concomitant of eccentricity.[1]

He goes on to give an account of such a gift discovered by accident and exercised with reluctance by a friend of his own. And he concludes,

Granted that these strange gifts of healing are not understood, yet if good can be done by their use it seems a serious thing to deprive patients of any possible benefit they might receive. Tennyson possessed this gift, but never linked it with religion, although he was a deeply religious man. Yet he laid his hands on the sick and a number recovered.[2]

Doris Collins is a lady who has been exercising such psychic gifts for almost 70 years. This is how she describes her experience:

As far as I remember, it was when I was only five or six that I first made contact with someone who was physically dead— another little girl, the daughter of one of my father's relations— but it was not until I was about sixteen, after apparently meeting my sister Emmie, who had died some three years earlier, that I was told by the mother of a schoolfriend that I had the psychic gift and also the great power of healing. Earlier experiences began to make sense when I talked to this woman, who was the first acknowledged psychic I had met, and from that time forward I began to investigate spiritualism and to cultivate my gifts.... Whatever people may think of me, they can hardly question my experience, the fruits of which I seek to convey to my readers in this book.... I have been called an extraordinary woman. I like that. I regard myself as ordinary.... If there is anything extraordinary about me, it is in my gifts—my clairvoyant gift and my healing gift—which are really all part of one.... The only extraordinary thing about me is that, when faced with the slightly unsettling knowledge that I had psychic power, I did not run a mile but instead sought to investigate it and use it for what I see as good purposes—to bring comfort where I can to those in physical or mental pain (pp. 13, 14).

It does not lie within the purpose of this work to investigate such a situation in depth. Mrs. Collins is an unapologetic necromancer who engages in activities which are clearly and categorically forbidden in the Scriptures upon pain of divine judgment (Deut. 18:11). But, as we shall see (pp. 252–3), much of her work bears such resemblance to that of some professed Christian faith-healers as to call for the utmost caution lest truth and counterfeit should be confused.

Then there are those who cure particular maladies by means of 'charms'. A charm is a spell or something used to influence people, circumstances or events, for good or ill, by means of supernatural or occult power. Magic is used universally. 'Black' magic attempts to produce evil results through such means as curses, spells, the destruction of models of those whom it is intended to harm or injure, and alliance with evil spirits. 'White' magic seeks to undo curses and spells and to use occult forces for the good of oneself or others. The magician or sorcerer (Exod. 7:11; Acts 13:6) tries to use or compel a demon or evil spirit to work for him; or he performs a rite with or without some form of mumbo-jumbo to make psychic forces fulfil his purposes. Both forms of magic or sorcery depend upon fear and superstition for their effectiveness, but they are much more than mere superstition. They are the use and manifestation of the spiritual powers and resources of witchcraft, astrologers, spiritists and spiritual mediums.

There are those who claim to have 'charms' for specific purposes including healing for particular maladies. Often the capacity to effect such charms is said to be relayed from generation to generation and particularly through a seventh generation, for example, a seventh son of a seventh son or seventh daughter of a seventh daughter. And there can be no doubt that the exercise of such 'gifts' or charms is often effective. The question remains, however, from what source or by what authority they derive their effectiveness. And it is essential to note the categorical distinction between the exercise of such propensities and that of Christian faith-healing. To fail to do so is to fail to understand the very nature of the biblical concept and its operation.

The use of charms in healing usually entails the exchange or wearing of amulets, ornaments, stones or trinkets bearing an inscription or requiring an incantation to a god, goddess or spirit known or unknown, and the pronouncement of a good spell or evil spell (curse).

> The practice of wearing amulets was common throughout the ancient Near East, and the Hebrews were unique in condemning their use, which was thought to protect the owner from evil....
> The Hebrew *lahas* commonly denoting the whispering sound used to charm snakes (Ps. 58:5; Eccl. 10:11) is once applied to amulets (A.V. 'earrings') worn by women and condemned by Isaiah (3:18–20).[3]

Almost all ornaments or jewelry such as those used by Aaron to make the 'golden calf' at Sinai (Exod. 32:2) or buried by Jacob (Gen. 35:4) were regarded as charms. Such charms were also hung on animals to increase fertility (Judg. 8:21, 26).

But the Bible universally condemns and forbids the wearing of charms or the use of magic because they are seen to be contrary to the worship and fear of the 'One living and true God'.

> The most striking reference to Hebrew witchcraft is Ezekiel 13:17–23. Here Hebrew prophetesses were also practising magic arts for the preservation and destruction of individuals. In this they were going farther than the false prophets of Micah 3:5, who gave messages of good or ill to individuals according to whether they were prepared to pay.[4]

While the details of this passage are not easy to piece together, J. S. Wright notes two main interpretations,

> G. A. Cooke (ICC) thinks that bands were placed on the wrists of the client and a covering on the head of the witch. In verse 20 he emends the text to read, 'Their arms'. He thinks that the binding was a piece of sympathetic magic, and represented the binding of the client's enemy for destruction. The veil was for loosing someone from death. The other interpretation is that of J. G. Frazer in his *Folk-lore in the Old Testament*. This is that the women professed to catch souls and bind them up in cloth bands. The imprisonment would cause the owner of the soul to waste away. In return for money a wandering soul would be restored to a sick person.[5]

The whole procedure is to be utterly denounced by the prophet (Ezekiel), and the wrath of God is pronounced upon all who participate in such things. 'Therefore ye shall see no more vanity, nor divine divinations: for I will deliver my people out of your hand: and ye shall know that I am the Lord' (Ezek. 13:23).

There are a number of passages, however, in which magic and superstition might appear to be countenanced in Scripture. For example, the use of mandrakes to ensure conception (Gen. 30:14–18); the use by Jacob of 'peeled rods' for the purpose of affecting the result of reproduction among the flocks of Laban (Gen. 30:37–43); the story of the cutting of Samson's hair (Judg. 16) which was superstitiously believed to be the source of his extraordinary strength. But in each of these cases, and others too, a careful examination of the Scripture text will show clearly that there are different explanations of the events which do not in any way require the assumption of superstition.

In Exodus 7:10–13 the Egyptian magicians were able to produce the same 'miraculous' effects as Moses. Balaam too was some sort of 'diviner' (Num. 22:17, 18). Nebuchadnezzar used divination for military purposes to secure the conquest of Jerusalem (Ezek. 21:21, 22). And in the New Testament the existence of sorcerers and their art is recognised, but always as being in opposition to the work of Christ and the Apostles (Acts 8:11; 13:6; 16:16). It is clear that the ability of magicians and soothsayers to effect unnatural phenomena is not denied or called in question. But it is evident that their capacity to do their work is attributed directly to the power of Satan and to the defiance of God's intent and purposes.

> Magic is a rival to true religion, though it can be practised in conjunction with false religious ideas. True religion centres in the personal experience of the one God, with an attempt to live a life that is conformable to his will. The believer walks humbly with his God, prays to him, and is prepared to accept the circumstances of Life as the sphere in which to glorify him. Magic, on the other hand, deals with lower supernatural beings, or attempts to force issues by using psychic forces, irrespective of whether the issues are for the glory of God.[6]

Healing therefore by means of charms is clearly forbidden by Scripture (Deut. 18:9–12; Acts 8:9, 23; 13:8–11; 16:16–18). This, of course, would include the whole gamut of cures wrought by means of the use of relics or the superstitions connected with religious shrines and rituals to which we shall return later.

II. 'SPIRITUAL GIFTS'

The Scriptures speak of another category of gifts—'spiritual gifts' or *charismata*. The *charismata* were extraordinary gifts or abilities bestowed by the Holy Spirit upon believers for special kinds of service (Rom. 12:6).

> The word used for the gifts is *charismata* which in the singular *charisma* means a gift freely given, a gift which results from grace (*charis*).... About twenty different gifts are included in the six lists (see Table VI), and there is no suggestion that these lists are exhaustive.[7]

Moreover, each of the gifts mentioned may be inclusive of a variety of different expressions. For example, J. R. W. Stott says,

> Again, only one of the five lists includes 'evangelists'. Is this a comprehensive gift to be claimed by all who engage in any form of evangelism? Or does not our experience of the variety of evangelistic gifts from God suggest that there may be a gift of crusade evangelism, another of home evangelism, another of friendship evangelism, another of casual contact evangelism, another of teaching evangelism, another of literature evangelism, and many more kinds besides?[8]

Concerning the nature of a *charisma* Wilkinson notes,

> Bittlinger...warns us to beware of a twofold misunderstanding of

the *charismata*. The first is the 'enthusiastic' misunderstanding which regards them as purely supernatural and miraculous, and therefore an unnecessary addition to normal Christian life. The second is the 'activist' misunderstanding which treats the *charismata* as purely natural in character, consisting of the normal activities and capabilities of man so that a *charisma* is exercised whenever a Christian does anything within the church. The first type of misunderstanding does not give man his true dignity as created by God, whilst the second ignores the result of his Fall. The truth must be that *charismata* are both natural and supernatural. To quote Bittlinger's definition we may say that a *charisma* is a gracious 'manifestation of the Holy Spirit, working in and through, but going beyond, the believer's natural ability for the common good of the people of God'.[9]

Stott suggests that there may even be a close connection between the natural abilities of the believer before conversion and the spiritual gift or gifts that he exercises afterwards.

Surely then we cannot suppose that there was no bridge between the two halves of their life? Would it not be more in keeping with the God of the Bible to suppose that he gave them an actual endowment *before* their call (genetic conditioning, we might say in modern times), which came to life and came into use only after it?[10]

Moreover, some of the *charismata* listed in the New Testament are not miraculous in themselves (for example, 'wisdom', 'counsel', 'administration'), but in their exercise they are demonstrative of the enabling of the Holy Spirit (Rom. 12:8). Of course, it is also evident that God bestows on believers gifts of the Spirit which manifest hitherto absent abilities or traits of character. Witherow puts it this way,

Sometimes they consisted in the enlargement of capacities and tendencies already planted from birth, and which henceforth were directed to new objects; at others they were the bestowment of new powers that the subject of them did not possess before.[11]

And Wilkinson recalls,

When we discussed what the epistles had to say about healing we took the view that the gift of healing was neither wholly natural nor wholly supernatural, but shared the characteristics of both spheres. It was given by God to certain individuals as a natural endowment which was supernaturally enhanced by the Holy Spirit once they became Christians.... This natural endowment includes such characteristics as sympathy or the ability to enter into another person's difficulties, patience or the facility to listen to their story, wisdom to know how to advise them and what to do in their particular case, and confidence to encourage them to expect recovery and healing. To these natural characteristics the Holy Spirit adds a new dimension by intensifying them and including with them faith in God's promise to heal through the prayer of faith.[12]

These gifts are distributed by the Holy Spirit according to God's sovereign will, that is, he gives them to whomsoever he will (1 Cor. 12:11), and they include among many others the gift of healing (1 Cor. 12:9). An individual may receive one or more, but not everyone receives the same gifts, nor does any one individual have all the gifts (1 Cor. 12:28–30). The possession of a gift or gifts implies the privilege and duty to exercise it or them in accordance with the Word of God, the example of Christ and the Apostles, and the prompting of the Holy Spirit (Rom. 12:6–8).

The general purpose for which such gifts are given is twofold. Primarily it is the edification of the whole church. 'And he gave some apostles; and some prophets; and some evangelists; and some, pastors and teachers; for the perfecting of the saints for the work of the ministry, for the edifying of the body of Christ. Till we all come in the unity of the faith, and of the knowledge of the Son of God, unto a perfect man, unto the measure of the stature of the fulness of Christ' (Eph. 4:12, 13). And secondarily it is for the conversion of unbelievers (Acts 2:43, 44; 3:12–4:4; 5:12–15; Rom. 15:18, 19). They are not given as ends in themselves, nor are they to be used for the personal advantage of the possessor, or merely for the physical or material benefit of any (1 Pet. 4:10, 11). Unlike the exercise of the ministry of the Word, there is no precedent in the New Testament for anyone to be provided with a living in order to exercise the other gifts on a full-time basis. So that while there are full-time preachers, teachers, evangelists and pastors, there are no full-time healers.

An examination of Table VI reveals that twenty apparently distinctive gifts are mentioned, though we cannot be certain that, for example, 'prophecy', 'prophets' and 'speaking' refer precisely to the same gift. Indeed 'teaching' might also in certain circumstances involve 'prophecy' in the wider sense of that term. The frequency of mention of each of the gifts may also be to some extent misleading since, for example, the gifts listed in 1 Corinthians 12:29, 30 are really only a rhetorical reference to those mentioned in verse 28, so that it is not really strictly correct to count this as a separate mention. We might therefore on this basis conclude that fourteen are mentioned once; four are mentioned twice; one is mentioned three times; and one is mentioned four times.

Moreover from Table VI it should be noted that the 'miracle-working' gifts (11–16) have no specific mention in the New Testament outside of 1 Corinthians. And out of the thirty-six places altogether in the New Testament in which spiritual gifts are mentioned as such only eleven have reference to the 'miracle-working' gifts.

T. C. Edwards in his commentary on 1 Corinthians groups the gifts thus:

1. intellectual power (*logos sophias, logos gnoseos*)
2. miraculous power (*pistis, iamata, dunameis*)
3. teaching power (*propheteia*)
4. critical power (*diakriseis pneumaton*)
5. ecstatic power (*gene, hermeneia glosson*)[13]

He points out that there is progress from the most worthy (*logos sophias*, 'the power of the spiritual man to understand the divine philosophy of the revelation in Christ') to the least worthy (*glossais lalein*).

The precise designation of the gift of healing is of interest and importance. Wilkinson says,

> Literally it is 'the gifts of healings', for both nouns are in the plural. This is usually interpreted as meaning that there is specialisation amongst the gifts of healing with different gifts for different diseases, and that no one person could heal all diseases.[14]

It could also mean surely that a capacity to heal might be given to an individual not only for a particular disease, but also for a particular occasion or situation only, and that, in fact, that individual might not have been called to an ongoing ministry of healing.

But to return to Table VI, so far as the gift of healing is concerned, it is surely most significant that it is mentioned twice but only in one chapter, and only in the context of the Corinthian church. This may suggest a number of possibilities:

1. Was it mentioned in reference to the Corinthian church only because it had achieved particular prominence or had become, like the gift of tongues, a particular problem there? From all that we know of Corinth and the church there, the former would not be in the least surprising, but the latter would seem unlikely because Paul mentions it but does not, as in the case of the gift of tongues, make any special comment or criticism, or give any specific directions regarding its performance. Indeed, Paul does not expressly say that anyone in Corinth exercised a healing gift. He simply lists healing as one of the gifts bestowed by the Spirit upon individuals in accordance with God's will and purpose. It seems reasonable to assume that in the highly charged situation in Corinth such a gift was being exercised, but there is no clear word on the matter and certainly no mention of anyone having been miraculously healed.

2. Was it mentioned only in Corinth because it did not occur in any other place? Or might it be that it was so much a normal activity of

church life in other places that it did not require special mention there? It is certainly assumed by those who have a special interest in spiritual gifts that the gift of healing was an integral part of each church and fellowship, and was widely and commonly in evidence. But there would appear to be little real evidence for such a conjecture. The church at Corinth seems to have presented a great many problems of confusion or abuse arising from spiritual immaturity or extravagance. This would seem to make it the more difficult to be sure that any procedure which was unique to that church should be regarded as normative for the church as a whole.

3. It is noteworthy that in the only other place in the Epistles in which reference is made to the practice of healing, James 5, there is no mention whatever of the existence or recognition of anyone possessing a gift of healing, and indeed the procedure promulgated by James is altogether different.

4. The question also arises as to whether the gift of healing was possessed or exercised by the disciples of Jesus or the Apostles. We have already noted that the disciples did not individually perform miracles of healing but only corporately. And again, they apparently could only do so when they had a specific instruction or commission from the Lord. They would appear not to have been free to heal at their own discretion but only as a part of a particular mission to which they were assigned by the Lord.

Wilkinson observes,

> There is much more that we would like to know about the gift of healing, but we are left with many of our questions unanswered. Why is the gift mentioned only in connection with the church at Corinth and not elsewhere? Why are those who healed the sick in the Acts not said to have a special gift of healing? Why is there no mention of such a gift in the Epistle of James? Why, when such a gift existed, were the leaders of the Christian community including the apostle Paul himself allowed to go unhealed? The existence of so many unanswered questions suggests that an understanding of the nature of the gift of healing is not necessary for the practice of healing. When we add to this the obscurity with which the gift of healing is described, and the fact that it is never associated with any act of healing in the New Testament record, and is not mentioned in the explicit description of the church's practice of healing given by James, it suggests that the gift of healing consists essentially of the application of earnest prayer and the enhanced natural endowments of the members of the Christian community.[15]

The conclusion of all this must be that while 'gifts of healings' are clearly listed by Paul among the gifts of the Spirit, there is no account anywhere in the New Testament of their operation.

From Table VI, then, we note that the special gifts and ministries appear to fall into two categories.

1. The first were permanent in their operation and became part of the constitutional and public function of the church—preachers, teachers, evangelists, prophets, and pastors who would, of course, follow the Apostles not in any historical or ecclesiastical succession but in the spiritual succession of the Apostles as those who 'continued steadfastly in the apostles' doctrine and fellowship' (Acts 2:47). Each and all of these would be essential to the basic requirement of the ministry of the Word both to the believers within the fellowship of the church and to those as yet within or without the church who had not received the truth of the Gospel to salvation.

2. The other gifts would appear to be of a more personal and occasional nature. That is to say, they would be used from time to time in particular circumstances or for particular purposes rather than have a continuous function, for example, 'giving', 'ruling', 'showing mercy', 'discerning spirits', 'counselling', 'working miracles' or 'helps' ('general helpfulness'). There is no indication that in the exercise of these gifts a person was to devote himself or herself to a full-time ministry, but rather that in particular needs or circumstances some person with an appropriate gift would either be called upon or would offer his or her services in dealing with the matter.

III. WITHDRAWN OR NOT?

Now we come to the crucial question, Did the spiritual gifts endure beyond the days of the Apostles or the church of the New Testament period? If not, when did they cease to be operative? And if they did continue are they available today, and in what circumstances? On the answers to these questions Christians have been and are deeply divided. Many Christians, especially Pentecostals and Charismatics, insist that at no time is there any indication that the gifts disappeared or were withdrawn. Whereas the churches of the Reformation, following Calvin, have largely adopted the view that the gifts of the Spirit—especially those related to miraculous powers—did not outlast the period of the Apostles and the New Testament church.

(i) The 'Reformed' view

B. B. Warfield is strongly representative of the Reformed view. He describes the origin of the *charismata* thus:

> His own [Christ's] divine power by which he began to found his church he continued in the Apostles whom he had chosen to complete his work. They transmitted it in turn, as part of their

own miracle-working and the crowning sign of their divine commission, to others, in the form of what the New Testament calls spiritual gifts in the sense of extraordinary capacities produced in the early Christian communities by direct gift of the Holy Spirit.[16]

Warfield describes these gifts of the Spirit as 'distinctively gracious' and 'distinctively miraculous'. The non-miraculous are regarded as 'the greatest gifts' and even among the miraculous gifts there is a distinction in favour of 'prophecy' and those others by which the body is edified. Among the 'extraordinary' he includes,

gifts of healings, workings of miracles, prophecy, discernings of spirits, kinds of tongues, the interpretation of tongues—all of which are appropriate to the worshipping assembly.[17]

The Apostolic church, he maintains, was characteristically a miracle-working church. But these gifts which the Apostles possessed,

were distinctively the authentication of the Apostles. They were part of the credentials of the Apostles as the authoritative agents of God in founding the church. Their function thus confined them to distinctively the Apostolic church, and they necessarily passed away with it.[18]

And he goes on,

The theologians of the post-Reformation era, a very clear-headed body of men, taught with great distinctness that the *charismata* ceased with the Apostolic age.'[19]

But this teaching gradually gave way in the Protestant Churches to the unreformed view that the gifts continued after the Apostolic age for three centuries down to the time of Constantine (323 A.D.) when Christianity came to be established by the civil power.

The widely held view was that,

miracles having been given for the purpose of founding the church, they continued so long as they were needed for that purpose; growing gradually fewer as they were less needed, and ceasing altogether when the church having, so to speak, been firmly put upon its feet, was able to stand on its own legs.[20]

But Warfield says,

if the evidence is worth anything at all, instead of a regularly progressing decrease, there was a steadily growing increase of miracle-working from the beginning on.... There is little or no evidence at all for miracle-working during the first fifty years of the post-Apostolic church; it is slight and unimportant for the next fifty years; it grows more abundant during the next century (the third); and it becomes abundant and precise only in the fourth century, to increase still further in the fifth and beyond.[21]

He goes on to assert that by the date of Polycarp's martyrdom in 155

A.D. the beginnings of the claim of the presence of miraculous powers
in the church were becoming evident; for example, in Justin Martyr
who mentions the gift of healing, and Irenaeus who mentions also
speaking with tongues and raising the dead. But their references are
only in general terms and are uncorroborated either by the citation of
any specific cases or by any contemporary writer. Origen, he says,
professes to have been an eye-witness of many instances of exorcism,
healing, and prophecy, though again he refuses to record any details.
Cyprian speaks of gifts of visions and exorcisms.

> And so we pass on to the fourth century in an ever-increasing
> stream, but without a single writer having claimed himself to
> have wrought a miracle of any kind or having ascribed miracle-
> working to any known name in the church, and without a single
> instance having been recorded in detail.[22]

He declares that the adoption of the apocryphal writings—'these wild
and miracle-laden documents'—by the Catholic Church became the
basis of belief in miracle-working.

> It is from these apocryphal miracle-stories and not from the
> miracles of the New Testament, that the luxuriant growth of the
> miraculous stories of later ecclesiastical writings draw their
> descent. And this is as much as to say that their ultimate
> parentage must be traced to those heathen wonder-tales.[23]

Warfield believes that the purpose for which the gifts were given was
not the extension of the church, but the authentication of the Apostles
as messengers from God,

> the *charismata* belonged, in a true sense, to the Apostles, and
> constituted one of the signs of an Apostle. Only in the two great
> initial instances of the descent of the Spirit at Pentecost and the
> reception of Cornelius are *charismata* recorded as conferred
> without the laying on of the hands of the Apostles (Acts 8:14–
> 17).[24]

He suggests that to restrict the *charismata* to the Apostles and those
on whom they conferred them explains the fact that their cessation was
gradual and unnoticed. There can be few of those who had received
them at the hands of the Apostles still living in the second century.
Justin Martyr and Irenaeus may have known of, if not actually witnessed, miracles wrought by those who had received the gifts from an
Apostle though they could not claim the power for themselves.

Miracles, Warfield maintains,

> belong to revelation periods, and appear only when God is
> speaking to his people through accredited messengers, declaring
> his gracious purposes. Their abundant display in the Apostolic
> church is the mark of the richness of the Apostolic age in
> revelation; and when this revelation period closed, the period of

miracle-working had passed by also, as a mere matter of course.[25] He goes on to show in great detail how the miracle-working which in Apostolic times was the evidence and effect of the working of the divine power of the Holy Spirit, systematically and progressively degenerated in the centuries of the Roman Catholic Church down to the Reformation into nothing more than the pagan idolatry and superstition of saint-worship and the magical use of charms. He writes,

> J. H. Newman...remarks that many miracles are ascribed to the tombs or relics of the saints, rather than to the saints themselves; and this is only an example of the uses to which they have been put. So many were wrought in connection with superstitions which grew up about the Eucharist, for instance, that 'wonders wrought by the Eucharist' is made one of the main divisions of the article.[26]

And Warfield asks,

> What are we to think of these miracles? There is but one historical answer which can be given. They represent an infusion of heathen modes of thought into the church.[27]

Weatherhead comes to the same conclusion. Speaking of the times after the Apostles he says,

> One reluctantly writes down the sentence—Christ's followers found that their power to heal had gone. As St Cyprian once wrote, 'The sins of Christians have weakened the power of the Church'; and though the early church rationalised and pretended that God had 'withdrawn the gift given to the Apostles', or that he no longer 'willed to heal' and that Christians 'had to bear their sufferings as Christ his Cross', and that illness was 'a punishment for sin and must not be interfered with', yet the grim truth was as stated.[28]

The result he says was that non-physical methods of healing were abandoned for the use of drugs. Exorcism and healing made no reference to the power of Christ and,

> Even Origen asserted, 'The force of the exorcism lies in the name of Jesus', and sometimes he seems to have taken a pagan view of the matter and encouraged superstition. The power of this superstition gradually displaced the power of faith and love. The sale of holy relics abounded, though it was hotly opposed by the authorities of the church, and even the devout followers of Jesus...must have been disturbed to find that pagan exorcists could obtain similar results to themselves.[29]

Weatherhead goes so far as to assert that the James 5 passage,

> was responsible for making all three methods (of healing— prayer, anointing with oil and laying on of hands) into a magical rite instead of a sacrament.[30]

Presumably he means the James passage quite wrongfully was made the pretext for magical rites. Eventually, he says,

> Finding that...treatments with oil—and sometimes with holy water—had fewer and fewer successes so far as the recovery of health was concerned, the very meaning of the service of anointing with oil insidiously altered[31]

and became, by Decree of the Council of Trent (1549), the sacrament of Extreme Unction which was not a means of healing but a preparation for death. With the progress and development of medical science, and the treatment of all kinds of disease, the care of the body became the responsibility of the medical profession and the care of the soul the responsibility of the church. And so for many it has remained.

We may summarise the arguments for the cessation of the *charismata* thus:

1. Christ's power to work miracles was transmitted by the Holy Spirit to the Apostles.

2. The *charismata* were the authentication of the Apostles as God's agents in establishing the church.

3. The Apostles transmitted the *charismata* to others through the laying on of hands. This was the only means of their transmission.

4. Since they related specifically to the Apostles the *charismata* ceased with the passing of the Apostles.

5. Since miracles belong to periods of revelation and revelation ceased with the passing of the Apostles, the *charismata* ceased with them.

6. While miracle-working continued in the church and progressively increased after the passing of the Apostles, it was to be attributed not to the power of the Holy Spirit, but to pagan superstition in the use of relics and false sacraments.

7. With the development of medicine and drugs the care of body and soul became divided between medical science and the church.

(ii) The 'Pentecostal' view

We have already noted that the *charismata* were 'extraordinary' abilities bestowed on believers by the Holy Spirit. Some, we said, were not miraculous in themselves, but rather, natural capacities quickened by the divine power. Bittlinger underlined the fact that they were neither purely natural nor purely supernatural. Wilkinson in specific reference to the gift of healing insisted that it was neither wholly natural nor wholly supernatural. And Edwards identified the expressly 'miraculous' gifts as faith, healing, and miracles. We also saw that while Warfield distinguished between the 'gracious' and the 'miraculous' gifts he nevertheless grouped the *charismata* together in his assertion that they ceased with the Apostles.

We now must examine the contrary view that the *charismata* at no time were withdrawn. But here opinion is divided as to whether the 'miraculous' gifts were included in the continuation of the *charismata*. J. R. W. Stott asks,

> 'The working of miracles' and 'workers of miracles' proclaim themselves as involving miracles, and so probably do 'gifts of healing' and 'healers', together with 'various kinds of tongues', and 'the interpretation of tongues'. Assuming these to be miraculous gifts, are they still bestowed today?[32]

He notes that some Christians see the activity of God only in the miraculous whereas, in fact, he normally works in and through the regular processes of the natural world. Others are convinced that God,

> intends miracles to be as regular a feature of our life and ministry today as they were in the ministry of our Lord and his apostles. But this also cannot be seriously maintained by those whose doctrine of miracles is derived from Scripture.[33]

He goes on to show that miracle-working in Scripture centred around Moses, Elijah and Elisha, the Lord himself and the Apostles, corresponding to,

> the four main epochs of revelation—the law, the prophets, the Lord and the Apostles. And the major purpose of miracles was to authenticate each fresh stage of revelation.[34]

And he concludes therefore that our position ought to be,

> I don't expect miracles as a commonplace today, because the special revelation they were given to authenticate is complete; but of course God is sovereign and God is free, and there may well be particular situations in which he pleases to perform them.[35]

With regard to the other *charismata* Stott says,

> [Some] Christians tend to say and write that there is 'no biblical evidence whatever' that any gifts would ever be withdrawn. But, on the contrary, there *is* evidence for the very thing for which they say there is none.[36]

And he goes on to show, for example, that the *charisma* of 'apostle' was limited to the original twelve (omitting Judas Iscariot who lost his apostleship) (Luke 6:12, 13), together with Paul (Gal. 1:1), probably James the Lord's brother (Gal. 1:19) and possibly one or two others. Since the essential qualification of an Apostle was to have seen Jesus (Acts 1:21, 22; 1 Cor. 9:1, 15; 8:9) they could have no successors. Prophets too were distinguished by the fact that they were agents of divine revelation of whom Christ himself was the last of the line (Heb. 1:1–3).

> So in the primary sense of 'prophets', as vehicles of direct and fresh revelation, it seems we must say that the *charisma* is no

longer given.[37]

Even in the sense of not adding to revelation but foretelling future events, the evidence of the failure of the predictions of those who have claimed to possess the gift to be fulfilled, denies the reality of the *charisma*. The continuance of the remaining *charismata* seems to present no difficulty whatever, indeed, they would appear to be necessary to the ongoing edification and extension of the church as is expressly stated to have been their purpose in the first place (1 Cor. 14:12).

J. O. Sanders takes a similar view:

> Once the credibility of the witness of the apostles had been established, and the canon of the New Testament had been completed, there was not the same necessity for the exercise of the miraculous gifts which gradually became less prominent. Bishop H. C. G. Moule said in this connection: 'It is not ours to be decisive where the Scripture is reticent. But on the whole Scripture points to a cessation of *charismata* in the normal life of the church.... In 1 Cor. 13:8 there is the intimation of a certain transiency in these manifestations, in contrast to the permanency of grace'. There are those who contend that the miraculous gifts completely passed away, but this would be difficult to maintain in the light of church and missionary history.[38]

But A. B. Simpson, who takes an extreme view, confidently asserts,

> the dear Master never contemplated or proposed any post-apostolic gulf of impotence or failure. Man's unbelief and sin have made it. The church's own corruption has caused it.... He said: 'All power is given unto me in heaven and earth, and lo, I am with you all the days, even unto the end of the age'. It was to be one age, not two, and his 'all power' has never been withdrawn.... The age of miracles is not past. The Word of God never indicated a hint of such a fact. On the contrary, they are to be among the signs of the last days; and the very adversary himself is to counterfeit them.[39]

And F. L. Wyman with reference not merely to the healing of the sick but to the raising of the dead writes,

> One cannot but be frankly amazed at the fact that the church, having been Divinely committed to the task of raising the dead, and having the promise that Christ's followers would be permitted to perform even greater works than Christ himself performed during his earthly Ministry, that with such a Divinely bequeathed passport, the church through sheer fearfulness and unpardonable doubt, if not unbelief, wanders through the shallows, seeking to find contentment and satisfaction with such things as completely stagger spiritual sensitiveness.[40]

We may summarise the arguments for the continuance of the *charismata* thus:

1. While God who is sovereign in all things normally works through natural processes he may at any time manifest his power in miracle.

2. While there is evidence that the *charismata* related to Apostleship and prophecy necessarily ceased with the passing of the Apostles and the completion of Divine revelation, it is equally evident in the history and experience of the church that the other *charismata* have continued to be exercised.

3. The apparent absence of the charismata is the result of the faithlessness, error, and disobedience of the members of the church.

(iii) The 'middle' view

The two views, however, concerning the cessation or continuance of the *charismata* are not totally exclusive of each other. There is, as we have seen, a distinction between those *charismata* which are evidenced by supernatural effects (*e.g.* tongues, miraculous healing and other supernatural phenomena) and those which are evidenced by natural procedures (*e.g.* preaching, administration, counsel, sympathy, generosity, *etc.*).

Those who regard them as bestowed permanently on the church attribute their early disappearance to a decline of faith and spirituality, and claim that they have been rediscovered in later times, especially during religious revivals.... The popular view, that the *charismata* were given for the founding of the church and ceased during the 4th century when it became strong enough to continue without their assistance is contrary to historical evidence.[41]

IV. SUMMARY

We may draw the following general conclusions regarding the nature and purposes of the 'gifts of the Spirit' including the 'gifts of healings':

1. They are to be distinguished from natural gifts or talents of human personality, character and ability.

2. They are to be distinguished from the possession or use of 'charms' which is expressly forbidden in Scripture.

3. They are to be distinguished from the superstitious use of ritual or relics which is contrary to the Word of God.

4. They are among the *charismata* listed in the New Testament as being a manifestation of the power of the Holy Spirit in and through the believer who possesses them.

5. They can be either a supernatural capacity to work miracles or a natural capacity quickened and heightened by the power of the Holy

Spirit.

6. They are possessed in accordance with the sovereign will and purpose of God and are neither attainable otherwise nor universally bestowed on all believers.

7. They may take a variety of forms and have specifically different applications in different people or circumstances.

8. They were not attributed to the disciples or Apostles, though they did heal the sick by express commission of the Lord.

9. There is no recorded instance of their use in the New Testament.

10. Some of the gifts of the Spirit were intended to be permanent in their operation, while others were occasional in their use.

11. The view that the *charismata* as a whole were withdrawn is untenable in the light of the history and experience of the church.

12. Their absence may, though not necessarily, be the result of the faithlessness or disobedience of church members.

13. They are given not for individual or personal advantage but for the edification and betterment of the Body of Christ.

14. They are not marks of the spiritual superiority of those who possess them, but capacities for witness to Christ and service to others.

15. They continue to be manifested in the edification and extension of the Body of Christ.

NOTES

1   L. D. Weatherhead, *Psychology, Religion and Healing,* Hodder and Stoughton, London, 1951, p. 144.
2   *Ibid.,* p. 146.
3   D. J. Wiseman, *New Bible Dictionary,* IVF, London, 1962, p. 34.
4   J. S. Wright, *New Bible Dictionary,* IVF, London, 1962, p. 767.
5   *Ibid.,* p. 767.
6   *Ibid.,* p. 766.
7   J. Wilkinson, *Health and Healing,* Handsel Press, Edinburgh, 1980, p. 107.
8   J. R. W. Stott, *Baptism and Fullness,* IVP, Leicester, 1977, p. 89.
9   J. Wilkinson, *Health and Healing,* Handsel Press, Edinburgh, 1980, p. 108.
10   J. R. W. Stott, *Baptism and Fullness,* IVP, Leicester, 1977, p. 91.
11   T. Witherow, *The Form of the Christian Temple,* T. & T. Clark, Edinburgh, 1889, p. 45.
12   J. Wilkinson, *Health and Healing,* Handsel Press, Edinburgh, 1980 pp. 175f.
13   T. C. Edwards, *Commentary on First Corinthians,* 1885, p. 314.
14   J. Wilkinson, *Health and Healing,* Handsel Press, Edinburgh, 1980, p. 108.

15 *Ibid.,* pp. 109f.
16 B. B. Warfield, *Counterfeit Miracles,* Banner of Truth Trust, London, 1972, p. 3.
17 *Ibid.,* p. 5.
18 *Ibid.,* p. 6.
19 *Ibid.,* p. 6.
20 *Ibid.,* p. 9.
21 *Ibid.,* p. 10.
22 *Ibid.,* p. 12.
23 *Ibid.,* p. 18.
24 *Ibid.,* pp. 21f.
25 *Ibid.,* p. 26.
26 *Ibid.,* p. 51.
27 *Ibid.,* p. 61.
28 L. D. Weatherhead, *Psychology, Religion and Healing,* Hodder and Stoughton, London, 1951, p. 89.
29 *Ibid.,* pp. 89f.
30 *Ibid.,* p. 91.
31 *Ibid.,* p. 93.
32 J. R. W. Stott, *Baptism and Fullness,* IVP, Leicester, 1977, p. 96.
33 *Ibid.,* p. 97.
34 *Ibid.,* p. 97.
35 *Ibid.,* pp. 98f.
36 *Ibid.,* p. 99.
37 *Ibid.,* p. 101.
38 J. O. Sanders, *The Holy Spirit and His Gifts,* Marshall, Morgan and Scott, London, 1970, p. 111.
39 A. B. Simpson, *The Gospel of Healing,* Morgan and Scott, London, 1915, pp. 52f.
40 F. L. Wyman, *The Dead Are Raised Up,* Ken-Pax Publishing Co., Minehead, 1954, p. 18.
41 W. G. Putman, *New Bible Dictionary,* IVF, London, 1962, p. 1213.

6

THE CALL FOR HEALING

It is surely most remarkable that the passage of Scripture which springs most readily and most adamantly to the lips of faith-healers as the basis for their practice is James 5:14–18. For, with all its difficulty and variety of interpretation, the one thing that it cannot be said to justify is the exercise of the power to heal by an individual whether priest with his counterfeit sacrament or evangelist with his laying on of hands.

James 5:14–18 has been used in many ways. Wilkinson remarks,

> It has been the main proof text for auricular confession to a priest, unction, extreme unction and so-called faith-healing. It would be tragic if the church continued to treat this passage as it has treated it in the past and missed what we believe to be its clear teaching.[1]

We shall consider the passage under the three main ways in which it has been construed namely: (1) as referring to spiritual rather than physical healing (2) as referring to sacramental preparation for death, and (3) as referring to physical healing in answer to prayer.

I. SPIRITUAL OR PHYSICAL?

Some things in the passage may appear to suggest that the healing in question is spiritual rather than physical. For example,

(i) The involvement of 'the elders'

It is the 'elders of the Church' who are to be called rather than someone with the gift of physical healing, and nowhere else in the New Testament is the exercise of the gift of healing attributed to, or required of, the elders. Wilkinson notes,

> In so far as the office of elder is defined in the New Testament there is no suggestion that healing the sick was a specific function of this office. There is no reference to healing as a function of elders or bishops in the Pastoral Epistles although these terms describe the same office. In the Corinthian church healing gifts were not associated with the elders, but were given to those to whom the Holy Spirit willed to give them (1 Cor. 12:9, 28, 30).[2]

The particular responsibility of the elders was pastoral care of the flock and spiritual discipline. They should therefore have a special interest in and concern for those who for one reason or another (not necessarily specific sin) were spiritually sick. Surely nothing could be better calculated to provide spiritual comfort and restoration of such a stricken believer than the sympathy, concern, support and prayer of the more spiritually mature and experienced elders. Tasker makes the point well,

> While it is true that they could intercede for the sick man without being present at his bedside, nevertheless, by coming to the actual scene of suffering and by praying within sight and hearing of the sufferer himself, not only is their prayer likely to be more heartfelt and fervid, but the stricken man may well become more conscious of the effective power of prayer uttered in faith, by which, even in moments of the most acute physical weakness, communion with God can be maintained.[3]

Such is the practice of all normal 'pastoral' ministry in the church, especially that of the elders whether clergy or laity, and has been so since the times of the New Testament church. Mayor commenting on *presbuteros* says,

> We need not of course suppose the word to be used in its later hierarchical sense.... It seems better, however, to regard it as an official title, denoting the leaders of the local Christian society...who would exercise a general superintendence over the activity of the individual members and over the use to be made of the *charismata*. Those who possessed these gifts in the largest measure would doubtless be themselves included in the council of elders (*to presbuterion* 1 Tim. 4:14).[4]

We have already noted the fact that no such qualification was required in the New Testament Epistles for the eldership. But Mayor goes on to speculate,

> On notification of a case of sickness, the council would, we may suppose, consider whether it was a fit case for the exercise of the

charisma, and would depute some of their body to attend to the case and unite in prayer for the sick person (Matt. 18:20).[5]
Ropes goes even further and regards the procedure as a formal and 'solemn visit' based on the precedence of the visitation of the sick by Jewish rabbis.[6]

(ii) The terms used

The spiritual nature of the exercise might also be construed from a number of the terms used. For example, *astheneo* (v. 13) basically means 'to be weak' and *kamno* (v. 15) which basically means 'to be weary' and only secondarily came to refer to physical sickness. *Kamno,* both Wilkinson and Mayor note, is used outside the New Testament in participle form to refer to 'dying'. But both commentators fail to see any reason for making any distinction between them in the present context,[7] and conclude that they both refer to physical sickness.

   sozo (v. 15) certainly is used with reference both
to physical healing and spiritual salvation.

> The verb *sozo*...includes both healing and salvation in the gospels. When we come to the epistles, however, we find that Paul deliberately limits the application of both the noun and the verb to man's relationship to God as the main area where *soteria* is required and it was this usage which came to predominate in theological writing.... Salvation in the New Testament sense is total and includes the whole man producing in him that condition of safety and soundness which forms part of the New Testament concept of health.[8]

But Wilkinson further notes,

> The verb *sozo* is used only in James 5:15 in a sense which clearly includes the healing of the sick.[9]

iathete (v. 16) also is used with reference to both physical and spiritual sickness.

> For the use of *iasthai* in reference to the diseases of the soul *cf.* Hebrews 12:13; 1 Peter 2:24; Matthew 13:15; *etc.*[10]

But Mayor goes on to say,

> If the word is understood literally of bodily disease...as by De Wette, Huther, and Spitta, the connection of thought is perhaps closer, keeping to the subject of the miraculous cure, which is spoken of in the preceding verse and seems to be referred to in the words which follow, dwelling on the miraculous power of the prayer of Elijah.[11]

Plummer agrees that the context demands this construction.

> It is not quite certain that the word rendered 'ye may be healed' (*iathete*) ought to be limited to bodily healing; but the context seems to imply that the cure of bodily disorders is still in the

mind of St James. If, however, with various commentators, we take it to mean 'that your *souls* may be healed', then there is no need to supply any such thought as 'when sickness comes upon you'.[12]

Moreover, while intercessory prayer for others with a view to their repentance and forgiveness is widely advocated in Scripture, there is no ground for believing that their salvation can be effected by any means other than their own personal exercise of saving faith in Christ, whereas it is plainly asserted that 'the prayer of faith shall save the sick'.

> We are never told in the New Testament that a man will be saved in a spiritual sense by prayer. Furthermore, physical healing would naturally precede the raising up which forms the second part of the definition. The first part of the definition means, therefore, the healing of physical disease.[13]

egerei (v. 15) certainly is used with reference to resurrection from the dead and therefore might well be construed with a spiritual significance, but evidently not in the present context.

> The word *egeiro* is the usual one used for the physical resurrection of our Lord from the dead, but it is plainly not used of raising from the dead in our paragraph.... The Lord not only heals the sick of his disease, he also raises him up from his bed and puts him on his feet again with new strength and vitality (Matt. 9:6).[14]

Ropes is categoric about the meaning of the word. He says,

> The word means 'raise from the bed of sickness to health', and is a virtual repetition of *sosei...egerei* cannot refer either to the awakening of the dead to life or to the resurrection.[15]

Taken together with *kamnonta* ('the sick'), *egerei* might be understood to have reference to resurrection, but Tasker comments,

> In its past tense it (*kamno*) was sometimes used as a description of 'the dead'; but as there is no instance of the present participle conveying the meaning of 'the dying', it is most improbable that that is the sense here, and that the writer means to suggest that the sufferer is 'in extremis'. Similarly, the expression 'shall raise him up' cannot be interpreted in a spiritual sense, but must mean 'shall enable him to stand on his feet'. The verb *egerei* used here in a transitive sense with 'the Lord' as the subject, is used intransitively at the beginning of the command given by Jesus to the paralytic 'Arise, take up thy bed and walk' (Mark 2:9).[16]

(iii) 'Anointing'

The spiritual nature of the exercise might also be implied from the use of anointing oil and the references to confession and forgiveness of sin.

We shall return to these matters later, but for the moment we must consider whether they indicate that the exercise is to be understood as that of the healing of physical or spiritual sickness.

Anointing with oil was already widely accepted and practised among the Jews as symbolic of spiritual healing and anointing with grace (Heb. 1:9). Ropes comments,

> The use of oil for healing was combined with the appeal to spiritual forces, as we can see in James 5:14 and as is hinted in Mark 6:13. The reference in James is to an accepted popular custom, and the writer would hardly have been able to distinguish the parts played in the recovery by the two elements, or perhaps even to give any theory of the function of the oil. It is possible, as has often been suggested, that one motive for James' exhortation is to counteract the habit of seeking aid from superstitious, often heathenish, incantations and charms. The verse is often quoted to that end by later Christian writers.[17]

While, as we shall see, the anointing with oil later came to be given an entirely new and unwarranted meaning, in the counterfeit sacrament of Extreme Unction, with specific reference to spiritual rather than physical healing, here it was clearly intended, if not expressly to have medicinal effect, at least to reinforce the expectation of physical healing.

(iv) 'Confession'

The spiritual nature of the exercise might also be inferred from the references to confession and forgiveness of sin. At this stage it is sufficient to note that in verse 15 it is to be assumed that the forgiveness of sin is related to the possible cause, direct or indirect, of the physical sickness. Tasker says,

> The meaning seems to be that, if God should effect a miraculous cure in answer to the elders' prayer of faith accompanied by anointing with oil in the name of the Lord, that would be a clear indication that any sins of the sufferer, which might have been responsible for this particular illness, were forgiven.[18]

The most obvious and impressive examples to be found in the New Testament are those of the paralytic man brought to Jesus on his mattress (Mark 2:5–11) and the man healed at the pool of Bethesda (John 5:1–9, 14).

The reference to mutual confession and intercession (v. 16) might also suggest a spiritual rather than a physical need.

> We need not, however, suppose any reference here to a formal confession of sin, but merely to such mutual confidences as would give a right direction to the prayers offered by one for the other.[19]

What is being dealt with is not a spiritual problem as such, but rather the effective application of spiritual resources to physical and temporal needs by means of mutual understanding and support in prayer.

The connecting link between all the verses in this section would appear to be the power of prayer. In verse 16 James seems to be insisting that if 'the prayer of faith' can have such a miraculous result as that mentioned in the previous verse, Christians should always pray for one another, not only in times of illness but in all the vicissitudes of their lives, so that healing, in the fullest and widest sense of that word, may be bestowed upon them. And in order that their prayers may be intelligent and based on specific knowledge, they should not hesitate to confess to one another their 'faults', so that their brethren may bring these faults to the throne of grace.[20]

The reference to confession and intercession also indicates that healing whether of bodily or mental sickness inevitably has a spiritual dimension. Man's threefold nature, spirit, soul and body, as Paul describes it in 1 Thessalonians 5:23, is inseparable. As the Apostle taught, when one part is affected then the whole person is affected too. Hence physical healing ought not to be seen in isolation. Just as the cause of physical affliction may lie in the mind or the soul, so the healing of the body has necessary mental and spiritual implications. This is why James in dealing with healing so closely interlinks them.

Sickness has always more than a physical dimension even if it be so minor as the common cold. It always has mental, social and spiritual dimensions, and this paragraph of James reminds us of all of these. Similarly healing cannot be confined to the physical or medical dimension, but must include the other dimensions too.[21]

We may conclude then that while spiritual factors are necessarily involved, the subject being dealt with by James in this passage is physical healing not spiritual sickness.

II. 'EXTREME UNCTION'

It is not difficult then to see how the false construction of the Roman Catholic Church came to be imposed upon this passage of James. Mayor comments,

it may probably be inferred that, the anointing with simple oil having ceased to be effective in the healing of the sick, some endeavoured to add fresh virtue to the oil either by special consecration, or by combining it with the relics of saints, while others...supposed it to retain a purely spiritual efficacy, thus changing a hypothetical appendage to the injunction into the essence of the injunction itself. There is, I believe, no recorded instance (except one) during the first eight centuries of the anointing of the sick being deferred, as having only a spiritual efficacy.[22]

It was in the eighth century that,

> the use of oil was transformed into an anointing of those about to die, not as a means of their recovery, but with a view to the remission of their sins, and in connection with the giving of the 'viaticum'.[23]

But it was the twelfth century before Extreme Unction was mentioned by name as one of the seven sacraments of the Roman Church. The Council of Trent (1545) which formulated and established the doctrines of the Roman Church, in setting forth its Decrees on Extreme Unction, falsely declared that it was ordained as a sacrament by Christ in Mark 6:13 and promulgated by James 5:14. The Decrees also anathematised any who refused to believe in the effectiveness of the sacrament *ex opere operato*, opposed or neglected it, or who denied that the elders referred to by James were episcopally ordained priests. The Roman Catechism, we are told,

> adds that it is only to be administered to those who are dangerously ill.... Pastors must instruct their people that by this sacrament venial sins are remitted, the soul is freed from the weakness contracted by sin, and filled with courage, hope and joy. If bodily health does not follow from it, this is to be ascribed to the want of faith of those who administer or receive the sacrament.[24]

Of course we know that in practice not only is the administration of Extreme Unction deferred until the latest possible moment in the life of the sufferer, but that in fact often it is administered after death has actually taken place. So there can be no doubt whatever that in Roman doctrine it relates in reality to the expectation of death (or even death itself) and its consequences rather than to the expectation of recovery and life as in the intention of James.

In the post-Vatican II era we are told, however, that as a result of that Council's Decrees,

> a sacrament which, in recent centuries, was used primarily to prepare a person for death and only secondarily and condition-ally, to lead to healing, has been changed so that its primary purpose is now to heal the whole man who is suffering the special trial of sickness. As Pope Paul VI writes, 'We thought fit to modify the sacramental formula in such a way that, in view of the words of James, the effects of the sacrament might be fully expressed'.[25]

What this means, of course, is not that the original doctrine is in any way changed, but that the 'sacramental formula' has been 'modified' with a form of words which enables what *is still* primarily intended and administered as Extreme Unction that is, anointing with oil at the extremity of life, to be used in other circumstances for the purpose of offering relief to the suffering. Francis MacNutt notes the following apparent changes in the meaning and administration of the sacrament since Vatican II:

1. It is no longer called 'Extreme Unction' but 'anointing of the sick'. The Vatican II Decree on the Sacred Liturgy section 73 says,

> Extreme Unction which may also and more fittingly be called 'anointing of the sick' is not a sacrament for those only who are at the point of death. Hence, as soon as any one of the faithful begins to be in danger of death from sickness or old age, the appropriate time for him to receive this sacrament has certainly already arrived.[26]

It should be noted, however, that Extreme Unction as such is in no way diminished or replaced by the Vatican II Decree. On the contrary, it still relates to those who 'begin to be in danger of death from sickness or old age', and in fact it thus serves only to make the administration of the sacrament more urgent without in any way altering its purpose except to extend it beyond sickness to 'old age'. But it is still very much to be a preparation for death.

2. The essential form has been changed to appear to emphasise *healing* whereas the previous form stressed *forgiveness of sin*. But what healing is there for 'old age'?

3. The sacrament is to be administered to those who are *seriously ill*, rather than merely to those who are *in danger of death*. But this is not necessarily so. The question still remains as to when the person is 'in danger of death'. All that is permitted is that the administration of the sacrament need no longer be postponed till the last possible moment, or even till death may have taken place.

4. Ideally the anointing is to be a communal prayer involving the patient's family, doctor, nurses and other members of the people of God whereas Extreme Unction was usually administered in private because of its connection with the confession of sin. *Ideally* this may have been made possible, but this does not mean that it is necessarily or usually so, and, in fact, it need not be so at all.

5. The oil may now be blessed by a priest if necessary and not just by a bishop. Since such 'blessing' is nowhere contemplated or required by Scripture, this 'change' would appear to be purely a matter of convenience and totally irrelevant to the meaning or value of the rite.[27]

We may conclude then that while certain accommodations have been made by Vatican II to the more 'charismatic' approach to healing that has come about in the Roman Catholic Church, the misinterpretation of the James passage as a basis for the false sacrament of Extreme Unction remains.

III. PROCEDURES

The passage has been taken by many to refer to the exercise of the gift of healing, and as such it merits close examination. We note the procedure laid down by James thus:

(i) The initiative

The initiative is to be taken by the sick person, or presumably by others at his request or on his behalf (as often in the ministry of the Lord).

There is an interesting grammatical point to be considered. James changes the tense of the verbs (*proskalesastho, proseuxasthosan*) from the present imperative to the aorist imperative which would suggest that the action should be taken immediately and once only.[28] This would appear decisively to conflict with the common practice of seeking such help only after all other means of healing have been tried and failed; or indeed the tendency to seek the help of one spiritual agent of healing after another when there appears to be no effect forthcoming.

It is for the elders to come to the sufferer. His calling for them would seem to imply either his membership of the church as a believer, or, at least, his acknowledgment of the spiritual prerogative of the elders of the church for this purpose. It would appear also that the ministry of healing was to be exercised in private rather than in public, unless, of course, all that is implied is that the sufferer is bedridden.

(ii) The 'elders'

The elders of the church are to be called, and it is *they* who are to pray. Nowhere in the New Testament other than in this passage is healing designated as part of the function of 'eldership'. Elders in the Jewish Synagogue were a body of senior men (senior presumably either in age or experience) who were chosen to have oversight of its worship and wellbeing.[29] In the New Testament church this pattern was followed and those chosen were charged with responsibility for teaching and ruling ('oversight') and hence were referred to either as 'presbyters' ('elders') or 'bishops' ('overseers') (Acts 11:30; 15:2; 16:4; 20:17; 21:18; Phil. 1:1; 1 Tim. 5:17; Tit. 1:5).

Moreover, the Apostle Paul does not relate the 'gifts of healing' (1 Cor. 12:9, 28, 30) to the elders but simply to members of the church so endowed by the Holy Spirit. Calvin says,

> Since it was the practice to choose those endowed with more outstanding gifts, he [James] tells them to summon the elders,

being those in whom the power and grace of the Holy Spirit were most exerted.[30]

But James also recognises that any or all of the members of the church may be, and indeed should be, involved in the work of healing by means of prayer and intercession (5:16). What then is the particular function of the elders in the matter? Wilkinson says,

> The most probable view is that the elders were called in as representatives of the congregation and not because of any healing function which was inherent in their office. Intercession for others was part of their pastoral care and duty certainly, but it was a duty which was shared by every member of the congregation.[31]

We note that the call is not addressed to one person or to an individual healer. It is noteworthy also that when Jesus commissioned the disciples to heal, it was not to be done individually. So in James,

> The elders were to be commissioned as a body, and it is of interest to note that Luke always refers to the elders in Acts as a body and never as individuals. James does not envisage an individual elder acting as a healer in private, but only of healing as a corporate function of the body of elders of a congregation.[32]

Thus, a faith-healer acting on his own cannot be said to be fulfilling the pattern of James 5.

But it is also interesting that James does not assume that there would be a member or members of the local church who possessed the gifts of healing and who might be called in in such a situation. Surely if such a person were assumed to be available the obvious instruction to the sick would have been to 'call for the local healer'. The procedure, however, which he here promulgates would imply rather that the care of the sick, and especially the application of healing should be a matter for the congregation as represented by the elders.

It has been suggested, amongst Pentecostal Churches (see pp. 189f) that James' instruction that the elders should be called for, rather than a church member exercising the gift of healing, represents a distinction between dealing with the problem of sickness in the case of those who were church members and those who were not. That is to say, the exercise of the healing gifts by individual church members was intended for the benefit of non-Christians or non-church members, whereas the ministry of the elders was directed towards those in full membership. But there is nothing in this passage, or any other, to indicate such a distinction. The whole emphasis of this passage would appear to be on the ministry of intercession as the special means whereby the church can claim and exert the divine power in such a personal crisis.

(iii) The 'prayer of faith'

Prayer was to be offered by the elders. They were not to be mere spectators, but were each to be engaged in the healing process. It is to be believing prayer (*euche*), that is, prayer that is based not on the faith of the patient but of the elders who are praying. It is to be specific prayer (*deesis*), that is, addressed to the particular need and circumstance of the moment, not general intercession for all and sundry. It is to be fervent prayer (*proseuche proseuxato*), that is, intense and concentrated upon the need and condition of the sufferer.

(iv) Anointing

The sufferer was to be anointed with oil, probably, but not necessarily, before or during the prayer. It was not the anointing oil that would provide the healing, however, but the Lord would heal in response to the 'prayer of faith'.

As we have seen, it is difficult to know whether the anointing was simply a traditional Jewish practice used in a Christian context, or whether the oil was to be symbolic of the healing. We noted that when our Lord healed, he did not use symbolic additions, but simply spoke the word of power.

Two words are used by James for anointing, *aleipho* which usually refers to the use of oil for toilet or medicinal purposes (Matt. 6:17; Luke 7:46) and *chrio* which connates ritual or official anointing (Luke 4:18; Acts 4:27; 10:38; 2 Cor. 1:21; Heb. 1:9). Robertson says,

> It is clear both in Mark 6:13 and here that medicinal value is attached to the use of the oil and emphasis is placed on the worth of prayer. There is nothing here of the pagan magic of the later practice of 'extreme unction' (after the eighth century). It is by no means certain that *aleipho* here and in Mark 6:13 means 'anoint' in a ceremonial fashion rather than 'rub' as it commonly does in medical treatises. Trench (N.T. Synonyms) says: '*aleiphein* is the mundane and profane, *chriein* the sacred and religious word'. At bottom in James we have God and medicine, God and the doctor, and that is precisely where we are today. The best physicians believe in God and want the help of prayer.[33]

Thus there are two views of the anointing referred to by James. The one is that it was a normal medical procedure used specifically in the name of the Lord and supported by believing prayer. The second is that the procedure indicated was a religious and symbolic act with no medical significance. Wilkinson comments,

> There is probably not enough evidence in this passage to allow us to decide which of these two views is correct. However, an analysis of the usage of the verb *aleipho* in the New Testament

appears to support the medical view rather than the religious one.... Further, if anointing with oil had only religious significance and not medical, it is difficult to explain why it was so often omitted, and in particular why it was never practised by Jesus himself, but only by his disciples.[34]

On the other hand, Tasker takes the other view.

> It is therefore probable that the mention of oil in this passage is to be regarded as one of the accompaniments of that *miraculous* healing which was no infrequent occurrence in the apostolic age, and is regarded in the New Testament as a supernatural sign vindicating the truth of the Christian gospel in the early days of its proclamation.[35]

He therefore does regard the use of oil as symbolic with no medical significance. He goes on, however, to observe,

> this verse cannot be appealed to as evidence that the Lord committed to his church for all time the power of miraculous healing. Nor can we deduce from it that anointing of the sick with oil consecrated by priests should for Christians either supplement as a matter of course the work of medical practitioners in the healing of disease, or be regarded as a means of sacramental benediction when hope of a cure through ordinary channels has been abandoned.... The only unction of which the New Testament speaks as a permanent possession of the Christian in every age, by which he is continually invigorated and enlightened, is the unction of the Holy Spirit (1 John 2:20, 27).[36]

Wilkinson adds an interesting observation which, if correct, would call in question the Scriptural basis of a whole range of healing activity.

> We cannot escape the feeling that a reference by James to contemporary medical practice to illustrate a principle has been mistaken for a binding instruction on the church. James held that healing should be by a combination of medical and non-medical methods, and in illustration referred to the contemporary medical method of anointing sick people with oil which he said the elders should now do in the name of the Lord Jesus Christ and with prayer.... The fact is not without significance that the church did not appear to understand the practice of anointing, and eventually came to change its meaning from that of a prelude to healing to that of preparation for death. This would explain why the modern church commonly neglects the practice altogether, and commonly shows some embarrassment when the subject is raised.[37]

(v) Confession of sins

If the sickness of body or mind were the direct result of sin, then healing will require confession of the sin in question with a willingness to repent and a desire for forgiveness. If the sickness is the indirect result of sin (*e.g.* depression, anxiety, guilt arising from unfaithfulness or wrong done to others) then readiness for reconciliation or even restitution may also be necessary.

The importance of the word 'if' should be noted. As we have already established, in the Scriptures while some sicknesses are the direct result of some sins, and all sickness is the consequence of sin in the world through the Fall of our first parents, James is not teaching that every sickness is directly related to a particular sin committed by the sufferer.

Members of the church are exhorted to confess their faults one to another 'that ye may be healed'.

We note that there is no instruction to the sufferer to confess his sins to the elders as a requirement for healing, much less to a priest for absolution:

> there is no justification here for the practice of 'auricular confession' to a priest. The fact that the prayer of faith will result in healing for the sick man shows that it is not offered in anticipation of his death but of his recovery.[38]

The purpose of mutual confession of the members of the church to each other

> is an indication of the close sympathy and fellowship which existed betwen members of the early Christian community. It is noteworthy that there is no mention of anointing the sick with oil in this verse. That appears to be reserved for the elders to do.[39]

Calvin comments here,

> Many believe that James is presenting them here with a way of fraternal reconciliation, by mutual admission of sins: however, he had a different object, as we have stated. He puts mutual prayer together with mutual confession, and he means that the advantage of confession is to find assistance from the prayers of our brethren in the sight of God.[40]

He seems to be saying that mutual acknowledgment of failings and needs would help them better to understand and sympathise with each other's circumstances and therefore pray the more intelligently and effectively. The mutual 'confession' therefore is not so much a request for forgiveness as an acknowledgment of equality or similarity of need for healing.

(vi) Important omissions

There are several important omissions from the instructions given by James in this passage.

1. There is no reference to the 'laying on of hands' which was specifically mentioned in the Lord's 'commission' to the disciples in

Mark 16:18 where among the 'signs following' their preaching and teaching of the Word he promised 'they shall lay hands on the sick and they shall recover'. The 'laying on of hands', as we have seen, is certainly more frequently mentioned in the Gospels and Acts than 'anointing with oil', as James must have been well aware. No explanation of the omission is apparent. Did James regard Mark 16:18 as a 'commission' to all believers? The omission must surely call in question the claim of modern-day faith-healers who insist on the necessity of the practice to be acting on the basis of this passage. Yet in the modern ministry of healing it seems almost indispensable. For example, Maddocks writes,

> In any teaching about this ministry, it is important to emphasise that it is the touch of the Lord people are seeking. It is he who heals and adopts the sufferer into the health-giving body of his Son. We are his unworthy instruments. We can however rejoice that in this ministry, particularly in regard to touch, the renewal movement in the church has brought a welcome informality and loss of embarrassment that has led to the unfreezing of some ecclesial inhibitions. In this context we may hope for a more regular use of this ministry.[41]

2. There is no reference to exorcism of demons. The verb *astheneo* is never used in the New Testament in reference to demon-possession.

3. There is no reference to the exercise of the 'gift of healing' such as is spoken of by Paul in 1 Corinthians 12:9, *etc.* Wilkinson says,

> James does not mention such gifts, but assumes that all elders and even all members of the church can heal. His emphasis is on the place of prayer in healing rather than on special gifts. There need be no real contradiction here. The presence of some with a special gift of healing does not mean that healing is necessarily confined to them, nor that all cannot share in healing. In any case we do not know how extensively these gifts were present in the apostolic church, for they are only mentioned in connection with the church at Corinth. The fact is that James does not mention them here.[42]

This raises a number of questions. Were the 'gifts' still operative? If they were what was the point of calling for the elders? Should not James have recognised the ministry of those who were endowed with the gifts and commended their ministry to those in need of healing? Could they not have 'prayed, laid hands on and anointed' the sick with equal effect?

IV. CHANGING PATTERN

Now it is evident from all this that we have here a situation very different from that of our Lord's ministry or that of the Apostolic church. If we are to take it that James is laying down the procedure for the practice of healing in the church then we must take note of the main differences thus:

1. It is an exhortation, not a command given in the name of the Lord (Compare the example of Paul in 1 Corinthians 7:25) (v. 14).

2. The healing is to be effected not by a word of divine authority spoken in the name of the Lord Jesus Christ, but by intercessory prayer (v. 14).

3. Faith, confession of sin (where appropriate) and righteousness are all required for the effectiveness of the healing prayer (v. 16).

4. May the possibility of failure at least be implied by the expression 'the prayer of faith' suggesting that without faith the prayer may be ineffective and therefore responsibility for failure would rest upon lack of faith on the part of those concerned? Certainly not, as is indicated by the use of the word *energoumene*. Mayor (commentary, pp. 177–179) takes it to have 'the passive meaning that the prayer of a righteous man is powerful when it is made effective by the Holy Spirit' (Wilkinson, p. 147). But the active meaning which is preferred by most translations is that the prayer of a righteous man is powerful in its effect as evidenced by the example of Elijah. Either way, rather than providing for the possibility of failure, James is asserting total confidence in the reliability of God's power in response to believing prayer.

5. The use of oil is required. This is contrary to the practice of the Lord himself and of the Apostles except in one reference in Mark 6:13.

6. It would appear that the procedure laid down here is intended to be effected in private rather than in public. It would seem to be a matter for the church in fellowship rather than a public display to the world of the power or authority of those engaged in the healing.

V. WHY THE CHANGE?

It would appear then that the procedure set forth in James 5 has little or no connection with that of the Lord or of the Apostles. How are these changes to be accounted for? A number of possibilities come to mind:

1. The development of the church's constitution, assuming the Epistle was written about 60 A.D. as seems likely. Pastoral care of the members has now become the responsibility of the duly appointed elders, that is, teaching elders (ministers) and ruling elders, and the exercise of spiritual authority and power is vested in them rather than in any individual member of the church.

2. The absence of any member of the Christian community who

either claimed or exercised the healing gifts since the passing away of the Apostles.

3. The basic purpose of the whole exercise. There is nothing in the context of this chapter to indicate that James is laying down a new pattern for the ministry of divine healing in the church. On the contrary, he is in fact dealing with the general problem both of joys and afflictions in the life of the believer in the context of prayer. Amongst such vicissitudes physical sickness and its consequences are all too obvious.

> Instead of resorting to mutual recrimination under the trials of their earthly life, or impetuously breaking out into oaths, Christians are here bidden to turn constantly to prayer, whatever the circumstances of their life may be.[43]

So that what we have here is not the sacrament of Extreme Unction, which is repulsive to every principle of Scripture, nor is it the charismatic exercise of the gifts of healing, if such there be, but rather the church's ministry of intercession applied to a particular kind of need.

We must therefore conclude that what we have in James 5:14–18 is a challenge to the Christian believer, faced with the trial of physical sickness, or any other affliction for that matter, to seek God's will and help in prayer himself (v. 13), and then, if he feels the need of further help or encouragement, to call upon the spiritual overseers of the Christian fellowship to which he belongs, to visit him, assuming he is unable to leave his sickroom, and to share with him the ministry of intercession on his behalf, in the assurance that such a ministry would 'save' him from doubt and despair, enable him to accept God's will with faith and courage, as in the case of Paul's 'thorn', or bring relief or cure for his illness according to the sovereign purpose of God. The rightness and effectiveness of such a pattern of events has been demonstrated consistently in the history of the church and the experience of believers of every age and circumstance.

NOTES

1   J. Wilkinson, *Health and Healing*, Handsel Press, Edinburgh, 1980, p. 157.
2   *Ibid.*, p. 150.
3   R. V. G. Tasker, *Tyndale NT Commentaries Epistle of James*, Tyndale Press, London, 1957, p. 129.
4   J. B. Mayor, *The Epistle of St James*, Macmillan and Co., London, 1910, p. 169.
5   *Ibid.*, p. 169.

6 J. H. Ropes, *ICC Commentary Epistle of St James*, T. & T. Clark, Edinburgh, 1948, p. 304.

7 *cf.* J. Wilkinson, *Health and Healing*, Handsel Press, Edinburgh, 1980, p. 148; J. B. Mayor, *The Epistle of St. James*, Macmillan and Co., London, 1910, p. 174.

8 J. Wilkinson, *Health and Healing*, Handsel Press, Edinburgh, 1980, p. 11f.

9 *Ibid.,* p. 104.

10 J. B. Mayor, *The Epistle of St. James*, Macmillan and Co., London, 1910, p. 176.

11 *Ibid.,* p. 176.

12 A. Plummer, *Expositor's Bible St James and St Jude*, Hodder and Stoughton, London, 1891, p. 336.

13 J. Wilkinson, *Health and Healing*, Handsel Press, Edinburgh, 1980, p. 149.

14 *Ibid.,* p. 149.

15 J. H. Ropes, *ICC Commentary Epistle of St James*, T. & T. Clark, Edinburgh, 1948, p. 308.

16 R. V. G. Tasker, *Tyndale NT Commentaries Epistle of James*, Tyndale Press, London, 1957, p. 133.

17 J. H. Ropes, *ICC Commentary Epistle of St James*, T. & T. Clark, Edinburgh, 1948, p. 305.

18 R. V. G. Tasker, *Tyndale NT Commentaries Epistle of James*, Tyndale Press, London, 1957, p. 133.

19 J. B. Mayor, *The Epistle of St James*, Macmillan and Co., London, 1910, p. 175.

20 R. V. G. Tasker, *Tyndale NT Commentaries Epistle of James*, Tyndale Press, London, 1957, p. 134.

21 J. Wilkinson, *Health and Healing*, Handsel Press, Edinburgh, 1980, p. 157.

22 J. B. Mayor, *The Epistle of St James*, Macmillan and Co., London, 1910, p. 171.

23 J. H. Ropes, *ICC Commentary Epistle of St James*, T. & T. Clark, Edinburgh, 1948, p. 306.

24 J. B. Mayor, *The Epistle of St James*, Macmillan and Co., London, 1910, p. 172.

25 F. MacNutt, *Healing*, Ave Maria Press, Indiana, 1975, p. 277.

26 W. M. Abbott, *Documents of Vatican II* (73), G. Chapman, London, 1967, p. 161.

27 F. MacNutt, *Healing*, Ave Maria Press, Indiana, 1975, p. 277f.

28 *cf.* J. Wilkinson, *Health and Healing*, Handsel Press, Edinburgh, 1980, p. 146.

29 *cf. Ibid.,* p. 150.

30   J. Calvin, *Calvin's Commentaries Epistle of James,* Saint Andrew Press, Edinburgh, 1972, p. 315.
31   J. Wilkinson, *Health and Healing,* Handsel Press, Edinburgh, 1980, p. 150.
32   *Ibid.,* p. 151.
33   A. T. Robertson, *Word Pictures in the NT VI Epistle of James,* Broadman Press, Nashville, 1933, p. 64.
34   J. Wilkinson, *Health and Healing,* Handsel Press, Edinburgh, 1980, p. 153.
35   R. V. G. Tasker, *Tyndale NT Commentaries Epistle of James,* Tyndale Press, London, 1957, p. 130.
36   *Ibid.,* p. 133
37   J. Wilkinson, *Health and Healing,* Handsel Press, Edinburgh, 1980, p. 154.
38   *Ibid.,* p. 146.
39   *Ibid.,* p. 146.
40   J. Calvin, *Calvin's Commentaries Epistle of James,* Saint Andrew Press, Edinburgh, 1972, p. 316.
41   M. Maddocks, *The Christian Healing Ministry,* SPCK, London, 1981, p. 123.
42   J. Wilkinson, *Health and Healing,* Handsel Press, Edinburgh, 1980, p. 155.
43   R. V. G. Tasker, *Tyndale NT Commentaries Epistle of James,* Tyndale Press, London, 1957, p. 126.

7

TO HEAL OR NOT TO HEAL

To conclude our survey of the biblical evidence of 'faith-healing', we turn again to some matters which have already been examined but would appear to require some further comment. The healings effected by Jesus and the Apostles in the New Testament, as by the prophets in the Old Testament, were miraculous. That is to say, they were the result not of the use of human knowledge or skill, but directly of the intervention of divine power. We noted how in all the instances recorded in Scripture the healing was instantaneous, requiring no convalescence and without failure or relapse, and included the power to restore life to the dead. The exercise of faith was evident in some instances while in others it was not. And there were instances where healing did not take place as might have been expected or was even categorically refused. We must therefore give some further consideration to (1) the nature of faith-healing especially as it involves miracle or the supernatural; (2) the nature and relevance of faith; and (3) the implications of the failure or refusal of healing.

I. THE NATURE OF FAITH-HEALING

Sickness is the condition resulting from the disease or malfunction of any organ, sense or faculty of the body, physical or mental, or their interaction. Healing is the process by which such an organ, sense or faculty is restored to soundness or normal function. God has built into the human organism a natural capacity for healing which can be assisted (or impeded) by means of physical or psychological treatment. Medical science does not yet fully understand all the factors involved in the healing process, but it can be said to come about normally as the result of (a) medical treatment (b) remission, that is, temporary cessation of the progress of the disease or malfunction, or (c) spontaneous cure, that is, complete restoration (verified, of course, by medical evidence and investigation) without any kind of physical or psychiatric treatment or any process understood, or capable of explanation by, medical science.

In any attempt to account for healing it is important to recognise each and all of these factors. Remission and spontaneous cures, however inexplicable they may be, are well attested phenomena and may not be irrelevant to the discussion of faith-healing. This is not in the least to suggest that a claim to faith-healing may be summarily explained or dismissed either as remission or spontaneous cure. But equally care must be taken not to confuse instances of remission or spontaneous cure with the result of faith-healing.

At the outset we noted the difficulty of the use of the term 'faith-healing'. As Christians we believe that all healing, whether by natural or supernatural means, is divine healing (except such as is said to be effected in the name or by the activity of evil spirits or magic of any kind). But we understand faith-healing to refer to healing which takes place apart from all the normal processes including treatment, remission and spontaneous cure. It is effected by divine power and is experienced by the sufferer as the result of the divine intervention, sought or unsought, and either with or without the mediation of a human agent, doctor or faith-healer. In other words, it is a 'miraculous' event. But this raises the question, What constitutes a 'miracle'?

Weatherhead defines a miracle thus:

> A miracle is a law-abiding event by which God accomplishes his redemptive purposes through the release of energies which belong to a plane of being higher than any with which we are normally familiar[1]

all of which just means that it is a divine intervention in human affairs. In the case of faith healing it is not so much an interference with the natural laws governing the function of human life as the provision of divine resources in a particular situation in accordance with the will of God and the fulfilment of his promise to hear the cry of his believing children. When a cancer sufferer who is beyond the help of medical skill is healed in response to prayer, none of the laws of the universe or of healing are broken or upset. What happens is that new and divine resources are set in motion which, under God's direction, enable the normal and healthy functions of the body to be resumed.

For our purposes it is not necessary to discuss the philosophical or metaphysical aspects of miracle. It will be sufficient to consider them in their biblical context.

A great deal of confusion on the subject of miracles has been caused by a failure to observe that Scripture does not sharply distinguish between God's constant sovereign providence and his particular acts. Belief in miracles is set in the context of a world-view which regards the whole of creation as continuously dependent upon the sustaining activity of God and subject to his sovereign will (*cf.* Col. 1:16, 17). All three aspects of divine activity—wonder, power, significance (as indicated by the Hebrew *nipla ot*, Exod. 15:11; *gebura*, Pss 106:2; 145:4; *ot*, Num. 14:11; and the Greek *teras*, Acts 4:30; *dunameis*, Matt. 11:20; *semeion*, John 2:11)—are present not only in special acts but also in the whole created order (Rom. 1:20).... Miracles are events which dramatically reveal this living, personal nature of God, active in history not as mere Destiny but as a Redeemer who saves and guides his people.[2]

Since we accept the principle of the divine sovereignty of the creator and the revelation given to us in the Scriptures of his providential involvement in the affairs of his creatures, the question for us really amounts to understanding whether, and in what circumstances, we may expect him to intervene in the normal processes of health or sickness, life or death.

Warfield puts the question quite starkly thus:

The question at issue is distinctly whether God has pledged Himself to heal the sick miraculously, and does heal them miraculously, on the call of His children—that is to say without means—any means—and apart from means, and above means; and this so ordinarily that Christian people may be encouraged, if not required, to discard all means as either unnecessary or even a mark of lack of faith and sinful distrust, and to depend on God alone for the healing of all their sicknesses.[3]

A miracle is not simply something extraordinary, strange or unexpected, though often such events are loosely described as miraculous. Nor is it necessarily something which violates the course of nature or constitutes a suspension of it. It may indeed involve one or other or all of these characteristics, but the essential aspect of it lies not in this fact, but in its revelation of the presence and activity of God.

Miracles, signs and wonders always result from a divine intervention. Their supernatural character resides precisely in this divine origin and not in the astonishment, more or less considerable, which they are capable of producing in the human spirit. It should be said again and again: a divine action of quite ordinary appearance, visible only to the believer, is a miracle. On the contrary, a phenomenon which is extraordinary, amazing, inexplicable, but unrelated to faith, is not one.[4]

Magicians can work 'wonders'. In the Old Testament, for example, the magicians of Egypt were able to effect some of the wonders which Moses did (Exod. 7:11, 12, 22; 8:17, 18) and in the New Testament we have references to those who practised magic and sorcery (Acts 8:9, 11; 13:6, 8). Wonder-working can be effected by the power of evil spirits, superstition and the occult, and indeed the Lord himself warned of a time when 'false Christs and false prophets shall arise; and shall show signs and wonders, to seduce, if it were possible, even the elect' (Mark 13:22). So that mere wonder-working is not adequate as proof of the divine activity or intervention. True miracle must be based on, obedient to, and in fulfilment of the revelation of God in his Word.

Speaking of the 'wonder-life', as he calls it, of the Church of Rome, Warfield says:

> With all the hundred and more examples, however, it is after all, a small place which stigmatization takes in the wonder-life of the church of Rome. The centre about which this life revolves lies, rather, in the veneration of relics, which was in a very definite sense a derivation from heathenism.... There is certainly a true sense in which the saints are the successors of the gods, and the whole body of superstitious practices which cluster around the cult of relics is a development in Christian circles of usages which parallel very closely those of the old heathenism.... In point of fact the great majority of the miracles of healing which have been wrought throughout the history of the church, have been wrought through the agency of relics.[5]

It is precisely in this respect that much modern-day spiritualistic and 'charismatic' activity is open to question and danger. There are other spirits besides the Holy Spirit. There are the 'principalities and powers' of which Paul speaks (Eph. 6:12) and of whose malicious activities he was constantly aware. There are the 'demons' whose malignant activities Jesus himself confronted and who continue to exercise their pernicious influence upon the world and human affairs (Acts 5:16; 8:6, 7). Hence the exhortation from John, 'believe not every spirit, but test the spirits whether they are of God; because many false prophets are gone into the world' (1 John 4:1). The only means by which we can test the spirits is by the authentic revelation of the Word of God.

Faith-healing, then, is not to be confused with mere wonder-working. Nor is it to be confused with the effects of psychological therapy which may indeed present 'extraordinary' features, but must nevertheless be seen as the fruit of natural rather than supernatural gifts or activities. They are the result of scientific investigation of the workings of the mind and the application of its findings to mental or psychological disorders just as medicine or surgery are developed and applied to the physical. They depend for their effectiveness not upon the intervention of divine power in a supernatural way, but on the human discovery and application of natural laws and principles. Hence faith-healing is not to be identified with, nor explained by, such devices as 'mind-cure', theosophy, Christian Science, animal magnetism, or spiritualism.

As Leslie Weatherhead put it:

We do not understand the significance of the miracles while we concentrate on their wonder or think of them as only in the same category as modern therapeutic achievements. They may throw light on the latter and the latter on them, but running through the miracle stories is a divine light but infrequently seen in a purely therapeutic treatment today.... I would therefore argue that even if by psychological means we learnt to do the things that Jesus did, there would be an essential difference between our activities and his.... This comes home to us very vividly when we compare the long laborious methods of psychoanalysis with the speedy way in which his patients were restored to health. Nor can we suppose that the commission to his disciples was a commission to study medicine or surgery or psychology, or any other science.... It was a commission calling upon them, through faith and prayer and character, to enter his world, which he called the Kingdom of Heaven, and use the energies available therein.[6]

We would not accept, of course, for a moment that it might be possible by psychological means to do the things which Jesus did, and that for the very reason that Dr Weatherhead himself submits—'there would be an essential difference between our activities and his'. Moreover, further advance in the science of psychology in recent years has itself called in question the value and validity of psychoanalysis.

Psychic phenomena too have no place whatever in the explanation or performance of faith-healing in the Christian sense. They are indeed clearly among the methods expressly forbidden by God. 'Regard not them that have familiar spirits, neither seek after wizards, to be defiled by them. I am the Lord your God.... And the soul that turneth after such as have familiar spirits, and after wizards, to go a whoring after them, I will even set my face against that soul, and will cast him off from among his people.... A man also or woman that hath a familiar spirit, or that is a wizard, shall surely be put to death' (Lev. 19:31; 20:6, 27). They are thus regarded in God's Word in the same way as the practice of magic or charms (see pp. 62–3).

Weatherhead, who was not averse to acknowledging the possibility that,

Spiritualism, and other phases of psychical research, like some

of the Yoga practices, more common in the East, will gradually show us how to direct those energies (*i.e.* of prayer and meditation) towards the alleviation of our ills. That is in the future.[7]
nevertheless concludes,

But the explanation of the phenomena of Spiritualism which suggests that, through a medium, the spirits of doctors long since dead can be called up to diagnose the pain of a person living today is difficult for the mind to accept, especially in view of the fact that there is an alternative view which would take us just as far.[7]

To the mind redeemed by the grace of Christ and dedicated to obedience to the Word of God and the sanctifying power of the Holy Spirit such a resort would seem to be nothing less than repugnant and even blasphemous. This is not to deny the existence or power of psychic forces, but rather to subscribe to the view that they are a Satanic perversion of the God-given mental facilities which in fallen mankind have been corrupted and used by the unregenerate who refuse to believe in God, or to worship him according to his commandments, for the worship and glorification of Satan, thus bringing them into the thraldom of those 'principalities and powers' from which the regenerate have been delivered and which they have been commanded to resist by means of the divine power of the Holy Spirit (Eph. 6:10–20).

II. THE NATURE AND RELEVANCE OF 'FAITH'

Faith-healing, then, as distinct from either medical or psychic operations, implies the exercise of 'faith'. But the question is, What is the nature of the faith that is involved? By whom is it to be exercised or manifested? And how does its exercise impinge on or affect the healing operation?

It may be helpful to recall what we have already discerned about the question of faith and its part in healing. With reference to the healings of Jesus we noted that in some instances he called for faith on the part of the sufferer or those seeking help on the sufferer's behalf, but in the vast majority the issue of faith did not arise (Tables I and II). Nor, while on one occasion it is said that Jesus 'could do no mighty work because of their unbelief' (p. 14), do we anywhere read that a person's failure to be healed (if indeed there were such) was attributed to a failure of faith (p. 24: 11, 12) The failure of some of the disciples, in the absence of Jesus, to heal the epileptic boy seemed to be due, to some extent at least, to a failure on their part of that degree of commitment to and reliance upon him which could not fail (p. 29f).

In the conclusions drawn with reference to the healings effected by the Apostles, it was noted that the issue of faith either on the part of the healer or the patient was not mentioned (p. 41). In the survey of healing in the Old Testament the issue of faith received no mention though it would probably be fair to say that, in at least some of those instances where healing was sought, some kind of faith must have been implied (p. 44). The pattern for healing set forth in James 5 specifically demands the 'prayer of faith' as the essential requirement for the efficacious practice of healing by the 'elders' (p. 92: 3, 4). On the other hand, J. C. Peddie writes,

> Many humble and good folk feel that they have not enough faith to receive benefit from the ministry, but I cannot write too emphatically that they need have no such fear. While faith at its highest and best is essential in the one who ministers, and while patients who have great and simple faith are more responsive and easier to heal, those who have no faith in God, or in this form of ministry, can most surprisingly be healed. It seemed as if, in his infinite compassion, he cannot resist even the crude unbeliever.[8]

But all of this leaves some important questions still to be considered. For example, did the absence of faith on the part of the patients hinder or prevent the Lord or the Apostles from healing? Certainly it is clear from Tables I and II that he and they healed many without even raising the question, and in cases where he indicated the importance of faith, for example when he said, 'Go in faith', or 'Thy faith hath saved thee', or 'According to your faith be it unto you', none is said to have gone away unhealed. In the instance of the saying regarding Nazareth, 'he could do no mighty work there because of their unbelief', it is clear that some were in fact healed and that he was prevented from healing others not because of their personal lack of faith, but rather because the opposition which arose as a result of the general antagonism of the people of the town drove him to withdraw from the place altogether and thus resulted in only a few benefiting from his power to heal. The lack of faith was not directly related to the matter of healing, but to the larger issue of the rejection by 'his own' of his claim to be not merely the Son of the carpenter, but the Son of God.

> Jesus looked for faith as the right response to his saving presence and deeds; it was faith which 'made whole', which made the difference between the mere creation of an impression and a saving communication of his revelation of God. It is important to observe that faith on the part of human participants is not a necessary condition of a miracle in the sense that God is of himself unable to act without human faith.[9]

This leaves the question, Why did Jesus demand faith on some occasions and not on others? From Table I we see that Jesus demanded faith on only five occasions. In three of them (Jairus' daughter, the epileptic boy, and the raising of Lazarus) it was not so much a demand of faith as an encouragement or challenge to them not to be disheartened by the faithlessness or scepticism of others. In the other two cases (two blind men, and the man born blind), the two blind men had already expressed their belief that he was the 'Son of David' and he was therefore simply testing the depth of their faith which he immediately recognised by saying 'according to your faith be it unto you'. In the case of the man born blind it is interesting that Jesus did not question his faith at the point where he anointed his eyes with clay and sent him to wash in the Pool of Siloam. It was when he later found him cast out of the synagogue that Jesus asked him, 'Do you (still) believe on the Son of God', not questioning his original faith but rather confirming the depth and courage of his commitment in view of the shameful and intimidating treatment he had received.

So that while the evidence of some kind of faith on the part of a sufferer, or someone requesting healing on his behalf, must have given warm satisfaction to Jesus, nevertheless, in no recorded case of his healing, or of that of the Apostles, was it a decisive issue. In five of the twenty-six instances recorded of Jesus' healing faith was recognised by him; in nine it was expressed by those seeking help; and in fourteen the issue of faith was not even mentioned.

Perhaps one of the most interesting incidents of Jesus' healing was that of the man at the Pool of Bethesda (John 5:1–9). The circumstances were remarkable. That Jesus should have travelled to this place on the Sabbath Day, seen the crowds of sufferers waiting in the expectation of a chance to find healing, selected just one of them, healed him on the spot without any question concerning the man's faith in God or even recognition of himself, and departed never to return there, surely makes the case unique. Much time has been spent by the commentators seeking to establish the precise location of the sheep-pool or the particular feast which was referred to. Much has been made of the debate on the Sabbath to which the healing gave rise. But little attention apparently has been given to explaining the reasons for, or implications of, what Jesus did.

It would appear that the reason for the paralysed man, and all the other sufferers being there was a superstitious belief in the magical capacity of the 'troubled' waters to heal due to the presence of an 'angel' at certain times. Discussing the fact that verses 3 and 4 are omitted in many of the most ancient manuscripts and regarded as doubtful in others, Hoskyns says,

> The passage is either a gloss added to explain verse 7, or it belongs to the original text of the gospel and was struck out in order to avoid giving support to popular pagan practices

connected with sacred pools and streams.[10]

So could this be it? What Jesus intended to do by his visit to the pool-side was to show the folly of seeking for healing by means of superstition or magic however pious or well-intentioned. When Jesus asked the poor man 'Do you really want to be made whole?' was he really saying, 'If you do you're going the wrong way about it. Surely after thirty-eight years (or as much of that time as he had spent waiting by the pool) you must realise that your hope is vain.' Had Jesus not come to this 'shrine' for the very purpose of revealing to all who were there the emptiness of their misplaced hopes, and to show that he could do by his word and power what all their pilgrimages and religious devotions could never achieve? To make his point most effectively he chose to deal with the one person present who had been waiting longest; the one who was known to everyone and the subject of so much sympathy or ridicule; the one who seemed to have the least likelihood of being healed; and the one whose sudden cure would therefore become the cause of the widest possible interest and reaction. What better way to convince all who were present not only that he was the person whom he claimed to be—the Son of God—but also to demonstrate the power of God to heal and save, and to confound apparent faith which amounts to nothing more than superstition or mistaken piety.

A novel suggestion has been made that Jesus only healed the one man because he alone was unable to get into the water at the appropriate time, whereas the others had the opportunity of divine healing at the time when the water was disturbed. From this it is argued that the case illustrates God's healing by 'medicine' as well as 'miracle'.

> The key passage for our right understanding of the theological position of medicine is John 5:1–17…. There is one verse in the account which is sometimes omitted in early manuscripts, suggesting that some scribes had difficulty with it! It is John's profound insight, 'the angel of the Lord came down into the pool, and the water was disturbed' (v. 4)…. This is not angelology but theology! What John is saying is that when Christ was at the Pool God was actively healing in *two* ways.
>
> 1. In Christ God was healing through the Son.
>
> 2. In the Pool God was healing through his creation…. Jesus ministered to the one person who—for thirty-eight years—had *not* been able to avail himself of God's healing in the Pool. In leaving the crowd Jesus does not leave them God-forsaken, but leaves them to partake of his Father's 'divine healing' in and through his creation! This is not just first century mythology, but it is highly relevant today.[11]

Nor is faith to be confused with credulity or suggestibility. No doubt both may produce psychological effects for either good or ill, injury or healing. But they cannot be identified with, or substituted for, real faith in God.

> Suggestibility is almost wholly an emotional response to a powerful stimulus, with the reasoning and volitional sides of personality inhibited. But 'faith' is the response of the whole person, emotion, reason and will. In suggestion, the person is *acted upon, compelled,* by a strong personality or mass feeling. In faith the person *acts,* intelligently and deliberately, towards another person or towards a certain end.[12]

But neither is faith in the Christian sense a mere 'attitude' like 'positive thinking' or 'optimistic expectation'. And certainly, as we have seen already, it can have nothing to do with belief in sorcery, witchcraft, magic or any other form of the occult, although, again, as we have seen, this is not to deny that these powers can produce results both bad and good.

> Faith means abandoning all trust in one's own resources. Faith means casting oneself unreservedly on the mercy of God. Faith means laying hold on the promises of God in Christ, relying entirely on the finished work of Christ for salvation, and on the power of the indwelling Holy Spirit of God for daily strength. Faith implies complete reliance on God and full obedience to God.[13]

Thus 'faith' in Scripture takes a variety of forms characterised by both 'belief' and 'trust':

1. Sincere acceptance of the truth of someone's statement (Matt. 21:32).

2. Simple, unquestioning, though not 'blind', confidence in the ability of someone to do what they claim to be able to do or have been seen or known to do (Mark 5:36; Luke 8:50).

3. Abandonment of oneself to the mercy and power of God on the basis of the promises and pronouncements of his Word (Matt. 9:28; 15:21–25; Mark 9:24).

4. Reliance on the finished work of Christ on Calvary as the sole and sufficient ground of salvation (Acts 16:31).

5. Constant dependence upon the power and grace of God supplied through the indwelling presence of the Holy Spirit in the heart of the believer (Eph. 4:20–30).

Evidently 'faith' as used by Christ in reference to healing was either 1, 2 or 3 and could be 4 but not necessarily so.

In all healing there must be an element of faith in some sense or other. The sufferer, for example, must exercise faith in the sense of 'confidence' in both the physician and the treatment. The absence or failure of such confidence (or faith) will often render all efforts towards healing utterly useless. The presence of such confidence, on the other hand, can make the most innocuous treatment potent and effective.

The exercise of such a faith would seem to have been required by Jesus on occasions, for he specifically asked some who sought healing, 'Believe ye that I am able to do this?' (Matt. 9:28; Mark 9:23; Luke 8:50). Such faith need not, of course, have any spiritual content. It would equally apply to the watchmaker to whom one would entrust a valuable timepiece for repair. We would surely require to believe that he was a trustworthy person whose knowledge and skill there was no reason to question. It has even been suggested by some that this may have been all that was involved in Christ's assurance to some who had received healing that their 'faith' had saved them. Leslie Weatherhead says,

> the faith required for healing is not, and never has been, theological in its character. That is to say it has not been a faith in the truth of creedal statements. It has rather been expectant trust in a person. Such faith is necessary in all treatments, and Jesus seems to have evoked it again and again and to have been unable to work without it.[14]

While there are several things in this statement which are open to question, it must be accepted that for many this must have been the level or extent of their 'faith' at least when they approached the Lord.

But it would seem that the question of Jesus demanded more than this. To believe that he was able to restore sight to the blind, power to the paralysed, cleansing to the leper, *etc.*, implied surely, in however embryonic form, the acknowledgment at least that he was the person he claimed to be—the Son of God—and that his ability to heal was the exercise and manifestation not of human but of divine power and resources. Thus his inability to do any mighty work in Nazareth was not because of the people's failure to recognise and acknowledge his capacity to heal (for some in fact did and were healed), but rather because, as a whole, they were unwilling to accept him as anything more than the son of the carpenter.

There are those, however, who insist that the 'faith' which Jesus demanded or referred to had to be nothing less than faith in him as Saviour, that is, personal and saving faith in Christ. But this is difficult to prove.

> Christian faith for healing...is confidence intelligently and deliberately placed in Christ himself, either by the patient or the patient's friends, or both. It is a confidence which persists through rebuffs and obstacles and delays and apparent denials.... Not only the Bible itself, but wider human experience exemplifies the power of such faith.[15]

Wilkinson says,

> The object of the faith to which Jesus responded by healing is not usually explicitly stated. The sick or their relatives are exhorted to believe, but it is not commonly stated in what they are to believe, as we can see in such references as Mark 5:36; 9:23; John 4:48, *etc....* The faith which was answered by healing was faith in the power and ability of Jesus to heal. A faith which was sometimes expressed in the title by which Jesus was addressed by the sick...but more often was implied in the approach of the sick or their relatives to Jesus that they might be healed.[16]

On the other hand, in some instances the question of faith did not arise at all. It was neither asked for nor expressed. For example, the man at the pool of Bethesda evidently did not recognise who it was had healed him, and certainly he gave no indication of any kind of faith in Christ. Similarly, in the case of the man born blind, Jesus took the initiative without any challenge to the sufferer. And in the case of the Gadarene demoniac, the sufferer being 'out of his mind' was presumably incapable of giving expression to intelligent faith in Christ, although the demons within him did. So that in these and other instances the healing was a sovereign act of mercy on the part of the Lord, for the purposes of revealing his power and glory, and his love and concern for suffering humanity, and did not involve any indication of faith on the part of the sufferer.

Faith is frequently spoken of as the result rather than the precondition of the healing power of the Lord when either they experienced that power for themselves or witnessed others experiencing it (Matt. 9:8; 15:31; Luke 18:43; 19:37, 38; John 6:14). The ultimate expression of such faith lies not even in the realisation of healing, but in the spiritual capacity to accept the denial of healing or the phenomenon of apparently 'unanswered' prayer which may be not the evidence of lack of faith, but the display of victorious faith. And that leads to the question of the failure or refusal of healing.

III. FAILURE OR REFUSAL

In the New Testament we found only two cases in which an attempt to heal failed (pp. 28–30). One was the occasion when the father brought his epileptic son to some of the disciples while Jesus was absent from them on the Mount of Transfiguration. The healing failed not because of any default on the part of the patient or the father but because of the lack of faith and obedience on the part of the disciples, as is seen by the fact that later the boy was healed by Jesus (Matt. 17:18). The other was the incident when the sons of Sceva attempted exorcism in the name of Jesus (Acts 19:13–18) but with disastrous results because of the sin of those who attempted the healing.

In the Old Testament we found one attempt at healing by Gehazi the servant of Elisha which failed, the raising of a dead boy to life (2 Kgs 4:31). This again was the result of the sinfulness of Gehazi. The boy was later restored to life by the prophet. But also in the Old Testament we found three cases of healing expressly refused by God (Table V:15–17 also pp. 70f.).

In the New Testament we found three instances (p. 36f) namely those of Timothy (1 Tim. 5:23), Trophimus (2 Tim. 4:20) and Epaphroditus (Phil. 2:27) in which if faith-healing was sought it must have failed or been refused and the patients had to resort to medicinal help. There is also the case of Gaius mentioned in 3 John verse 2 which is specially interesting because of the fact that his spiritual health was strong while his physical health was weak, thus directly challenging the false idea of some that there is any promise in the Scriptures to the effect that spiritual excellence carries a guarantee or even a prospect of physical health or vigour. And in the case of Paul's 'thorn in the flesh' (2 Cor. 12:7–9) there was a categorical refusal by God to grant healing. There is, in fact, nothing to indicate either failure or refusal of healing in the case of the former four, but in the case of the latter not only was healing refused but it was clearly established by God that the 'thorn', while being a 'messenger of Satan', was specifically intended and used to provide spiritual benefit and blessing through the discipline it imposed and the grace it evoked.

What conclusions, then, are we to draw from these incidents?

> Anyone who has witnessed the procession of 'the lame and the halt and the blind' at a healing service, many of whom are persistently there, cannot but ponder the matter in his heart. Some there are who have sought every available means of divine Healing—anointing with oil, consecrated handkerchiefs, laying on of hands, by one 'healer' after another—for years, but still they are not healed. A boy of our acquaintance, for example, a pathetic case of mental and physical infirmity, has sought healing along these channels for years. His church has continually interceded for him, and one lady of deep piety and strong faith once fasted for three weeks on his behalf. He is still unhealed.[17]

These words were written not by one who doubts or denies the validity of faith-healing but by a Pentecostalist. As we noted earlier, Christ did not heal all whom he might have done. Moreover, there is nothing in Scripture to warrant a belief that what happens to one person must necessarily or inevitably happen to another in regard to healing. All of this raises a number of questions regarding both the problem of suffering and its implications for Christian life and witness, and the will of God in the matter of suffering.

(i) 'Sickness' and 'suffering'

It is asserted by some that in the New Testament 'sickness' is not to be confused with 'suffering'.

> The meaning of 'suffering' in the New Testament, as far as the Christian is concerned, is the persecution that comes from being a Christian. This is the broad and consistent theme and there are no exceptions. There are other meanings to the word 'suffer', such as 'to hold up', 'to permit', *etc.*, but they do not affect the issue. As with the suffering of Christ, the use of the word in relation to the Christian is not in any way a reference to sickness...sickness is always sickness; it is never described as suffering. And we are to react to it quite differently. When he said, 'Is any among you suffering? Let him pray.... Is any among you sick? Let him call for the elders of the church.' He saw them as different matters and said that we are to react to them in different ways.[18]

But is this distinction real? There can be no doubt that suffering is a more general and comprehensive word than sickness. Physical sickness is certainly a form of suffering, but suffering takes a variety of forms and may not necessarily be physical sickness. For example,

> The Bible in speaking of suffering never emphasises the aspect of physical pain. Often suffering is moral; it is the suffering aroused by scorn, calumny, desolation or the hardness of heart of others (Ps. 55; Jer. 15:18; Matt. 27:39–44; Gal. 4:19). But, far from being considered simply as a physical evil or a moral evil, suffering has always in Scripture a spiritual character: it represents a mortification in the presence of God, it is a sign of his reprobation and anger (Job 10:2; Ps. 107:12, 39; Matt. 27:45, 46; 2 Cor. 12:5–10).[19]

Now this is not to say that sickness cannot be suffering, but rather that suffering, even in the sense of physical pain can, and often does have a deeper and moral or spiritual dimension.

> Whether it speaks of the suffering of bodily sickness (Matt. 17:15; Jas 5:13) or of moral temptation (Heb. 2:18; Jas 1:12) or, as so often, of persecution (2 Tim. 3:10f.) the N.T. proclaims that suffering has been overcome by Christ but not yet done away; through the life of faith it becomes a state of grace in which the believer can rejoice here and now, for it is the pledge of future glory (Acts 5:41; Rom. 8:17ff.; Phil. 3:10; 1 Pet. 4:13).[20]

To suggest that the sufferings of Christ had no reference to his physical pain or weakness seems incredible, yet Glennon says,

> Jesus suffered but he was not sick.[21]

But it is one of the cardinal arguments of Glennon himself and many faith-healers that Isaiah 53:4, as quoted in Matthew 8:17 means that our Lord in his atoning work bore not only our sins but our 'sicknesses'.

This prophecy comes from the Suffering Servant passage in Isaiah 53 and in the view of some can only mean that healing (of sickness) is included in the atonement.[22]
But it must then also mean that 'sickness' is part of the 'suffering' process. Indeed when dealing with this passage it is claimed categorically by some that the reference is specifically to physical sickness, and hence to the fact that healing of the whole man in redemption requires healing of bodily sickness. If Christ could only deal with the physical consequences of our sin—death—by experiencing death for every man, then presumably he could only deal with the physical effects of sin—sickness—by experiencing sickness too.

But it is neither necessary nor desirable to press the point so far. The Scripture says, 'he was touched with the feeling of our infirmities and tempted and tried in *all points* as we are yet without sin' (Heb. 4:15). If words mean anything it is plain that the Lord Jesus did suffer all the frailties of our human existence—hunger, weariness, pain and distress of body and mind, so that while it is true there is no specific reference to his being sick in body there can be no doubt that 'the things which he suffered' and from which 'he learned obedience' included many of the afflictions which in human life are either the cause or consequence of bodily sickness. To limit the meaning of suffering in the New Testament to persecution is neither reasonable nor warrantable.

When Glennon wishes to illustrate Paul's assertion that suffering has a redemptive purpose, he in fact uses the Apostle's reference to his 'trouble' in Asia in which he says, 'we were pressed out of measure, above strength, insomuch that we despaired even of life' (2 Cor. 1:8, 9). It would appear that the strength and sentiment of the words used by the Apostle are not simply a reference to the riot in Ephesus where it is clear his life was not in danger, but rather to some grievous bodily sickness which brought him close to death. For example Alford says,

It is generally supposed that the tribulation here spoken of was the danger into which Paul was brought by the tumult at Ephesus, related in Acts xix.... I own, however, that the strong expressions here used do not seem to me to find their justification in any thing which we know of that tumult or its consequences. I am unable to assign *any other event* as in the Ap.'s mind: but the expressions seem rather to regard *a deadly sickness*, than a persecution.... Understanding it ('sentence of death') literally as above, I cannot see how it can be spoken with reference to the Ephesian tumult.... The whole verse (10) seems to favour the idea of *bodily sickness* being in the Ap.'s mind.[23]

Indeed the tenor of the whole passage is that of a man ill to the point of dying who was restored in answer to the prayers of God's people. Such an interpretation would seem to be substantiated by Paul's reference to his being 'troubled on every side' in 2 Corinthians 4:8 and his explanation in 4:10 as 'always bearing about in the body the dying of the Lord Jesus' and his further reference in 12:9 to his readiness to 'glory in his infirmities'.

From this particular example, chosen by Glennon himself, we can only conclude that the artificial distinction made between 'suffering' and 'sickness' is wrong and his statement,

> sickness is always sickness; it is never described as suffering and we are to react to it quite differently[24]

is quite wrong and misleading. If, as he claims,

> suffering is to be redemptive and sickness is to be healed[25]

there are many Christians who are getting the worst of both worlds, enduring both redemptive suffering and unhealed sickness. Of course the saving truth of the matter is that 'Whom the Lord loveth he chasteneth' (Heb. 12:6) and many a Christian tested in the fires of physical weakness, pain and distress has proved to be pure gold.

The point in seeking to make the distinction between 'sickness' and 'suffering' is, of course to make possible the conclusion that 'suffering' may be the will of God for the Christian but 'sickness' is not.

> Suffering for the Christian is intended to be a redemptive experience by which we learn the obedience of trusting not in ourselves, but in God. This is the value of suffering, and its importance cannot be overstressed. Nowhere does the New Testament speak of 'sickness' in the same way.[26]

But nothing has served more effectively in the lives of devoted Christian people to deepen trust in God and to prove the sureness of his grace and promises than having to battle, often over a long time, against physical pain or weakness, or mental stress, loneliness, anxiety or other affliction. And none more so than the Apostle Paul himself. 'I was with you in weakness (sickness), and in fear, and in much trembling' (1 Cor. 2:3). If suffering can be the will and purpose of God for the Christian, then so also can sickness.

(ii) 'Thy will be done'

There remain to be considered the cases of Trophimus, Timothy, Epaphroditus (and Gaius) who were certainly not cured by faith-healing, and that of Paul's 'thorn in the flesh'.

It is contended that Epaphroditus (Phil. 2:25–30) was in fact healed and therefore there is no case to answer. But of course the question is not whether he was healed but rather why Paul or no one else exercised the power of healing. With regard to Trophimus and Timothy, Glennon comments,

There is nothing to say that Trophimus and Timothy had been
prayed for, and there is nothing to say they were not subsequently
healed.[27]
But this will just not do. For one thing, Paul actually recommended
medicine to Timothy for what appears to have been a recurring
complaint, 'frequent ailments' (1 Tim. 5:23). Such advice seems
eminently sensible but it clearly shows that, for whatever reason, the
Apostle made no attempt to heal his 'own son' nor did he suggest any
way by which effective faith-healing might have been obtained for
him. Such a situation seems nothing short of incredible if, as the faith-
healers contend, the practice of faith-healing was common in the
church and essential to the commission of the Apostle. But to suggest,
as Glennon does, that these friends of Paul were not even 'prayed for'
is so outrageous as to be absurd, especially in view of Paul's statement
in 2 Timothy 1:3, 'without ceasing I have remembrance of thee in my
prayers night and day'. Or was the Apostle's prayer not a 'prayer of
faith'?

So far as Paul's 'thorn' is concerned, much time and effort has been
devoted to attempting to discover the nature of the affliction. Whether
it was physical or mental in its nature or effects; whether it was an
organic disease or a neurosis; whether it was a form of religious
opposition or of spiritual temptation; whether it was a painful disorder
or a nervous complaint, have all been canvassed. As Wilkinson says,
> A list of all the conditions which have been suggested for the
> diagnosis of the thorn reads like the index of a textbook of
> medicine.[28]
But our concern is simply to deal with the fact that whatever it was,
it was not healed.

Faced with the problem, the faith-healer replies that either Paul's
thorn is the one exception that proves the rule—
> one instance where healing was not available in response to
> faith.[29]
Or else it is not an exception at all in the sense that the assumption that
it was a sickness was wrong. Glennon, for example, believes,
> As there is no reason to think the 'thorn' was a sickness, this
> further identifies it with the 'suffering' syndrome.... The thorn
> in the flesh was a figurative way of describing a messenger or
> angel of Satan who continually harassed him.[30]
But even if this were so it is difficult to understand why such a person,
or the harassment being caused, could not have been removed. He
concludes,
> the circumstances which led to the thorn and which prevented its
> removal were obviously unique to Paul and therefore cannot be
> applied generally to others.[31]

Having said this, however, he goes on,

> Notwithstanding what has been argued so far, the traditional approach should be reckoned with in its strongest form. For that reason we would accept that it is possible for a 'messenger of Satan', in the shape of sickness, not to be removed by God.... This means that if the person is not to be healed, this fact will be revealed by God. It also means that, up to this point, the prayer of faith will be acted upon in full expectancy of healing. Furthermore, if it is then revealed that healing is not to take place, it means that the sick person will 'all the more gladly boast of (his or her) weaknesses' as did St Paul, and will not continue to seek their removal.[32]

Surely a complete '*volte face*', by all of which it would appear to be established, in direct conflict with his former assertion,

> Nowhere in the New Testament is sickness shown to be suffering which is beneficial,[33]

that sickness may indeed be used by God for the discipline and spiritual development of his faithful servant.

What makes the difference between sickness which is beneficial and that which is not is often the readiness of the sufferer to accept God's will in the matter. That is what made the agony of Gethsemane and the tragedy of the cross the way of fulfilment and victory for the Master. 'O my Father, if it be possible', he prayed, 'let this cup pass from me' (Matt. 26:39). In the will of God it was not possible, therefore he could add 'nevertheless not as I will but as thou wilt'. To pray, 'if it be Thy will', is neither to doubt God's promises nor to question his goodness and love. It is rather, like the Master himself, to acknowledge God's sovereign wisdom and trust his sufficient grace. To say as Glennon does,

> It is agreed that we must pray according to God's will. But his will is revealed to us in his promises; his promises reveal his will. So as we accept his promises by faith, we are praying according to his will.... In James 5:14, 15...*there is a most clear promise of healing*. And this is part of a *wholly consistent revelation of this matter in the New Testament*.[34]

is true, but it totally begs the question in this context. Of course there is a promise of healing but it is not, as we have seen again and again, a universal and unconditional promise. Like every other promise of God it is subject to his sovereign and eternal purposes working in and through the circumstances of a fallen world to the glory of his grace and the fulfilment of his eternal design. For Christ that meant victory through suffering; so too may it mean for his servants.

IV. SUMMARY

We may summarise our observations on all these matters thus:

1. Healing may be a purely sovereign act of God's love and power without reference either to the faith or want of faith of the sufferer or the mediation of any human agent.

2. 'Wonders' may be effected by human agencies under the inspiration and enabling of demons, evil spirits or occult powers, but true miracle is based on, obedient to, and a fulfilment of, the Word of God.

3. Psychic phenomena belong to the natural rather than the supernatural realm and may involve procedures forbidden by the Word of God.

4. The exercise of prior faith is not in all cases essential to the experience of faith-healing nor did its absence render healing by the Lord or the Apostles impossible or ineffective.

5. The exercise of faith may be effected not only by the sufferer, but by others on his behalf.

6. Faith is not to be confused with superstition, credulity, suggestibility or with mere psychological phenomena such as 'positive thinking' or 'optimistic expectation'.

7. The faith required by Christ (where it was required) involved anything from simple confidence in his ability to heal to the acceptance and acknowledgment of his person as the Son of God and Saviour of men.

8. Faith may be the result rather than the pre-condition of healing.

9. The deepest faith may be that which can accept 'unanswered prayer'.

10. Healing can be refused in the will of God.

11. Healing by means of medicine is approved in Scripture.

12. Sickness is not to be distinguished from suffering as being permitted or willed by God.

13. Sickness can be the instrument of divine grace and blessing.

14. 'If it be thy will' is both a worthy and valid dimension of the prayer for healing.

NOTES

1   L. D. Weatherhead, *Psychology, Religion and Healing,* Hodder and Stoughton, London, 1951, p. 47.

2   M. Gray, *New Bible Dictionary,* IVF, London, 1962, p. 829.

3   B. B. Warfield, *Counterfeit Miracles,* Banner of Truth Trust, London, 1972, p. 192.

4   M. Carez, *Vocabulary of the Bible Von-Allmen,* Lutterworth

Press, London, 1958, p. 270.

5   B. B. Warfield, *Counterfeit Miracles,* Banner of Truth, Trust, London, 1972, pp. 92,98.

6   L. D. Weatherhead, *Psychology, Religion and Healing,* Hodder and Stoughton, London, 1951, p. 49.

7   *Ibid.,* p. 219.

8   J. C. Peddie, *The Forgotten Talent,* Fontana Books, London, 1966, p. 66.

9   M. H. Cressey, *New Bible Dictionary,* IVF, London, 1962, p. 830.

10 Hoskyns and Davey, *The Fourth Gospel,* Faber and Faber, London, 1948, p. 265.

11 J. Richards, *The Question of Healing Services,* Daybreak, London, 1989, pp. 61f.

12 N. Brooks, *Sickness, Health and God,* Advocate Press, USA, 1965, p. 25.

13 L. L. Morris, *New Bible Dictionary,* IVF, London, 1962, p. 413.

14 L. D. Weatherhead, *Psychology, Religion and Healing,* Hodder and Stoughton, London, 1951, p. 36.

15 N. Brooks, *Sickness, Health and God,* Advocate Press, USA, 1965, p. 31.

16 J. Wilkinson, *Health and Healing,* Handsel Press, Edinburgh, 1980, p. 43.

17 N. Brooks, *Sickness, Health and God,* Advocate Press, USA, 1965, p. 19.

18 J. Glennon, *Your Healing is Within You,* Hodder and Stoughton, London, 1979, pp. 156f.

19 S. Amsler, *Vocabulary of the Bible Von-Allmen,* Lutterworth Press, London, 1958, p. 412.

20 *Ibid.,* p. 414.

21 J. Glennon, *Your Healing is Within You,* Hodder and Stoughton, London 1979, p. 155.

22 *Ibid.,* p. 136.

23 H. Alford, *The Greek Testament Vol. II,* Rivingtons, London, 1857, p. 598.

24 J. Glennon, *Your Healing is Within You,* Hodder and Stoughton, London, 1979, p. 156.

25 *Ibid.,* p. 156.

26 *Ibid.,* p. 156.

27 *Ibid.,* p. 163.

28 J. Wilkinson, *Health and Healing,* Handsel Press, Edinburgh, 1980, p. 120.

29 J. Glennon, *Your Healing is Within You,* Hodder and Stoughton, London, 1979, p. 157.

30 *Ibid.,* p. 159.

31　*Ibid.*, p. 161.
32　*Ibid.*, p. 161.
33　*Ibid.*, p. 156.
34　*Ibid.*, pp. 164f.

8

THE ULTIMATE SOLUTION

I. DEATH—FRIEND OR FOE?

It is surely true to say that the most frequent and pressing reason for which the help of the faith-healer is sought is either the fact or the fear of incurable illness which threatens, or is thought to threaten, early death. It is certainly true to say that many who seek the help of the faith-healer in such circumstances would not do so, and would not feel the need to do so, under any other circumstances. This raises serious problems both for the healer and for the sufferer.

Now, of course, none of us wants to die, whether we are Christians or not. Even the great Apostle was 'in a strait betwixt two, having a desire to depart and be with Christ, which is far better. Nevertheless, to abide in the flesh is more needful for you' (Phil. 1:23, 24). Who wants to die? What parent wants to leave behind a family, or what child wants to lose a parent? On the level of human relationships—kinship, neighbourhood, friendship—and their emotional involvements, the answer is, of course, None.

As C. S. Lewis puts it,

> There are two attitudes towards Death which the human mind naturally adopts.... On the one hand Death is the triumph of Satan, the punishment of the Fall, and the last enemy. Christ shed tears at the grave of Lazarus and sweated blood in Gethsemane: the Life of Lives that was in Him detested this penal obscenity not less than we do, but more. On the other hand, only he who

loses his life will save it. We are baptised into the *death* of Christ, and it is the remedy for the Fall. Death is, in fact, what some modern people call 'ambivalent'. It is Satan's great weapon and also God's great weapon: it is holy and unholy; our supreme disgrace and our only hope; the thing Christ came to conquer and the means by which He conquered.[1]

As Christians we profess to believe with Paul that 'to depart and be with Christ is far better' (Phil. 1:23). R. P. Martin comments thus,

> Any idea of an unconscious state following death or of a purgatorial discipline in the next world is denied by the sheer simplicity of Paul's expectation. Many things about the future beyond the grave are veiled from us; but what has been revealed (Deut. 29:29) is all we want to know. 'So shall we ever be with the Lord' (1 Thes. 4:17; *cf.* 1 Thes. 5:10).[2]

(i) 'Reformed' teaching

The teaching of the Reformed churches in regard to death and what lies beyond may be represented by the statements of the Westminster Confession of Faith thus,

> I. The bodies of men after death return to dust, and see corruption (Gen. 3:19; Acts 13:36); but their souls (which neither die nor sleep), having an immortal subsistence, immediately return to God who gave them (Luke 23:43; Eccl. 12:7). The souls of the righteous, being then made perfect in holiness are received into the highest heavens, where they behold the face of God in light and glory, waiting for the full redemption of their bodies (Heb. 12:23; 2 Cor. 5:1, 6, 8; Phil. 1:23; Acts 3:21; Eph. 4:10); and the souls of the wicked are cast into hell, where they remain in torments and utter darkness, reserved to the judgment of the great day (Luke 16:23, 24; Acts 1:25; Jude 6, 7; 1 Pet. 3:19). Besides these two places for souls separated from their bodies, the Scripture acknowledgeth none.
>
> II. At the last day such as are found alive shall not die, but be changed (1 Thes. 4:17; 1 Cor. 15:51, 52): and all the dead shall be raised up with the selfsame bodies, and none other, although with different qualities, which shall be united again to their souls for ever (Job 19:26, 27; 1 Cor. 15:42–44).
>
> III. The bodies of the unjust shall, by the power of Christ, be raised to dishonour; the bodies of the just, by his Spirit, unto honour, and be made conformable to his own glorious body (Acts 24:15; John 5:28, 29; 1 Cor. 15:43; Phil. 3:21).[3]

In his Commentary on the Confession A. A. Hodge says,

> We know that when the soul leaves it the body is resolved into its original chemical elements, which are gradually incorporated

with the shifting currents of matter in the surface of the Earth. The Scriptures teach us, however, that, in spite of this flux of their material constituents, the real identity of our bodies is preserved; and that, as members of Christ, all that is essential to them will be ultimately preserved and brought to a glorious resurrection.... During the interval between the death of each individual and the general resurrection.... The souls of both believers and the reprobate continue after death conscious and active, although they remain until the resurrection separate from their bodies...the souls of believers are made perfect in holiness...(and) are immediately introduced into the presence of Christ, and continue to enjoy bright revelations of God and the society of the holy angels.... The souls of the reprobate are at once introduced into the place provided for the devil and his angels, and continue in unutterable misery.... Our Standards declare that there is no foundation whatever, in Scripture, for the Romish doctrine as to the intermediate state of deceased men (*i.e.* purgatory).[4] pp. 381ff.

(ii) 'Adventist' teaching

Seventh-day Adventism, however, takes a different view. Commenting on Philippians 1:23 Questions on Doctrine (the Statement of Doctrine of the Seventh-day Adventist Church) says,

> Of course it will be better to be with Christ. But why, it must be asked, should we conclude from this remark that the apostle expects, immediately upon death, to go at once into the presence of Christ? The Bible does not say so. It merely states his desire to depart, and to be with Christ.[5]

Nor does Adventism believe in the separation of soul and body.

> It should be observed that Paul does not tell us that it is his soul or his spirit that will depart. He merely says (in 2 Tim. 4:6) 'I' have a desire; the time of 'my' departure is at hand.... When the time of leaving comes, *he* departs, and *the whole person* goes; there is no separation of body and soul.... There is a time when Paul could go to be with his Lord as a whole man—body, soul, and spirit—*and that is at the time of the coming of the Lord*. This he stresses in 1 Thessalonians 5:23.[6]

Moreover, in commenting on 2 Corinthians 5:8 Adventism insists that there is no reason for concluding that being 'present with the Lord' need be immediately consequent upon being 'absent from the body'. Thus,

> It must be recognised that there is nothing in this text to justify our coming to the conclusion that being 'present with the Lord' will occur immediately upon being 'absent from the body'.[7]

In fact, Adventism believes that the fulfilment of the hope of the Christian lies not at death but at the resurrection.

> *Rewards are given to the saints, not at death but at the second advent.* The resurrection of the righteous takes place at the time of our Saviour's return from heaven to gather His people (Matt. 16:27; Isa. 40:10; 2 Tim. 4:8; *etc.*)... At death the saints go to the grave. They will live again, but they come to life and live with Jesus after they are raised from the dead. While asleep in the tomb the child of God knows nothing. Time matters not to him. If he should be there a thousand years, the time would be to him as but a moment. One who serves God closes his eyes in death, and whether one day or a thousand years elapse, the next instant in his consciousness will be when he opens his eyes and beholds his blessed Lord. To him it is death—then sudden glory.[8]

Speaking of those who in the Scriptures were raised from the dead— the widow of Zarephath's son (1 Kgs 17), the Shunamite's son (2 Kgs 4), the widow of Nain's son (Luke 7), the daughter of Jairus (Luke 8), Tabitha (Acts 9), Eutychus (Acts 20), Lazarus (John 11)—Adventism says,

> If the soul goes to either heaven or hell at death, surely those who have been resurrected would talk of the glories of the heavenly land, or they would warn sinners in no uncertain tones of the torments of the damned. Yet there is no record of their having said a single word. How strange, if the soul or spirit survives death as a conscious entity, that we have no word at all from any of the aforementioned individuals concerning what happened during the period they were dead![9]

But, however it is perceived, to be 'absent from the body' and 'present with the Lord' must, for the believer, mean 'to die is gain'.

(iii) To be or not to be

Moreover, when others die we turn for our comfort and consolation to the words of Christ, 'I go to prepare a place for you, and if I go and prepare a place for you, I will come again and receive you unto myself, that where I am ye may be also' (John 14:2, 3).

If, then, all this is really true, surely death is not the worst thing that can happen to those who are Christ's, but rather the best. Why should the answer to terminal illness be a search for faith-healing (and if one attempt fails, another, and another!) in order to avoid death? And why should anyone in the name of Jesus Christ think that he is offering 'hope' or 'consolation' by promising or attempting to prolong the sin and strife of life in this 'present evil world' as an alternative to the glory and joy of being 'with Christ'?

But, it may be said, why then should the Christian believer seek healing at any time or in any form—even through the doctor or the normal medical means? The answer is clear. It is, according to Scripture, our duty to preserve life by all normal and natural means. The command, 'Thou shalt not kill' teaches this, as the Shorter Catechism points out, 'The sixth commandment requireth all lawful endeavours to preserve our own life, and the life of others'.[10] It is for this reason we believe that murder, suicide, abortion (except for the preservation of the life of the mother) or euthanasia, whether with the consent of the person concerned or not, are contrary to God's Word and therefore unacceptable to the Christian conscience. It is our duty to preserve our own or our neighbour's life by all normal means and not to endanger it either by harmful or injurious activity on the one hand, or by neglect on the other.

In the matter of faith-healing, however, we are discussing not the normal preservation of life, but the abnormal prolongation of it when all the normal resources have failed or are thought to be unavailing. Nor are we suggesting that there need be anything wrong with seeking divine help in such circumstances provided it is on the Scriptural basis of 'not my will but thine be done', as our Lord himself prayed in those very circumstances. What we believe to be in question is the view that death is the worst enemy of the believer and to be evaded so long as possible by the exercise of faith-healing when all other means have failed, for this undoubtedly is the frame of mind in which much of the appeal to faith-healers is made. The position of the Christian believer must surely be that of the Apostle Paul, 'To me to live is Christ and to die is gain' (Phil. 1:21), and for the very good reason that 'with all boldness, as always, so now also Christ shall be magnified in my body, whether it be by life or by death' (Phil. 1:20).

What then are we to believe concerning death? And what has it to do with regard to the issue of faith-healing?

II. CAUSE OF DEATH

The life of an individual in this world comes to an end, according to the Scriptures, either by physical death or by translation into the presence of God at the return of the Lord Jesus Christ. 'It is appointed unto men once to die' (Heb. 9:27). Or again, 'Then we which are alive and remain unto the coming of the Lord shall be caught up together with them (the resurrected saints) in the clouds to meet the Lord in the air' (1 Thes. 4:17). Since time began there have been only two exceptions spoken of in the Scriptures. Enoch was translated into the presence of God without death, and the prophet Elijah was transported to heaven without dying (Gen. 5:21ff.; 2 Kgs 2:5–13). Death, therefore, is to be expected as the normal termination of life in this world.

It is the inevitable end of that process of 'change and decay' which is characteristic of all God's creation. As the wise widow-woman said to king David in an attempt to prevent further bloodshed in his violent land, 'We must needs die, and are as water spilt on the ground, which cannot be gathered up again; neither doth God respect any person: yet doth he devise means, that his banished be not expelled from him' (2 Sam. 14:14). Even the normal span of life is declared to be 'three score years and ten' (Ps. 90:10). But, of course, under the sovereign providences of God it may be longer or shorter, and the end may be directly effected by natural decline of strength, by accident, crime, famine, war, by self-inflicted injury or suicide, or by the process of physical disease. It can, of course, come about in different ways or circumstances, for example, with instant and unexpected suddenness; as the result of a long and distressing process of increasing pain or weakness; or as the peaceful climax of a gradual and contented approach to the fulfilment of the earthly mission and the realisation of the heavenly reward.

However it comes, it comes, by God's decree, as a biological necessity. But, in the Scriptures, it comes also as the result of the fall of mankind from that state in which our first parents were created 'in the likeness and image' of God, and from which they, and we as their natural progeny, were estranged by their submission to the will and power of Satan, and consequent separation from God in judgment. Thus, in Christian and biblical perspective, death is not merely a physical phenomenon but rather the physical result of the spiritual breakdown through sin of mankind's original relationship with God. Hence the Apostle could say, 'the wages of sin is death' (Rom. 6:23). Death is the penalty for sin which affects the whole human race, 'as by one man sin entered into the world, and death by sin, so death passed upon all men, for that all have sinned' (Rom. 5:12). As C. S. Lewis puts it,

> Spirit and Nature have quarrelled in us; that is our disease. Nothing we can yet do enables us to imagine its complete healing. Some glimpses and faint hints we have: in the Sacraments, in the use made of sensuous imagery by the great poets, in the best instances of sexual love, in our experiences of the earth's beauty. But the full healing is utterly beyond our present conceptions.[11]

Thus, from the physical point of view, death is seen by most people in purely negative and pessimistic perspectives. It represents the dissolution of life in terms of physical strength, and its resources of energy, vision, wisdom, concentration and perseverance; the disruption, if not the end, of the closest and most sacred relationships both of kinship and friendship; the destruction of skills, dreams and purposes without which the world becomes an even darker, poorer and more hopeless place. Death is so final. There is no filling of the vacant place it leaves. There is no hearing again the voice that is stilled. There is no undoing of the things which caused estrangement or pain. There is no bridging of the gulf that divides eternal darkness from eternal joy. Of all the enemies of mankind's peace and prosperity that Christ had to face and conquer, surely death was indeed the last and greatest. Speaking of the ultimate triumph of the Lord when 'He shall have put down all rule and authority and power' of the Evil One, Paul says, 'For he must reign till he hath put all enemies under his feet. The last enemy that shall be destroyed is death' (1 Cor. 15:25, 26). So death is the great enemy of man's peace and hope.

No wonder, then, that death is to be feared and avoided or postponed if possible. No wonder life is so sweet and to be preserved or held on to almost at any cost in terms of frailty, pain or need. That is a perfectly understandable position for the atheist or the heathen worshipper to be in. But not for the Christian believer.

III. THE HOPE OF LIFE

But it is the very epitome of the glory and victory of the Christian faith that 'death is swallowed up in victory' (1 Cor. 15:54–57). The sting of death has been drawn. The apparent victory of the grave has been reversed. Alford in reference to 1 Corinthians 15:25, 26 puts it thus,

> Death is 'the last enemy', as being the *consequence of sin:* when he is overcome and done away with, the whole end of Redemption is shown to have been accomplished.[12]

The consequence of sin in terms of God's judgment has been put away already for the believer, but when Christ comes to reign the very experience of death itself will be no more. In that sense the last enemy will itself have been finally destroyed. As the Seer of Patmos saw in his vision, 'death and hell were cast into the lake of fire. This is the second death' (Rev. 21:14). Leon Morris expresses it this way,

> Paul's thought is that Christ will at the last have full and complete authority over all things and all men, and that He will then 'deliver up' this authority, this rule, to His Father. When Christ comes back it will be to reign in majesty (*cf.* 2 Thes. 1:7ff.). All that opposes God will then be subdued.... Death will be robbed of all its power. At present no man can resist the touch of death. Then death will be able to touch no man.[13]

The bodily death and resurrection of Christ is both the means and the ground of the believer's confidence, and the guarantee of the Christian's hope and assurance for, 'as in Adam all die, even so in Christ shall all be made alive' (1 Cor. 15:22). With the Psalmist the believer can sing 'Though I walk through the valley of the shadow of death, I will fear no evil: for thou art with me.... Surely goodness and mercy shall follow me all the days of my life and I shall dwell in the house of the Lord for ever' (Ps. 23:4, 6); and with the Apostle can affirm 'We know that if our earthly house of this tabernacle were dissolved, we have a building of God, an house not made with hands eternal in the heavens' (2 Cor. 5:1). This in face of the fact that in our earthly condition, 'we groan, earnestly desiring to be clothed upon with our house which is from heaven' (2 Cor. 5:2).

Tasker sees Paul's refusal to be dismayed by the growing consciousness of his failing faculties and the increasing awareness that his sufferings will ultimately result in his death, as the result of his conviction that

> 'His human body, as he is becoming more and more conscious, is a temporary structure, adequate to shelter him during the few brief years of his earthly pilgrimage, but as vulnerable to the winds of circumstance and the wear and tear of everyday life as a "tabernacle" or tent'. But, 'he is convinced that the shelter that awaits him after death is as superior to that provided by the present body as the protection of a solid well-built house is superior to that of a tent. That better shelter already exists.... It was this "eternal" shelter, described as "mansions" or dwelling-places that Jesus told His disciples He was going on ahead to make ready for them.'[14]

But it has been suggested that Paul's use of the double compound verb *ependusasthai* ('clothed upon with') may mean

> that Paul longed to have this resurrection body put on over his present body as an additional vesture. In other words, he wanted to be alive when the Lord returned, so that his earthly body could be changed into a spiritual body without the dissolution of death.[15]

But, as Tasker submits, it is more likely that Paul's intention is that his sufferings

> are accompanied by groanings because he longs for the more permanent, heavenly (the meaning of 'from heaven') shelter which awaits him after death.[16]

But not only does the Christian believer possess that assurance of life beyond the grave, but also the prospect of a new quality of life to match the glory and perfection of that land which is 'fairer than day'. The resurrected body in heaven will be perfectly restored and, like the body of Christ, the church, will be 'without spot or wrinkle' (Eph. 5:27). Is not this the implication of Paul's words, 'It is sown in corruption; it is raised in incorruption; it is sown in dishonour; it is raised in glory: it is sown in weakness; it is raised in power: it is sown a natural body; it is raised a spiritual body' (1 Cor. 15:42–44)? Alford says of Paul's phrase 'in weakness' (*en astheneia*),

> Chrysostum understands *asth.* of its 'inability to resist corruption': De Wette would refer it to the previous state of pain and disease; but it seems better to understand it of the 'powerlessness' of the corpse, contrasted with *en dun.* 'in vigour', viz. the fresh and eternal energy of the new body free from disease and pain.[17]

The need for such a metamorphosis is expressed thus by Leon Morris,

> the body we now have is a body suited for the present life. It is adapted to the *psuche*, the rational principle of life. But such a body is ill-adapted for life in the world to come. For that a body is needed which is attuned to the spirit, in fact, 'a spiritual body'. This does not necessarily mean 'composed of spirit', but rather 'which expresses spirit', 'which answers to the needs of spirit'.[18]

In the same vein John in his vision of life in the eternal city says, 'God shall wipe away all tears from their eyes; and there shall be no more death, neither sorrow, nor crying, neither shall there be any more pain: for the former things are passed away' (Rev. 21:4). And in his vision of the consequences of the return of Christ in glory Paul is able to say that he shall 'change our vile body, that it may be fashioned like unto his glorious body, according to the working whereby he is able even to subdue all things unto himself' (Phil. 3:21). Here the 'vile' body is taken by Lightfoot to mean,

> the body which we bear in our present low estate, which is exposed to all the passions, sufferings, and indignities of this life.[19]

The JFB Commentary notes,

> Our spiritual resurrection now is the pledge of our bodily resurrection to glory hereafter (v. 20; Rom. 8:11). As Christ's glorified body was essentially identical with His body of humiliation; so our resurrection bodies as believers, since they shall be like His, shall be identical essentially with our present bodies, and yet 'spiritual bodies' (1 Cor. 15:42–44). Our 'hope' is that Christ, by His rising from the dead, hath obtained the power, and is become the pattern of our resurrection (Mic. 2:13).[20]

Not much detail is given in the New Testament regarding the form of our 'spiritual bodies'. Leon Morris sums up what is said thus,

> Our Lord's risen body appears to have been in some sense like the natural body and in some sense different.... It would seem that the risen Lord could conform to the limitations of this physical life or not as He chose, and this may indicate that when we rise we shall have a similar power.[21]

Salmond says that while Paul furnishes us with few answers to the many questions which have arisen regarding the nature of the 'spiritual body' of the believer after the resurrection, he does give us to understand,

> that the new body will be *our* body, and yet will be different from that of which we have experience, superior to it in incorruptibility, in honour, and in power, in freedom from waste, decay, and death, in the glory of perfection, in ability to discharge its function.... It is to be related to the former body, and yet is to be different from it and superior to it, as the golden grain with its rich increase is related to the buried seed, yet different from it and superior to it.[22]

Strangely, in speaking of Christ's 'body of his glory', the commentators make no reference to the fact that his post-resurrection body retained the wounds and nail-prints of his crucifixion. It was therefore not 'made perfect'. The question arises, therefore, as to whether this was an accommodation to the disciples' recognition of his identity (with particular reference to Thomas) while he remained on the earth, or whether, as the hymn-writer suggests, we shall recognise him in heaven by these very imperfections. Such a concept seems difficult for a number of reasons. For example, in the visions of the Lamb given to the Seer of Patmos there would appear to be a reference to such distinguishing scars in the figure of 'a lamb *as it had been slain*' (Rev. 5:6). But the lamb is also spoken of within the same verse as having 'seven horns' indicative of great dignity and power (and that in perfection as indicated by the 'seven'), which would suggest a purely figurative representation of the sacrifice and victory of Christ, rather than a description of his actual appearance. Nor would such marks of identification be necessary for one seated upon a throne. Moreover, if the 'body of his glory' retained the scars and blemishes of his earthly sufferings, and we are to be made 'like him', then, presumably, all the defects and mutilations of our terrestrial bodies would be reproduced in our celestial, and this would scarcely be congruous in the perfect environment of God's presence and glory. Nor would such imperfect reproductions appear to comply with the vision of our celestial bodies as described by the Apostle in 1 Corinthians 15:42–44 or with his declaration that 'flesh and blood cannot inherit the kingdom of God; neither doth corruption inherit incorruption.... For this corruptible must put on incorruption, and this mortal must put on immortality...then shall be brought to pass the saying that is written, "Death is swallowed up in victory"' (vv. 51, 53, 54).

That the bodies of the saints are restored to perfection in the resurrection is also necessitated by the very nature of the heavenly presence of God himself: 'there shall no wise enter into it anything that

defileth, neither whatsoever worketh abomination, or maketh a lie'
(Rev. 21:27).

Not only, however, does resurrection promise healing from all
physical pain, weakness, handicap and disease of mortal life, but also
of release from that mental ignorance, blindness, or handicap which is
the cause of so much distress, anxiety, fear and despair in the terrestrial
sphere. The Apostle Paul could, in the face of all the uncertainties and
perplexities of life that baffled human understanding or insight,
confidently look forward to a time when all that was dark and
mysterious would no longer threaten his peace and happiness. 'We
know in part, and we prophesy in part. But when that which is perfect
is come, then that which is in part shall be done away.... For now we
see through a glass darkly; but then face to face: now I know in part;
but then shall I know even as also I am known' (1 Cor. 13:9, 10, 12).

This assurance was the consequence of the resurrection and
ascension of the Lord Jesus Christ. Speaking of the power of Christ to
work miracles, C. S. Lewis says,

> it is a possible view that if Man had never fallen all men would
> have been able to do the like.... Whatever may have been the
> powers of unfallen man, it appears that those of redeemed Man
> will be almost unlimited. Christ, re-ascending from his great dive,
> is bringing up Human Nature with him. Where he goes, it goes
> too. It will be made 'like him'. If in his miracles he is not acting
> as the Old Man might have done before his Fall, then he is acting
> as the New Man, every new man, will do after his redemption.[23]

Death, then, has been transformed by the death and resurrection of
Christ and the prospect it provides for those whose faith and hope are
in him. For them death is no longer the great destroyer, but rather the
great healer. The measure of the transformation that is involved is
stated thus by C. S. Lewis,

> God is not merely mending, not simply restoring a *status quo*.
> Redeemed humanity is to be something more glorious than
> unfallen humanity would have been, more glorious than any
> unfallen race now is (if at this moment the night sky conceals any
> such). The greater the sin, the greater the mercy: the deeper the
> death the brighter the re-birth. And this super-added glory will,
> with true vicariousness, exalt all creatures and those who have
> never fallen will thus bless Adam's fall.[24]

The great hope of the Christian believer lies in that world where the
pain, weakness and weariness of earthly sorrow, suffering and sin are
past and gone for ever, and perfect health of body, mind and spirit are
the undisturbed possession of all who share the life of the Celestial City
where flows 'a pure river of water of life, clear as crystal, proceeding
out of the throne of God and of the Lamb. In the midst of the street

of it, and on either side of the river, was there the tree of life...and the leaves of the tree were for the healing of the nations' (Rev. 22:1, 2).

IV. BODY AND SOUL

How then does death and the life beyond relate to the health or sickness of the body? It is clear from the teaching of the Scriptures concerning the nature and effect of resurrection, that the body is an integral part of God's design for man's eternal destiny.

In the Old Testament the general word used for 'flesh' is *basar* (Gen. 2:21). *Tibchah* ('slaughtered food') occurs once (1 Sam. 25:11). *Lechem* ('flesh', 'meat', 'bread') occurs once (Zeph. 1:17). And *she'er* ('flesh', 'remains') occurs seven times. *Basar* represents the principal constituent of the body both human (Gen. 2:23) and animal (Gen. 8:17). From this it becomes flesh eaten as food (Exod. 12:8) or offered in sacrifice (Exod. 29:14). It also comes to be used to refer to the whole person (Ps. 16:9), thus man and wife are 'one flesh' (Gen. 2:24). And it is used to refer to the race of mankind as a whole, 'all flesh' (Ps. 145:21).

The New Testament reflects the same uses of 'flesh' as the Old. The general word is *sarx*, but the word *kreas* ('flesh' in the sense of 'meat') occurs twice (Rom. 14:21; 1 Cor. 8:13). In Matthew 16:17 *sarx* refers to human nature; in 1 Corinthians 1:29 it refers to the whole individual or person (Rom. 7:18); in 2 Corinthians 7:5 it refers to the whole body; in 1 Peter 1:24 it refers to mankind as a whole. But in the New Testament it has additional connotations. For example, 'the flesh' is said to have in itself 'lusts' and 'desires' (Ephesians 2:3), and these are said to be in conflict with those of 'the spirit'. That is, the 'flesh' is taken to represent the sinful human nature of fallen man as distinct from the new nature of his 'spirit' as the result of the work of regeneration in Christ effected by the Holy Spirit. Consequently, 'the flesh' represents the seat of man's moral weakness and corruption.

The concept of the 'body' then is, in both Old and New Testaments, an integral part of human personality, morality and destiny. In the Old Testament several words are used for 'body'—*beten* ('belly'); *basar* ('flesh'); *gab* and its derivatives ('back'); *nebelah* ('carcase'); *nephesh* ('soul'); *etsem* ('bone', 'substance'); *she'er* ('flesh'); *nidneh* ('sheath'). All of these refer to the physical entity in which man resides. No distinction is made in these terms between the physical and spiritual nature of mankind. The words simply refer to his physical nature. In the New Testament, the general word used is *soma*, the word *chros* ('frame') occurs once (Acts 19:12). In the New Testament, by contrast with the Old, clear distinction is made between the 'body' and the 'spirit' (Rom. 8:10). And while, as we have seen, the 'body' ('the flesh') is seen as the earthly, corruptible part of man's being, it is nevertheless inseparable from the person as a whole.

Thus, the body is said to be 'dead' because of sin (Rom. 8:10), but the spirit is alive in the Christian believer because of the righteousness of Christ imputed to it by faith (Rom. 4:11). Physical death is the temporary separation of spirit and body; resurrection is their reunion beyond the limitations of time and space. As earthly life requires both body and soul to constitute the whole person, so eternal life equally requires both parts of man's nature and person to be reconstituted. This is the whole burden of Paul's lengthy argument in 1 Corinthians 15 concerning the nature and necessity of the 'resurrection body'.

> The Bible…knows nothing of an abstract immortality of the soul, as the schools speak of it; nor is its Redemption a Redemption of the soul only, but of the body as well. It is a Redemption of man in his whole complex personality—body and soul together. It was in the body that Christ rose from the dead; in the body that he ascended to heaven; in the body that he lives and reigns there for evermore. It is his promise that, if he lives, we shall live also (John 14:19); and this promise includes a pledge of the resurrection of the body. The truth which underlies this is, that death for man is an effect of sin. It did not lie in the Creator's original design for man that he should die,—that these two component parts of his nature, body and soul, should ever be violently disrupted and severed, as death now severs them. Death is an abnormal fact in the history of the race; and Redemption is, among other things, the undoing of this evil, and the restoration of man to his normal completeness as a personal being.[25]

While therefore, as Paul puts it, 'Flesh and blood cannot inherit the kingdom of God' (1 Cor. 15:50), he is equally adamant that the Kingdom of God is not peopled by 'disembodied spirits'! It is for this very reason that he goes on to describe the transformation or transfiguration that will take place at Christ's return. The bodies of the dead saints will be raised 'incorruptible' and those of the living will be changed into the new likeness of Christ (1 Cor. 15:51–53). He speaks not only of the whole creation waiting for the Day of Redemption, but also of the Christian believers waiting for the 'redemption of the body' at the Day of Christ (Rom. 8:23). The picture is clear. The body, as now constituted, has by sin been made subject to disease, destruction and death, and as such cannot have any place in the realm of God's holy presence and perfection. If the child of God is to enter into the eternal presence and Kingdom of God it will require not only the regeneration of his spirit, but also the reconstitution of his body 'without spot and without blemish'.

Thus the hope of the believer lies not merely in the eternal preservation of his spirit from ultimate separation from God in judgment, but also in the reconstitution of his body. The resurrection in Christ is the guarantee not only of spiritual salvation but also of bodily healing and renewal in perfect soundness of form and function. As the institution of the Kingdom of God by the return of Christ will mean the end of the consequences of man's sin in the chaos, conflict and corruption of the created world and its redemption and restoration to the perfection in which it was first appointed by God, so life beyond the resurrection for the believer will mean the end of bodily sickness, pain, affliction and death in the glory and perfection of Christ's immediate fellowship and service. This must involve and will accomplish that perfect healing which is integral to the life of the Kingdom of God (Rev. 21:3, 4).

V. DYING WELL

It is one thing, however, to contemplate the experience of death and its consequences when there is no immediate indication of its proximity. It is another when the sentence of death has been received in the form of a medical diagnosis of an incurable and advancing disease. It is one thing to boast assurance of the glories of heaven while the expectation of continued enjoyment of the good things of earth is still strong. It is another when pain, weakness and fear bring the 'valley of the shadow' nearer by the day. It is particularly useful, therefore, to be able to consider the matter in the light of the experience of one who has put on record in the most honest and lucid terms his own faith and feelings in this very situation.

Rev. David Watson was Vicar of St Michael-le-Belfry in York before moving to St. Michael's, Chester Square, London. In January, 1983 he was diagnosed as having cancer and died in February, 1984.

His account of his experiences, both physical and spiritual, during those twelve months is a very moving and remarkable story of faith, courage and Christian triumph which is humbling, challenging and extremely illuminating in many aspects both concerning the Christian concept of death and the often confused and confusing notions and practices of faith-healing. It is all the more interesting and important because David Watson was not only a distinguished and widely travelled preacher and teacher of the Word of God, but also the son of a Christian Scientist, an advocate and practitioner of charismaticism and faith-healing, and a chronic sufferer from asthma.

Not surprisingly then, having received the shock of the original diagnosis, he quickly sought the help of his friend John Wimber, the pastor of a church in Yorba Linda, California, where amongst the vast congregation and multifarious activities of the Church a notable ministry of faith-healing takes place with miracle cures happening regularly at the normal services. Wimber's immediate reaction on the telephone was strangely to declare,

> I don't accept this cancer and I believe that God wants to heal you.[26]

He also called his whole congregation (three thousand souls) to 'urgent prayer'. After Watson had undergone surgery and it had been established that the cancer had spread to the liver, Wimber and two of his associates flew from California to visit him in hospital. During the visit they engaged in prayer for Watson, laid hands on him, and declared that it might well be that the cancer might continue to spread for a time, but one of them confidently pronounced,

> I believe that the root of it has now been cut. And soon it will begin to die.[27]

Watson continued to be prayed for by vast numbers of people around the world and several times was anointed with oil. On one such occasion when visited by Bishop Maurice Maddocks a Communion Service was held in his home and

> at the appropriate moment, Maurice anointed me with oil, laying hands upon me and praying for me.... In many ways it was totally different from the style of John Wimber and his two friends, and yet both forms of ministries, however different, seemed to bring the healing power of God into our lives.[28]

When further scans revealed the continuing progress of the cancer the reaction of Wimber was,

> We really believe God *is* healing you.... We'll go on praying, and if necessary we'll come straight over and pray with you some more.[29]

Watson also recalls,

> Ever since the initial ministry from John Wimber and others I have welcomed every opportunity of being prayed for, often with hands laid upon me. Almost every night Anne (*i.e.* his wife) lays her hands on my liver, curses the cancer in the name of Jesus, and prays for healing.... I have no doubt about the cumulative effect of this 'soaking prayer'.[30]

His condition continued to decline during the twelve months and at the end of that time began to deteriorate rapidly. He flew to California

> for special prayer at John Wimber's Church, since I felt I was losing the battle.... I was there for only eight days.... Each day different teams of Christians, experienced in the healing ministry, prayed for me, for periods ranging from two to five hours a day. Yet, for whatever reason, everything seemed to get worse.... I looked more dead than alive.[31]

We shall later consider many of the perplexing problems raised by the faith-healing aspects of this amazing story. For the moment we are interested only in the reaction of David Watson to the fact and the implications of facing death as a Christian believer. And what an impressive story that is. It is the story of Christian faith and hope growing deeper and surer as the crisis deepened. It is the story of courage and confidence holding fast not only against the onslaught of Satan and the ravages of disease, but also in the face of unwarranted faith-healing claims and pronouncements proving at every turn of the road to be wrong. It is the story of a soul beset by unanswerable questions and unintelligible contradictions yet buttressed by the certainties of divine promises that could be trusted and the comfort of an unseen presence that never failed.

Of course there were times of doubt and dismay—every servant of God from the greatest of the patriarchs and prophets to the greatest of the Apostles had them. But there was confidence too. He writes,

I had preached the gospel all over the world with ringing conviction. I had told countless thousands of people that I was not afraid of death since through Christ I had already received God's gift of eternal life. For years I had not doubted these truths at all. But now the most fundamental questions were nagging away insistently especially in those long hours of the night. If I was soon on my way to heaven, how real was heaven? Was it anything more than a beautiful idea?... Did God himself really exist at all?... How could I be certain of anything apart from cancer and death?... But in the middle of these nightmare storms, with waves of doubt and fear lashing all around me, I found that my faith was secure on that immovable rock of Christ.[32]

Of course there was the possibility that healing might not be given. When asked in a radio interview, What happens if you find that healing is not coming, he replied,

If I found it was not coming, I hope I have got to the position of really trusting in Christ that the best is yet to be. You know, actually to be with Christ and free for ever from the pain and suffering...there is nothing more glorious than that.[33]

And even later he could write,

The future officially is bleak, and I am getting used to people looking at me as a dying man under sentence of death. Nothing is certain. I'm not out of the wood yet. Everything is a matter of faith...the difficulties are still with me. I am not writing from a position of comparative safety.... And yet in reality, my position is not fundamentally different from that of anyone else. No one knows what the future holds.[34]

As the weary months passed he willingly acknowledged,

I believe that God is in the process of healing me. Every day I
thank him that he is healing me. But, logically speaking, it is
possible that I am wrong. God only knows.[35]

Of course there was the problem of suffering and its place in the
purposes of a loving God. Job too had faced that one.

Of course we should always strive to heal the sick and relieve the
oppressed; and we should rejoice that in heaven we shall finally
be set free from all pains and tears. But suffering can make us
more like Christ.[36]

Referring to Paul's declaration 'For this slight momentary affliction is
preparing for us an eternal weight of glory beyond all comparison' (2
Cor. 4:17) and recalling Paul's account of his many and desperate
crises of danger, pain and distress in 2 Corinthians 11:24–27, Watson
says,

Once we know the love of God for ourselves and believe in life
after death—or life *through* death—our outlook on this life, with
all its pains and sorrows, can be transformed.[37]

Of course there was the mystery of death and what lies beyond.

Faced with terminal cancer and with the medical prognosis of an
early death, I thought carefully about the perpetually puzzling
question, What happens at death? When the moment comes—as
it will for every one of us sooner or later, whether we think about
it or not—what will be the experience of death and what, if
anything, lies beyond it?... We cannot know exactly what we
shall be like after death. The apostle John put it like this: 'It is
not yet clear what we shall become. But we know that when
Christ appears, we shall be like him, because we shall see him
as he is' (1 John 3:2). That should be sufficient for us.... When
I die it is my firm conviction that I shall be more alive than ever,
experiencing the full reality of all that God has prepared for us
in Christ. The actual moment of dying is still shrouded in
mystery, but as I keep my eyes on Jesus I am not afraid. Jesus
has already been through death for us, and will be with us when
we walk through it ourselves.[38]

These are not the declarations of a terrified man desperate to escape
from an ordeal that looms over him in stark panic. Rather they are, in
spite of all the things that are not yet plain, the foundation-stones of
that peace and confidence with which he can commit the future, both
for himself and those whom he loves, into the hands of the One whose
company and communion have become his daily and nightly source
of rest and hope. Thus he concludes his testimony,

Whatever else is happening to me physically, God is working
deeply in my life. His challenge to me can be summed up in three
words: 'Seek my face'. I am not now clinging to physical life

(though I still believe that God can heal and wants to heal); but I am clinging to the Lord. I am ready to go and to be with Christ for ever. That would be literally heaven. But I'm equally ready to stay, if that is what God wants. 'Father, not my will but yours be done'. In that position of security I have experienced once again his perfect love, a love that casts out all fear.[39]

David Watson died peacefully a few days later having said to a friend, I am completely at peace—there is nothing that I want more than to go to heaven. I know how good it is.[40]

'This is the victory that overcometh the world, even our faith.' (1 John 5:4).

VI. DESTROYER OR HEALER?

What then shall we say of physical death? Is it something to be avoided at all costs? Is it to be feared as the final assault of Satan, or to be eluded for so long as possible by means either natural or supernatural? We have certainly seen that in the theology of mankind's rebellion and redemption it represents both the inevitable consequence of sin; the inescapable judgment of the sinner; and the incomprehensible condescension of the Saviour who 'though he was in the form of God, thought it not robbery to be equal with God: but made himself of no reputation, and took upon him the form of a servant, and was made in the likeness of men: and...became obedient unto death, even the death of the cross' (Phil. 2:6–8). And in that sense death was (and is) the last enemy of mankind's eternal glory to be defeated and destroyed by the risen, triumphant, and exalted Lord of Heaven. But for the Christian believer death is but the doorway to life more abundant and eternal. Its sting has been drawn; its victory has been upstaged; its threat to the dignity and destiny for which mankind was created by God has been removed; its evil consequences have been reversed; and it is now the very way to Life.

For the unrepentant sinner and unbeliever it is the door that shuts off all that constitutes light and life and love, and therefore must remain the ultimate threat of darkness and doom and the beginning of those eternal woes that can only be visualised in terms of unrelieved anguish and remorse—the great Destroyer. But for the Christian believer it is the portal of that realm where pain and weakness, sorrow and separation, tears and trials are ended and gone for ever. Where all that has been broken is mended; all that has been imperfect is restored; all that has been scarred is healed; all that has been lost is made secure for 'neither death nor life, nor angels, nor principalities, nor powers, nor things present, nor things to come, nor height, nor depth, nor any other creature shall be able to separate us from the love of God which is in Christ Jesus our Lord' (Rom. 8:38, 39)—the great Healer.

NOTES

1 C. S. Lewis, *Miracles,* Fontana Books, London, 1947, p. 129.
2 R. P. Martin, *Commentary on Philippians,* Tyndale Press, London, 1960, p. 79.
3 *Westminster Confession of Faith,* J. G. Eccles, Inverness, 1981, pp. 123f.
4 A. A. Hodge, *Commentary on the Westminster Confession of Faith,* T. Nelson and Sons, London, 1870, pp. 381ff.
5 Seventh-Day Adventism, *Questions on Doctrine,* Review and Herald Publishing Co., Washington DC, 1957, p. 527.
6 *Ibid.,* p. 528.
7 *Ibid.,* p. 528.
8 *Ibid.,* pp. 523f.
9 *Ibid.,* p. 525.
10 *Shorter Catechism of Westminster Divines,* J. G. Eccles, Inverness, 1981, Question 68.
11 C. S. Lewis, *Miracles,* Fontana Books, London, 1947, p. 163.
12 H. Alford, *The Greek Testament Vol. II,* Rivingtons, London, 1857, p. 579.
13 Leon Morris, *Commentary on I Corinthians,* Tyndale Press, London, 1958, pp. 215, 216f.
14 R. V. G. Tasker, *Commentary on II Corinthians,* Tyndale Press, London, 1958, p. 78.
15 *Ibid.,* p. 79.
16 *Ibid.,* p. 79.
17 H. Alford, *The Greek Testament Vol. II,* Rivingtons, London, 1857, p. 585.
18 Leon Morris, *Commentary on I Corinthians,* Tyndale Press, London, 1958, p. 228.
19 J. B. Lightfoot, *Commentary on Philippians,* Macmillan and Co., London, 1881, p. 156.
20 Jamieson, Fausset and Brown, *Commentary on the Whole Bible,* Oliphants, USA, 1966, pp. 1310f.
21 Leon Morris, *New Bible Dictionary,* Inter-Varsity Fellowship, London, 1962, pp. 1088f.
22 S. D. F. Salmond, *Christian Doctrine of Immortality,* T. and T. Clark, Edinburgh, 1895, p. 571.
23 C. S. Lewis, *Miracles,* Fontana Books, London, 1947, p. 139.
24 *Ibid.,* p. 127.
25 James Orr, *The Christian View of God and the World,* Andrew Elliott, Edinburgh, 1902, pp. 196f.

26 David Watson, *Fear No Evil,* Hodder and Stoughton, London, 1984, p. 25.
27 *Ibid.,* p. 57.
28 *Ibid.,* p. 90.
29 *Ibid.,* p. 99.
30 *Ibid.,* p. 109.
31 *Ibid.,* p. 170.
32 *Ibid.,* pp. 43, 45.
33 *Ibid.,* p. 92.
34 *Ibid.,* p. 152.
35 *Ibid.,* p. 107.
36 *Ibid.,* p. 135.
37 *Ibid.,* p. 140.
38 *Ibid.,* pp. 160–168.
39 *Ibid.,* p. 171.
40 *Ibid.,* p. 172.

9

THE CHURCH OF THE 'FATHERS'

I. A NEW WORLD

When we turn from the New Testament to the church of the immediate post-Apostolic times we find ourselves, so far as faith-healing is concerned, in a new world altogether—a world of myth and legend; of saints and shrines; of ritual and relics; of mystery and magic; of superstition and spiritism. The change came about as the purity of the church's doctrine and the power of its spiritual life declined and were replaced by the growth of unbiblical 'tradition' and practice down through the centuries till the age of the Reformation and then on till the present day.

As we have seen (p. 69) opinions differ as to how and when the change came about. As B. B. Warfield puts it, the commonly accepted view is that the exercise of the *charismata* and the working of miracles continued, but decreasingly till the end of the third century. Gerhard Ulhorn declares,

> witnesses who are above suspicion leave no room for doubt that the miraculous powers of the Apostolic age continued to operate at least into the third century.[1]

Nathaniel Marshall wrote,

> there are successive evidences of them, which speak full and home to the point, from the beginning down to the age of Constantine, in whose time, when Christianity had acquired the support of human powers, these extraordinary assistances were

discontinued.[2]

Henry Dodwell concluded that they ceased with the conversion of the Roman Empire to Christianity. Daniel Waterland extended the limit to the end of the fourth century. John Chapman extended it further through the fifth. William Whiston set the date of their cessation at AD 381, the time of the final triumph of Athanasianism. John Wesley was not consistent about his view that miracles ceased when the Empire became Christian. But the general pattern is the same—a gradual decline in miracle-working as the age of the Apostles receded.

To sum up, an examination of the passages in the apostolic literature which treat of spiritual gifts inevitably brings us to the conclusion that the life of the early church was characterised by glowing enthusiasm, simple faith, and intensity of joy and wonder, all resulting from the consciousness of the power of the Holy Spirit; also that this phase of Spirit-effected ministries and service was temporary, as such 'tides of the Spirit' have since often proved, and gave way to a more rigid and disciplined Church Order, in which the official tended more and more to supersede the charismatic ministries.[3]

It is the contention of B. B. Warfield, however, that the *charismata* of the New Testament died with the Apostles and those on whom they directly conferred them. This would necessarily mean that evidence of the continued exercise of these gifts continued to be seen until the last of the generation of those who had received them passed away, and this period overlapped to some extent the time of the early Fathers and their writings. For example, Quadratus (AD 126 or 127) wrote,

But the works of our Saviour were always visible, because they were true. Those, namely, who were freed from disease, or who were called back from death to life, were not only seen of men whilst they were being healed or called back to life, but also were seen in the time that followed. Nor was this only for so long as our Saviour remained upon earth, but they survived long after his departure, so long indeed that some of them have lived on even to our own time.[4]

Warfield, quoting from Bishop Kaye, says,

As the number of these disciples gradually diminished, the instances of the exercise of miraculous powers became continually less frequent, and ceased entirely at the death of the last individual on whom the hands of the Apostles had been laid. That event would, in the natural course of things, take place before the middle of the second century.[5]

And his own conclusion is,

The writings of the so-called Apostolic Fathers contain no clear and certain allusions to miracle-working, or to the exercise of the

charismatic gifts, contemporaneously with themselves.[6]
He goes on to quote Bishop Kaye writing in reference to Justin Martyr,
  Living so nearly as Justin did to the Apostolic age, it will natu-
  rally be asked whether, among other causes of the diffusion of
  Christianity, he specifies the exercise of miraculous powers by
  the Christians. He says in general terms that such powers
  subsisted in the church (Dial. pp. 254ff.)—that Christians were
  endowed with the gift of prophecy (Dial. p. 308B, see also p.
  315B)—and in an examination of supernatural gifts conferred on
  Christians he mentions that of healing (Dial. p. 258A).... He
  ascribes to Christians the power of exorcising demons (chap.
  VIII). But he produces no particular instance of an exercise of
  miraculous power, and therefore affords no opportunity of
  applying those tests by which the credibility of miracles must be
  tried.[7]
Warfield goes on to make the same comment on Irenaeus who
mentions also speaking with tongues and raising the dead, though he
is not apparently speaking as one who had personally witnessed these
things. As Warfield puts it,
  A scrutiny of his language makes it plain enough that he has not
  done so. In the passages cited Irenaeus is contrasting the miracles
  performed by Christians with the power of the magical wonders
  to which alone the heretics he is engaged in refuting can appeal.
  In doing this he has in mind the whole miraculous attestation of
  Christianity, and not merely the particular miracles which could
  be witnessed in his own day.... The use of the past tense...
  implies, we may say, that Irenaeus had not witnessed an example
  with his own eyes, or at least that such occurrences were not
  usual when he is writing.[8]
Thus Warfield concludes that rather than a slow decline in miracle-
working after the manner of the Apostles, what in fact happened was
that the gifts and powers of the Apostles disappeared very quickly after
the last of the Apostles and those who had been commissioned by
them, and that miracle-working of a very different kind soon began to
take its place. He bases his conclusion on certain clear statements of
the Apostolic Fathers.

  Justin Martyr (AD 100–165) in his Dialogue with Trypho speaks of
supernatural gifts conferred on Christians including that of healing, but
he makes reference to no particular instance. For example, speaking
of the *charismata*, he says,
  For one receives the spirit of understanding, another of counsel,
  another of strength, another of healing, another of fore-
  knowledge, another of teaching, another of the fear of God.[9]
He also makes reference to exorcism in the Second Apology thus,

For numberless daemoniacs throughout the whole world, and in your city, many of our Christian men exorcising them in the name of Jesus Christ...have healed and do heal, rendering helpless and driving the possessing daemons out of the men, though they could not be cured by all the other exorcists and those who used incantations and drugs.[10]

Irenaeus (AD 120–202) in the same way speaks in general terms and refers to speaking with tongues and even raising of the dead, but again without mention of specific examples. Contrasting the gifts of heretics with those of true believers, he says,

They can neither give sight to the blind, nor hearing to the deaf, nor put to flight demons, except those which are sent into others by themselves, if they can, indeed do this. Nor can they cure the weak, or the lame, or the paralytic, or those that are troubled in any other part of the body, as often happens to be done in respect of bodily infirmity...and so far are they from raising the dead as the Lord raised them and the Apostles did by means of prayer, and as when frequently in the brotherhood, the whole church in the locality, having made petition with much fasting and prayer, the spirit of the dead one has returned...(so far are they from doing this) that they do not believe that it can possibly be done, and they think that resurrection from the dead means a rejection of the truth of their tenets.[11]

Tertullian (AD 155–230) speaks of exorcisms and of a woman with the gift of prophecy and of the exercise of healing including the raising of the dead. In his word *To Scapula* in the fifth chapter he gives the following account:

All this might be officially brought under your notice, and by the very advocates, who are themselves also under obligations to us, although in court they give their voice as it suits them. The clerk of one of them who was liable to be thrown upon the ground by an evil spirit, was set free from his affliction; as was also the relative of another and the little boy of a third. And how many men of rank (to say nothing of the common people) have been delivered from daemons and healed of diseases? Even Severus himself, the father of Antonine, was graciously mindful of the Christians, having himself been cured.[12]

Origen (AD 185–253) claims to have been an eye-witness of many instances of exorcism, healing and prophecy, but again fails to mention specific instances. For example,

And there are still preserved among Christians traces of that Holy Spirit which appeared in the form of a dove. They expel evil spirits, and perform many cures, and foresee certain events, according to the will of the Logos.[13]

And in response to the claims made on behalf of the faith-healing carried on for a long time in the temples of Aesculapius, he says,

> And some [Christians] give evidence of their having received through this faith a marvellous power by the cures which they perform, invoking no other name over those who need their help than that of the God of all things, and of Jesus, along with a mention of his history. For by these means we too have seen many persons freed from grievous calamities, and from distractions of mind [*ekstaseon*] and madness, and countless other ills, which could be cured neither by men nor daemons.[14]

Cyprian (AD 200–258) speaks of gifts of visions and exorcisms, although with some misgiving:

> Cyprian, bishop of Carthage in North Africa...sounded the first note of alarm. Although he declared that healing still took place in the church he complained that it lacked strength in prayer because the church was growing more worldly and so giving power to the enemy.[15]

But, as Warfield says by way of general comment,

> And so we pass on to the fourth century in an ever-increasing stream, but without a single writer having claimed himself to have wrought a miracle of any kind or having ascribed miracle-working to any known name in the church, and without a single instance having been recorded in detail.[16]

From all of this, in Warfield's view, we conclude not that miracle-working ceased with the passing of the Apostles, but that the nature of miracle-working changed from the exercise of the New Testament charismata to other methods and motivations, with the biblical type of miracles decreasing and the non-biblical increasing.

This is confirmed by Weatherhead's survey of matters in the fourth and fifth centuries. For example, he says,

> St Ambrose (AD 340–397), Bishop of Milan, records the incident of a blind man being healed through touching the border of the garments in which the bodies of two martyrs were discovered beneath the pavement of the church, and says, 'Is not this like what we read in the gospel?' as if it were unusual to find such a close similarity.[17]

Of course there is no similarity at all between this and the woman with the haemorrhage touching the garment of the living Christ. Again,

> St Chrysostum (AD 357–407)...refers to healing as being a matter of common occurrence, and reports that commonly patients 'put away their diseases by anointing themselves with oil in faith', the oil being taken from the sanctuary lamps hanging before the altars of the churches.[18]

Here again there is nothing comparable to this in the New Testament.

Or again,
   St Augustine (AD 354–430)...writes as follows, 'And for
miracles there are some wrought as yet, partly by sacraments,
partly by the commemorations and prayers of the saints, but they
are not so famous nor so glorious as the other.[19]
And Weatherhead sums up the situation thus:
   The fact is that in the first three centuries of our era the Church
   increasingly lost the gift of spiritual healing....
      1. When those who had known Jesus in the flesh passed away,
   faith diminished, and love weakened and the potential of healing
   power was lowered.
      2. The change in technique is sinister.... His followers became
   increasingly content to lay all the onus for recovery on the
   patient, and the formula 'in the name of Jesus' became a charm
   instead of the means of conveying a power possessed by the
   healer through his communion with the living Christ and the
   strength of the undivided fellowship of the Church.
      3. One reluctantly writes down the sentence—Christ's
   followers found that their power to heal had gone.
      4. ...confidence in drugs and material remedies detracted from
   'the pious acknowledgment of God'.
      5. Even Origen asserted, 'The force of the exorcism lies in the
   name of Jesus', and sometimes he seems to have taken a pagan
   view of the matter and encouraged superstition. The power of this
   superstition gradually displaced the power of faith and love. The
   sale of holy relics abounded...and even the devout followers of
   Jesus...must have been disturbed to find that pagan exorcists
   could obtain similar results to themselves.
      6. (With reference to the conversion of Constantine) Christi-
   anity became, in fact, a polite veneer without power or beauty.
   Paganism remained, but now it was labelled Christianity as it is
   today.
      7. By the end of the third century science was becoming
   established and faith driven out.[20]
It appears to be accepted that faith-healing, as it is displayed in the
New Testament, was decreasingly in evidence in the immediately post-
Apostolic church. Some, like Weatherhead, would explain this by a
combination of factors such as listed above. Others, mainly of the
Reformed school of theology, like B. B. Warfield, would explain the
fact in a more fundamental way. They would say that the faith-healing
of the New Testament was identified with the authentication of the
divine purposes of redemption revealed fully and finally in Jesus Christ
both by his words and his works (*e.g.* healing), and supremely in his
own suffering, death and resurrection. When therefore the revelation

of those purposes was complete, and no new revelation was to be added, the accompanying phenomenon of miracles in general and healing in particular was withdrawn as being no longer necessary.

Miracles do not appear on the stage of Scripture vagrantly, here, there and elsewhere indifferently, without assignable reason. They belong to revelation periods, and appear only when God is speaking to His people through accredited messengers, declaring His gracious purposes. Their abundant display in the Apostolic Church is the mark of the richness of the Apostolic age in revelation; and when this revelation period closed, the period of miracle-working had passed by also, as a mere matter of course.[21]

But it is acknowledged by Warfield not only that miracles did continue to be a feature of the church's life after the times of the Apostles and the New Testament. Indeed it is his contention that, far from ceasing they became greatly proliferated in the succeeding years and centuries.

And whereas few writers were to be found in the earlier period (*i.e.* the first three centuries) who professed to be eye-witnesses of miracles, and none who wrought them were named to us, in the later period everybody appears to have witnessed any number of them, and the workers of them are not only named but prove to be the most famous missionaries and saints of the Church.[22]

But of course he regards these miracles not as a continuation of the biblical phenomenon, but as counterfeit miracles as we shall see.

II. NEW DEVELOPMENTS

As we have seen (p. 82), the James 5 passage was soon to become the basis of healing by 'Unction' (*i.e.* 'anointing with oil') and later to be constituted as a sacrament of the church. This would appear clearly to be an unwarranted development of the teaching of James. It was further misdirected by being changed in purpose from the healing of the body to the remission of sins. Dearmer attributes the change from a mistaken substitution in the Latin Vulgate of *alleviabit* for the original *egerei* of James which gave the meaning 'comfort' rather than 'raise up', thus leading to the Roman interpretation of 'the Lord shall comfort the soul of the sick man', and ultimately to the doctrine and practice of 'Extreme Unction' as a preparation for death rather than a restoration to health. Coupled with the further reference in the James passage (5:15) to any who 'have committed sins', Dearmer says,

> When a sick man is in this condition he is to confess his sins in order that 'forgiveness may be imparted to him, *aphethesetai auto*, in accordance with the Lord's commission, 'whose soever sins ye forgive, they are forgiven unto them' (John 20:23), where the same word is used for forgiveness or remission. It is not the

Unction which conveys this remission, but the Absolution following on confession of the sin. Two separate things are therefore described here—Unction for the body and Absolution for the soul.[23]

There was still no reference, however, to preparation for death. It was not until AD 800 that the change began to take place, when Bishop Theodulph of Orleans issued a pastoral instruction in which he ordered Unction to be administered as a preparation for death.

> The Council of Trent, however, in 1551 went a step further, established Peter Lombard's view as binding upon the Roman Church, and laid almost all the stress on the medieval view that Unction exists to prepare the sick man's soul for death.[24]

We shall see more of this later.

When we pass to the fourth and succeeding centuries the pattern is clear. The Sacramentary of Serapion (c.AD 350) mentions water and bread as being consecrated as well as oil for ministration to the sick. In St Jerome's 'Life of St Hilarion' (c.390) we read,

> He therefore blessed some oil, with which all the husbandmen and shepherds touched their wounds, and found an infallible cure.... There used to congregate about him bishops, presbyters, crowds of clerics and monks, of Christian matrons also, and a rabble of unknown persons...and even judges and others holding high positions. These all came to him with the object of receiving at his hands the bread or oil which he had blessed.[25]

The consecrated water used at first became 'holy water' and the consecrated bread became the bread of the sacrament. As time went by these were augmented by oil from Sanctuary lamps, relics of dead saints, incubation (*i.e.* 'temple-sleep' in which the patient having resorted to some church stayed there for some days and nights and dreamt that he had been visited and touched by a saint or celestial visitor and awoke either cured or given advice as to a remedy for his complaint), visits to shrines, pilgrimages, and the work of living 'saints' (*i.e.* people of exceptional virtue who later were recognised and canonised by the church). For our purpose it is necessary only to note that the 'faith' which constituted faith-healing in the patristic and medieval times was no longer faith in the living power of the risen Saviour ministered by the Holy Spirit in answer to believing prayer, but now had degenerated into superstitious confidence in objects, rituals or people authorised or encouraged by the church.

III. THE MEDIEVAL PERIOD

The medieval period was but a continuation of the patristic scene.
Ecclesiastical miracles of every conceivable kind were alleged.

Every variety of miracle properly so called Chrysostum declares
to have ceased. It is the contrast between miracles as such and
wonders of grace that Gregory draws. No doubt we must
recognise that these Fathers realised that ecclesiastical miracles
were of a lower order than those of Scripture. It looks very much
as if, when they were not inflamed by enthusiasm, they did not
really think them to be miracles at all.[26]

It is not our purpose to discuss the validity of miracles. We are
concerned with them only to the extent that they represent the church's
expression of faith-healing during that period. We must therefore
examine them in that context.

(i) Symbols and relics

Percy Dearmer notes that the earliest references to healing outside of
the New Testament speak of the use of Christ's name and the laying
on of hands (by Justin Martyr and Irenaeus) and the use of Unction (by
Tertullian who referred to the healing of the Emperor Septimus Severus
by a Christian using Unction). The Sacramentary of Serapion added the
use of consecrated water and bread. St Jerome endorsed the use of
bread and oil, the Apostolic Constitutions of AD 375 and the
Testamentum Domini of AD 400 speak of the use of oil and water, St
Martin (c.AD 395) and St Theodore (c.AD 350) mention the drinking
of oil or water that has been 'blessed', St Cuthbert (c.AD 687) used
consecrated oil, water and bread. Dearmer comments,

> Thus we are always in the realm of healing by faith, and one
> symbol is as good as another.[27]

But of course we remember that only in the James 5 passage is there
any mention of symbol in regard to faith-healing. Dearmer considers
that oil and water were appropriate symbols because of their common
employment in medicine and surgery, and finds evidence that they were
sometimes used together with prayer for both physical and spiritual
effect. However, he adds,

> I have said that this had little to do with the 'sacrament of
> Unction' in the medieval and modern sense; but I do not suppose
> that in earlier times the distinction would have had any
> meaning—it seems that a Christian healer would have used in the
> same way either oil that had come from a sacred place or oil that
> had been blessed by a priest, bishop or by a charismatic.[28]

With regard to the use of relics, Dearmer says,

> their use as a means of faith-healing was not only of early origin,
> but was predominant in the Middle Ages, and has continued
> abundantly down to the present day.[29]

In a strange and seemingly irrelevant reference Dearmer appears
almost to justify belief in the efficacy of relics by recalling the incident

in 2 Kings 13:21 where the corpse of a dead man was restored to life
when it was hurriedly thrown into the grave of Elisha and touched his
bones (see p. 47). Even more strangely he seems to suggest some kind
of similarity in the incident of the 'sweat-cloths' sent by the Apostle
Paul to the sick, and perhaps strangest of all, while expressing some
personal reservations he argues thus,

> We need not be surprised that it had so much play in the Christian
> church. Had it not been so, the church would have lain open to
> the *graver accusation* that she was something less than human.[30]

But surely the essence of Christian faith is that the 'human' has been
transformed from its bondage to fear, ignorance and superstition by the
spirit 'of power, and of love and of a sound mind' (2 Tim. 1:7). So that
indeed we have good reason to be surprised that superstition should not
only have such a large place, but any place at all in the Christian
church. Dearmer, however, goes on,

> No doubt, again, there grew up a miserable traffic in spurious
> relics, which has left a grave moral legacy of falsehood and
> pretence in those countries where relics have not been swept
> away.... The authenticity of the relics is a side issue, the faith is
> the main point; and men went on frequenting shrines because
> they often found that their faith made them whole. It is with this
> fact that we are concerned: for the greater part of Christian
> history faith-healing was mainly centred in relics, so that
> probably more people have benefited in this way than in any
> other. Unction fell into abeyance as a means of healing, and
> saints were sporadic; but the shrines of the saints were permanent
> institutions.[31]

This view raises some fundamental issues which cannot appropriately
be dealt with here, but it must be said that while faith in the power of
relics, just like faith in any other kind of object or material substance,
may produce psychological effects in the suggestible type of person,
and may indeed constitute some kind of psychiatric medicine, it cannot
be identified with the faith in the living power of the living Christ
which constitutes faith-healing in the biblical and truly Christian sense.
The same may be said of belief in 'incubation', visits to shrines, or
pilgrimages, none of which have any warrant from Scripture.

(ii) Saints

With reference to healings by 'saintly persons' Dearmer says,

> In addition to all this, there is right through Christian history a
> continuous record of healing by means of the exceptional virtue
> which belongs to those who live very near to God, and whom we
> call saints.... These medieval miracles, therefore, deserve
> respectful treatment; and the cumulative evidence of so much

concurrent testimony by distinguished and upright men makes it impossible to think that they were all deluded and mistaken.[32] There is no need, however, on the basis of Scripture to come to such a conclusion. The error of Dearmer's position is, of course, that he starts off from the wrong premises and definitions. A 'saint' in biblical terms is not constituted such by his or her 'exceptional virtues', but only by the grace of God received by faith in Christ Jesus (Eph. 2:8, 9). Moreover, the power to heal is not to be found in the merit of the Christian believer but in the Spirit of God in response to his obedience to the Word of God. As we have seen so clearly already, the exercise of the gift of God's grace and power in the life of the believer has, in the mercy and sovereign purposes of God, and in every age since the institution of the church of Christ, been effective in providing healing both of spirit and body. The healing is not 'by saintly persons', but by the power of the living Christ in them who 'walk in the Spirit'.

(iii) An English legend

Finally, Dearmer makes reference to a peculiarly English version of faith-healing which he calls 'Touching for the King's Evil' which is supposed to have begun in the time of Edward the Confessor.

> James I wished to drop it as an outworn superstition, but was warned by his ministers that to do so would be to abate a prerogative of the Crown: so the rite continued as long as the Stuarts remained on the throne, and was still printed in the early part of George I's reign.... Englishmen no longer believed in the efficacy of the saints, but they had a redoubled faith in that of the monarch; and the Church of England in the age of the Stuarts spent herself over the Divine right of Kings. We are not concerned to defend the belief that supernatural power emanated from royal hands, any more than it emanated from canonised bones; but those who held that belief no doubt were able to obtain spiritual help even through so grotesque a medium as James I.[33]

The form of ritual used, however, on such occasions reveals that, in fact, the royal chaplain presented those seeking help to the monarch and, after the reading of Scripture (Mark 16:14–end) and prayer, the monarch laid hands upon them while the chaplain offered prayers for healing, concluding with the Benediction. It must therefore be concluded that the monarch, rightly or wrongly, was purporting to act in the name of God with prayer and the laying on of hands.

IV. SUMMARY

We may sum up the situation in the period of the Apostolic Fathers thus:

1. The exercise of the *charismata* continued to be evident so long as there remained alive those who had been commissioned by the Apostles to exercise such gifts (*i.e.* the latter half of the second century).

2. The early 'Fathers' (*e.g.* Justin Martyr, Irenaeus, Tertullian, Origen, Cyprian) continued to speak of the exercise of such gifts down to the latter part of the third century though they did not claim either to have exercised the gifts themselves or to have witnessed the exercise of them personally.

3. By the beginning of the fourth century miracle-working, particularly in reference to healing, by non-biblical means (*i.e.* the use of relics, consecrated oil, bread, *etc.*) was taking place.

4. Miracle-working by non-biblical means increased in inverse proportion to the decline in the spiritual quality and power of the life of the church.

5. 'Unction' ('anointing with oil') which began with the practice of healing as described by James for the healing of the body became corrupted into a sacrament for the remission of sins.

6. Faith in the power of the living Christ degenerated into superstitious confidence in material objects, rituals or saints.

NOTES

1   G. Ulhorn, *The Conflict of Christianity with Heathenism*, as cited by B. B. Warfield, *Counterfeit Miracles*, Banner of Truth, London, 1972, p. 8.

2   Nathaniel Marshall, as cited by B. B. Warfield, *Counterfeit Miracles*, p. 7.

3   R. M. Pope, *Hastings Dictionary of the Apostolic Church*, Vol. I, p. 451, cited by B. B. Warfield, *Counterfeit Miracles*, p. 235.

4   Quadratus c.126 cited by P. Dearmer, *Body and Soul*, Dutton, New York, 1923, p. 243.

5   John Kaye (Bishop of Lincoln), *The Ecclesiastical History of the Second and Third Centuries*, 1845, pp. 98ff. cited by B. B. Warfield, *Counterfeit Miracles*, pp. 23f.

6   B. B. Warfield, *Counterfeit Miracles*, Banner of Truth, London, 1972, p. 10.

7   John Kaye, *Justin Martyr*, 1853, p. 121 cited by B. B. Warfield, *Counterfeit Miracles*, p. 11.

8   B. B. Warfield, *Counterfeit Miracles*, p. 15.

9   Justin Martyr, *Dial. with Trypho* 39 as cited by P. Dearmer, *Body and Soul*, p. 243.

10   Justin Martyr, *Second Apology* 6 as cited by P. Dearmer, *Body*

and Soul, p. 244.

11   Irenaeus, *Adv. Haer. II* 31:2 as cited by B. B. Warfield, *Counterfeit Miracles*, p. 241.

12   P. Dearmer, *Body and Soul*, p. 252.

13   Origen, *Con. Celsius* Bk I chap. 46 as cited by P. Dearmer, *Body and Soul*, p. 247.

14   Origen, *Con. Celsius* Bk III chap. 24 as cited by P. Dearmer, *Body and Soul*, p. 248.

15   M. Maddocks, *The Christian Healing Ministry*, SPCK, London, 1981, p. 97.

16   B. B. Warfield, *Counterfeit Miracles*, p. 12.

17   L. D. Weatherhead, *Psychology, Religion and Healing*, Hodder and Stoughton, London, 1951, p. 86.

18   *Ibid.*, p. 86.

19   *Ibid.*, p. 86.

20   *Ibid.*, pp. 87–91.

21   B. B. Warfield, *Counterfeit Miracles*, pp. 25f.

22   *Ibid.*, p. 37.

23   P. Dearmer, *Body and Soul*, p. 229.

24   *Ibid.*, p. 231.

25   *Ibid.*, p. 258.

26   B. B. Warfield, *Counterfeit Miracles*, p. 48.

27   P. Dearmer, *Body and Soul*, p. 263.

28   *Ibid.*, p. 267.

29   *Ibid.*, p. 270.

30   *Ibid.*, p. 273.

31   *Ibid.*, p. 274.

32   *Ibid.*, pp. 286, 290.

33   *Ibid.*, p. 295.

10

THE ROMAN CATHOLIC CHURCH

The position of the Roman Catholic Church on the matter of healing or faith-healing is rather anomalous and confused. The official dogma and liturgy of the Church provide for the ministry of healing as a purely sacramental practice. But, in fact, the vast majority of those who seek healing from the Church, or through faith, do so not by means of the sacrament as such, but by resort to the use of relics or pilgrimages to religious shrines; to the mediation of the Virgin Mary or the 'saints'; or, in more recent times, to the ministry of charismatic healers. Moreover, the controversy as to whether the sacrament of 'anointing of the sick' (Unction or Extreme Unction), based erroneously on the James passage in the New Testament, should be administered for the purpose of recovery from physical sickness, or for the spiritual preparation of the soul for death and judgment, has never been resolved. Indeed, in spite of all that has been said or written, it seems clear that the real and ultimate purpose of the sacrament, even when administered as part of the ritual of the healing shrines such as Lourdes, or the ministry of charismatic healers, is still a spiritual preparation for death either apart from, or as a precaution against, the failure of physical healing to take place. We therefore must consider briefly the three strands of the Roman Catholic approach to healing.

I. SACRAMENTAL HEALING

The Apostolic Constitution of Pope Paul VI, November, 1972,

reiterating the Decree of the Council of Trent, declares,

> The Catholic Church professes that the anointing of the sick is one of the seven sacraments of the New Testament, that it was instituted by Christ our Lord, intimated in Mark (6:13) and through James, the apostle and brother of the Lord, recommended to the faithful and made known.[1]

The Council of Trent following on the Decree of the Council of Florence, explained the reality and effects of the sacrament thus,

> This reality is in fact the grace of the Holy Spirit whose anointing takes away sins, if any still remain, and the remnants of sin; this anointing also raises up and strengthens the soul of the sick person, arousing a great confidence in the divine mercy; thus sustained, the sick person may more easily bear the trials and hardships of sickness, more easily resist the temptations of the devil 'lying in wait for his heel' (Gen. 3:15), and sometimes regain bodily health, if this is expedient for the health of the soul.[2]

and the Council went on to declare,

> this anointing is to be given to the sick, especially those who are in such a serious condition as to appear to have reached the end of their life. For this reason it is also called the sacrament of the dying.[3]

It is clear, therefore, that the Church of Rome retains its commitment to the healing of the sick as a sacrament to be performed only by a 'presbyter' or 'bishop'. The practice is traced historically from the New Testament in Mark 6:7–13 and James 5. The James 5 passage, as we have already seen, is regarded as indicating,

> neither a purely eschatological spiritual healing (salvation in the life to come, the future resurrection of the dead), nor simply a bodily medicinal effect in the manner of faith-healing. This rite touches upon the salvific situation of the sick person: the religious powerlessness and the threat that sickness poses to faith and trust in God. As a result, the sick Christian shall be raised up from this weakness and saved from the obstacle that sickness constitutes toward salvation.[4]

Although the sevenfold number and nature of the sacraments was not declared until the twelfth century, in the western Church anointing was practised as a rite for the sick during the first eight centuries. The most important part of the rite was the blessing of the oil by the bishop. And although the blessing of the oil by the bishop was required, and the application of it properly was to be by a bishop, it could also be applied by lay people. Its purpose during the first eight hundred years was not as a preparation for death. Apparently it was in the ninth century that the process began which was to transform anointing as a rite for the sick into a sacrament for the dying.

The 'Carolingian Reform' took place between the ninth and twelfth centuries.

> From the ninth century on the 'anointing with sacred oil' appears to be one of the Church's last rites for the dying (the other two being the reconciliation and the viaticum; Palmer, p. 322). The implications of this legitimate development are certainly two: the anointing is meant for the sick in danger of death; and it intends (not a bodily cure which in the circumstances is no longer hoped for but) a spiritual effect. Thus its sacramental nature becomes manifest, and so does its proper grace: spiritual help for the sick in danger of death. The name Extreme Unction, the last anointing or, when misunderstood, the anointing for the last moments, was introduced at this time.[5]

Having become one of the seven sacraments of the Church in the twelfth century, 'anointing of the sick' began to be postponed until the point of death.

> An abuse originating in some fanciful concepts about the effects of the anointing for those who recovered and were considered as bound to a sort of penitential life (Kilker, pp. 151ff., Palmer, p. 330), or in a misunderstood theology of the anointing of the sick as complement of the sacrament of penance as though it entailed, of its nature, immediate entrance into heaven.[6]

The Council of Trent formally defined the anointing of the sick as one of the seven sacraments.

> By the providential substitution of 'especially' (*praesertim*) for 'only' (*dumtaxat*) in its text on the recipient of the sacrament (D 1698) it ushered in the distinction between the danger of death and point of death, and thus struck at the root of the abuse of unduly delaying the anointing of the sick—which, however, persists even today.[7]

Until Vatican II Extreme Unction was administered to

> 'Catholics who, after having attained the use of reason, incur a danger of death through sickness or old age' as Canon 940 of the 1918 Code of Canon Law defined the 'subject' of the sacrament. While the Code of 1918 spoke of 'danger of death', it did not say '*imminent* danger of death', and even before the Second Vatican Council Popes of this century, such as Benedict XV and Pius XI, pleaded that for pastoral reasons the anointing be given at the earliest possible time, as soon as there was a prudent or probable judgment regarding the danger of death.[8]

Vatican II brought about changes of form but not of substance.

> Extreme Unction, which may also and more properly be called 'anointing of the sick', is not a sacrament for those only who are

at the point of death. Hence, as soon as any one of the faithful begins to be in danger of death from sickness or old age, the fitting time for that person to receive the sacrament has certainly already arrived.[9]

The change of name is said to be,

the first step towards a more scriptural, historical and pastoral understanding of the sacrament.[10]

The instruction not to delay the sacrament until the point of death (or afterwards) is said to be a departure from the Code of 1918, (which stated that the presence of the danger of death was 'necessary'), in order to show concern about undue delay. It was evidently not intended to indicate a change in the nature or purpose of the sacrament as charismatics would claim. And again, it is said that the concern of the Council was to restore the order of the sacraments for the sick and dying so that anointing of the sick would not take precedence over the Eucharist or Mass,

so that it is clear that the most important sacrament of the dying is Viaticum, not the anointing of the sick. (Viaticum is normally given within the Eucharist)11

Thomas Marsh (Lecturer in Theology in Maynooth) sees the statement of Vatican II in the Constitution on the Liturgy as

ambiguous, confusing and illogical. While the description 'anointing of the sick' is allowed (note the subjunctive), the context of the sacrament firmly remains danger of death, the traditional *'periculum mortis'*. There is really no theological change envisaged here.[12]

But on the later Constitution on the Church sec. 11 he says,

This passage makes no reference to danger of death and speaks only of the sick.[13]

The matter, however, is finally settled, in the opinion of Thomas Marsh, in 'The Rite of Anointing and Pastoral Care of the Sick' in which he says,

The Introduction describes the subjects of the sacrament as 'those who are dangerously ill due to sickness or old age', it declares 'a prudent or probable judgment about the seriousness of the sickness' sufficient, and cautions against a scrupulous attitude. What is perhaps most striking is the complete absence of reference to danger of death, the consecrated phrase which for so long had described the context of this sacrament, and which still does so in the Liturgy Constitution. The absence of this traditional reference and the numerous other indications of the new Rite make it perfectly clear that this is a sacrament of the sick and not merely of the dying. There is, therefore, no room whatever for any further quibbling on this issue.[14]

But indeed there is! In fact, if words mean anything other than what the writer wishes, it must be obvious that no change has in reality taken place at all. The new Rite statement expressly says 'those who are *dangerously* ill due to sickness or old age'. What can 'dangerously ill' mean other than to be in danger? And what 'danger' can be in view other than the danger of death? Moreover, any judgment about 'the seriousness of the sickness' can only be a judgment as to how great the danger, or how near the event of death, is.

Marsh, in seeking to show how the healing of sickness calls for the administration of the sacrament, sets out the theology of man, evil and salvation in which basically his argument is that there is no duality between body and soul (man physical and spiritual); that sickness and death are manifestations of the power of evil that separate man from himself, from the world, and from God; that salvation is the undoing of this separation and the restoration of man in the likeness and image of God. The ministry of Jesus, and particularly his ministry to the sick, is the revelation and execution of God's plan for this restoration and for the ultimate destruction of the forces of evil. This salvation, begun in the present, is brought to its fulfilment in the future. The mission of the church is to continue the ministry of Jesus, including his ministry to the sick and this it does by means of the sacraments.

> The Church seeks to achieve this by addressing herself to the sick person and expressing her deepest nature as, in Christ, the community and sacrament of salvation. By thus expressing herself in this context of sickness, the Church enables the sick person to experience the power of salvation which is in her and which she exhibits. She accomplishes this by effectively announcing the gospel of salvation in the sick context.[15]

Thus, Marsh says, the church calls the sick member to accept sickness as a condition which can be lived positively as a particular form of taking up the cross and following Christ.

> Restoration to health may also take place and it may come about in either an ordinary or an extraordinary manner. But such restoration, while it may be hoped for and should be prayed for and while it is certainly a primary reference of the sacrament, yet it cannot be said to be the basic effect of this sacrament, as if the sacrament is a failure if such restoration does not occur.[16]

Marsh clearly defines the relationship between the sacrament of anointing and the Eucharist thus

> The sacrament of anointing the sick is meant to be a preparation of the sick person for a renewed, fruitful participation in the Eucharist which is thus the natural climax of this ministry. Here the re-established relationships with God, Christ and his community will be most profoundly experienced and celebrated.[17]

The 'laying on of hands' is seen to be most appropriate in the rite of anointing. It is said to indicate that the particular person is the object of the Church's prayer; it is a sign of blessing; it is an invocation of the Holy Spirit to come upon the sick person; it is the biblical gesture of healing demonstrated in Christ's own practice.

As in the case of each of the sacraments, the authority and power lies in the Church and its 'ministers' (*i.e.* clergy). Such faith as is required on the part of the sufferer is not faith in Christ as such, but rather confidence in the Church and its agents to control and exercise the divine power to pardon and heal. Moreover, in the case of sacramental healing, the power lies in the sacrament itself which works *ex opere operato*. Whatever may be said in respect of healing the sick, and the distinction between 'anointing with oil' and Viaticum, it is clear that the use of the sacrament of Unction, and particularly of Extreme Unction, normally relates not to the procurement of healing and restoration of health to the body, but rather to the preparation of the soul for death. Hence the prevalent practice of administering the sacrament even after any evidence of life has ceased.

P. de Letter sums up the doctrine of the anointing of the sick thus. (1) It is a spiritual remedy against sickness intended for spiritual healing. It does not always procure physical recovery but it always provides spiritual strength to overcome the maleffects of sickness. (2) It is not only meant for those at the point of death but those in danger of death. But even when death takes place it provides the grace of a Christian death in which the soul experiences immediate victory and the body the delayed victory of glorious resurrection later. (3) It may in some cases lead to the restoration of bodily health by a psychosomatic process in which the spiritual comfort of the soul reacts on the body and thus may affect its cure according to God's providential design. It should not be called the sacrament of healing since this may give false hope, and undermine its spiritual effects. (4) It prepares the soul for immediate entrance into heaven, depending on the spiritual condition of the recipient, but it cannot provide, as suggested by St. Thomas, Suarez and H. Kern, an easy escape from purgatory. (5) Because it is a complement to the sacrament of penance, it effects, as any sacrament does, the grace which is intended, that is, spiritual healing, through the remission of mortal sin.[18]

II. THE LOURDES PHENOMENON

However, notwithstanding the doctrine and practice laid down in the Decrees of the Ecumenical Councils of the Roman Church, healing is sought, and encouraged to be sought, by other means, and chiefly by resort to miraculous cures said to be procured by the use of relics; the pursuit of pilgrimages to shrines and 'holy places'; or appeal to the Virgin Mary or the 'saints'. As Warfield says,

> The Church of Rome, accordingly, can point to a body of miracles, wrought in our own day and generation, as large and striking as those of any earlier period of the church's history.... This continuous manifestation of supernatural powers in its bosom constitutes one of the proudest boasts of the church of Rome; by it, it conceives itself differentiated, say, from Protestants; and in it it finds one of its chief credentials as the sole organ of God Almighty for the saving of the wicked world.[19]

Warfield sees the preoccupation of the Church of Rome with such miracle-myth as the result of the process by which heathen legendary was taken over and transformed into 'Christian' folklore.

> In one word what we find, when we cast our eye over the whole body of Christian legends, growing up from the third century down through the Middle Ages, is merely a reproduction, in Christian form, of the motives, and even of the very incidents, which already meet us in the legends of heathendom.... It is this mass of legends, the Christianised form of the universal product of the human soul, working into concrete shape its sense of the other world, that the church of Rome has taken upon its shoulders. It is not clear that it has added anything of importance to it.[20]

The importance and prevalence of relics, apparitions, and pilgrimages in the process of healing cannot be overestimated. Probably the best known and most important shrine for healing is that at Lourdes in South-west France where in 1858 the Virgin Mary is said to have appeared some eighteen times to a peasant girl, Bernadette Soubirous, and instructed her, amongst other things, to search in a certain place where she uncovered a spring of water with miraculous, curative power.

In *The Catholic Encyclopedia* Georges Bertrin writes,

> There exists no natural cause capable of producing the cures witnessed at Lourdes which dispense an unbiassed mind from tracing them back to the particular agency of God. Those who refused to believe in a miraculous intervention sought at first the successful interpretation of the occurrences in the chemical composition of the water of the Grotto. But it was then declared by an eminent chemist...that the water contains no curative properties.... Then (it was claimed that)...the results obtained at Lourdes may be accounted for by bathing in cold water. However, everyone knows that hydrotherapy is practised elsewhere...and that it does not work the miracle of curing every kind of disease, from cancers to troubles which bring blindness...

Those who deny supernatural intervention attribute the wonderful results...to two other causes. The first is suggestion...It is not suggestion that operates at Lourdes; the cause which cures acts differently and is infinitely more powerful.... There remains the last resource of having recourse to some unknown law and of saying, for instance, 'How do we know that some natural force of which we are still ignorant does not operate the marvellous cures which are attributed directly to God?'...the hypothesis of unknown forces of nature cannot be brought forward to explain the instantaneous cures of Lourdes. It is logically untenable.... They can only be from the intervention of God.[21]

But Herbert Thurston, S. J., in the *Encyclopedia of Religion and Ethics*, says

This is the miraculous water which is the reputed source of so many miracles.[22]

Warfield, as one might expect, takes a different view.

The immense success of Lourdes as a place of pilgrimage has been achieved in spite of the meanness of its origin, and is to be attributed to the skill with which it has been exploited.[23]

He notes the opinion of Monsignor R. H. Benson to the effect that about 90% of those seeking cure go away unbenefited. He also claims that while stress is laid on the instantaneousness of the cures, many are not so; and indeed many are never completed. Summing up his judgment of the nature and validity of what goes on at Lourdes, he says,

Even though we should stand dumb before the wonders of Lourdes, and should be utterly incapable of suggesting a natural causation for them, we know right well they are not of God. The whole complex of circumstances of which they are a part; their origin in occurrences, the best that can be said of which is that they are silly; their intimate connection with a cult derogatory to the rights of God who alone is to be called upon in our distresses,—stamp them, prior to all examination of the mode of their occurrence, as not from God.... What Lourdes has to offer is the common property of the whole world, and may be had by men of all religions, calling upon their several gods.[24]

In other words, Warfield does not deny the claim that healings do take place at Lourdes, he simply concludes that they are of the same nature as those effected by heathen witch-doctors, Christian Scientists, and other non-Christian mediums; but are certainly not to be attributed to the power of God as revealed in the experience and requirements of the Scriptures.

A more liberal Protestant view of the activity of Lourdes is taken by Leslie Weatherhead who visited the shrine in 1949. In his report he spends much time seeking to establish the fact that proven cures do

take place there. Having reviewed the medical procedures used by the
Church to establish and certify the reality of cures effected, he says,
    In my opinion, there can be no possible doubt that the cures of
    physical illness take place in a remarkable way.[25]
This, of course, is not in question. Our concern is to establish how or
whether such cures (or treatments) bear any relation to the biblical
doctrine and pattern of faith-healing. Weatherhead remarks,
    the experiences of a peasant girl began a world-famous cult,
    authorised finally by the Pope as the cult of Our Lady of
    Lourdes.[26]
He goes on then to analyse the experience of the girl herself. Her
original experience, he reckons, was an hallucination based on her age
(fourteen years), her heightened religious fervour as she contemplated
her first communion, her membership of a Guild of Girls known as
'Les Enfants de Marie' and participation in its religious ceremonies,
the recent death of the Guild's President, and the proclamation four
years earlier by Pope Pius IX of the dogma of the 'Immaculate
Conception' as an Article of Faith. She may have had the gift of water-
divining which would have accounted for her finding the spring.
Nothing was said to her by the Virgin Mary about the cure of disease
and, in fact, Bernadette herself was a lifelong victim of chronic asthma
and was not cured but eventually died of the disease.
    In his assessment of the healing power of Lourdes, Weatherhead
notes that the percentage of cures is very low—about 2%.
    Many patients not only went back home with the last hope gone,
    but it must have been a severe shock to their Christian faith.
And he concludes,
    Lourdes can, no doubt, provide a great spiritual experience. As
    a healing agency its proportion of failures makes it negligible.
    Few of its cures brought to our notice could possibly be regarded
    as 'miracles'...and those few did not depend on the paraphernalia
    of Lourdes.[27]
Percy Dearmer, after the usual survey of the medical aspects of the
healings (or failures to heal) at Lourdes, comments on the 'spiritual'
aspects of the whole phenomenon thus,
    The religious causes at Lourdes are indeed both impressive and
    inadequate. They owe their strength to certain ancient and
    permanent elements of faith and fellowship which are sufficient
    to establish relations with the spiritual world, being concentrated
    and intensified by the associations of the place. That it all should
    be based upon a worthless hallucination and contaminated by
    much narrowness and superstition is regrettable; but it increases
    our wonder that, in spite of defects which do great harm to the
    Church in France, there should be as many cures as there are. If

so many sick persons (whose diseases have generally baffled the doctors) should be cured at Lourdes, what might not the result be in some holy place of future days, where the religious motive should be above criticism and the methods beyond praise; where the intimate sacramentalism of Christianity should be purified from all puerile accretions, while nothing was lost of the ancient and permanent forces which have brought such precious succour to the human race.[28]

III. CHARISMATIC HEALING

Since 1967 the Roman Catholic Church, like all others, has been affected by the growth of the Charismatic Movement.

A second charismatic upsurge with many precursors began in the USA in 1960. Beginning among Episcopalians and then in other Reformation churches, especially Lutheran and Reformed, it spread to the Catholic Church in 1967 and thereafter throughout the whole world.[29]

As a result, often where the ecumenical movement had failed to bridge the gulf between Reformed and non-Reformed Christians and churches, charismatic activity succeeded. A WCC study acknowledges,

Whereas in the past, charismatic Pentecostalist revivals usually tended to divide congregations, the Charismatic Renewal of the Congregation must be seen as a strongly unifying movement. Spiritual experience in the most widely divergent traditions is nothing less than the start of a common ecumenical tradition and gives every ground for high hopes.... The release of the Spirit has brought a great number of Christians nearer to Christ and thus nearer to each other. They have found a common vision and a common worship. A number of prayer groups are interdenominational. At the Dutch national convention, Protestants participate in the Catholic eucharist and Catholics in Holy Communion.... The charismatic movement, in the few years of its existence, has begun to bring together, in significant numbers, the Catholic stream, the main-line Protestant stream, the evangelical Protestant stream, and the Pentecostal stream.[30]

Amongst the leading Roman Catholic writers on the subject of healing is Rev. Dr Francis MacNutt, O. P., whose publication *Healing* is claimed by the publishers to be

the first comprehensive Catholic book on healing by the foremost authority on the healing ministry in the Roman Catholic Church today. He was one of the first Catholics involved in the charismatic renewal and in the practice of praying for healing in prayer groups. In 1967 he became acquainted with the work of

Agnes Sandford, Rev. Tommy Tyson and other Protestant leaders in the healing ministry, and immediately realised that the basic teachings on healing were very much in line with Roman Catholic tradition.[31]

His healing ministry has spanned the United States of America, Peru, Bolivia and Chile. He is on the advisory Committee of National Catholic Charismatic Services. His second publication, *The Power to Heal,* deals with the practical application of the principles laid down in *Healing,* the first volume, in which he deals with the theology and basic principles of healing in a thoroughly scientific way. At this point in our study we are interested particularly in his account of his ministry as it relates to the dogma and practice of the Roman Church. And in this regard he sees important changes having taken place in recent times.

'In the past few years,' he writes, 'an extraordinary change has been going on in the Roman Catholic Church—all the way from the grass-roots level to the most official pronouncements the healing ministry is being renewed.'[32]

He sees the most far-reaching of all the changes, so far as official pronouncements are concerned, in the promulgation on January 1, 1974, as a result of the Vatican II Constitution on the liturgy, section 73, of a new decree concerning the sacrament of 'Anointing of the Sick' (commonly known as the Last Rites or Extreme Unction) by which

it is to be administered not just to those in danger of death, but to anyone suffering from a severe illness.[33]

Dr MacNutt sees this as a re-establishment of the former practice which, he says, prevailed in the Church until the Middle Ages. The point is that the sacrament is now to be seen not as a sign of hopelessness and despair in regard to recovery, but rather as a means to healing and hope. This indeed may be how the change is seen by charismatics, but it is not, in fact, what Vatican II said. In fact, as we have already seen, it would appear rather that all that the change was intended to do was to attempt to ensure that the administration of Extreme Unction was not delayed too long. But it is clear that it still was intended to refer to the possibility of death rather than the likelihood of recovery.

Again, he believes,

healing is probably easier for Catholics to understand than for most Protestants, since we have grown up with a tradition of saints blessed with extraordinary gifts, including healing, the one that is still used as a test for canonisation. Consequently, most traditional Catholics have little difficulty in believing in divine healing.[34]

What Dr MacNutt fails to understand is that Protestants have no difficulty whatever in believing in divine healing since their confidence rests not upon legendary tales of 'saints' with miraculous powers, but rather upon the clear promises of the Word of God regarding the gifts of the Holy Spirit given to true believers.

Besides, writing with reference to a Conference in Bogota, Colombia, of twenty-three Catholic charismatic leaders from eight countries, he says,

> In relation to the ministry of healing, there were also many fears on the part of the participants, because of the superstition connected with healing in the minds of the people.[35]

And he goes on to identify these problems as arising from (1) miracle-mongering, fraudulent healers and shrines which have given the whole ministry a bad name; (2) an increasing fatalistic tendency to leave matters to God with no initiative on the part of the people (even such as to create sanitary conditions or to visit the doctor); (3) confusion in people's minds which associates healing with witch-doctors, curanderos and other forms of superstition; and (4) a general reaction against the old church piety with its emphasis on prayer, shrines and relics. He adds, however, that priests and sisters who have actually become involved in the healing ministry find such problems more theoretical than real. Protestants do not have such problems.

But, on the other hand, it would appear healing, in the mind of Roman Catholics, is still very much tied to the sacrament and the saints. He quotes from *The Holy Spirit and Seventy Priests* by Father John B. Healey the following account of what took place during seven days of retreat:

> Unquestionably the highlight of each day was the Eucharistic Liturgy celebrated in the evening. Inspired homilies were delivered amid manifest appreciation and joy on all sides. Inner gifts of healing took place during Mass, sometimes through the ministration of brother-priests. The Holy Spirit favoured me with a deep peace and joy which I have not previously known. It remains constant. I have experienced a greater love of prayer, of Mary, of the Scriptures and of the Eucharist. Other priests there received the same gifts.... In the final Eucharistic Liturgy a number of priests presented their physical ailments to Christ for healing through the ministering hands of brother-priests. In my own case, I was healed of a severe difficulty in swallowing food.... This difficulty disappeared immediately after the Mass. It has not returned.[36]

And again, in his own experience Dr. MacNutt relating his prayer in seeking deliverance from a demon for someone says,

> As the prayer begins it is wise to pray for protection. I pray that

the power of the blood of Christ surround and protect every
person in the room. Then I pray that Mary, the Mother of God,
St Michael the Archangel, all the angels and saints, and all the
court of heaven intercede with us for the person we are praying
for.[37]

Another of the difficulties for Roman Catholics in the way of believing
in divine healing is the fact that

most theologians and preachers in the Catholic Church have
emphasised with great certainty Christ's desire to save souls and
to take away sin, the sickness of the soul; but there has been no
corresponding certainty about Christ's desire to heal the sickness
of the body. In fact, quite the contrary, sickness has often been
presented not as evil, but as a blessing desired by God because
of the great good that comes to a person's soul as a result of
suffering. How then, he asks, are we to regard sickness basically?
Is God's will ordinarily sickness—or is it health?[38]

Indeed he declares in reference to the James passage,

the very texts of the Bible that would encourage the faithful to
pray for physical healing were translated (in the Vulgate, the RC
Bible) to emphasise the spiritual aspect alone.[39]

This attitude is confirmed by the process of history, he claims. For
example, he asks,

What happened to the simple gospel view of Christ healing the
whole man? The historical development can be traced from the
early Fathers of the Church (St Justin Martyr and St Irenaeus in
the second century) to a view that the body's suffering is
preferable for the sake of the soul (St Gregory the Great in the
fifth century).... Under the influence of the Desert Fathers, severe
asceticism was held up as the model of Christian perfection:
man's body is to be distrusted and not just tamed; it is to be put
to death through various mortifications and penances. The
Christian then looks forward to a time when his soul will be
released from the confines of the flesh.[40]

While Dr MacNutt recognises the value in some respects of the older
'spirituality' he concludes,

it did reflect, in part, a stoic, unchristian view of the body that
is still very much with many people.... Some saints, 'victim
souls', were genuinely inspired to mortify their bodies by self-
inflicted penances; for most of us, choosing extraordinary
penances was regarded as presumption since God might not have
called us to the heights of heroic sanctity. The least we could do
was not to try to escape those sufferings that were not self-chosen
but sent by God. Sickness was generally regarded as a gift from
God to help men to grow spiritually. To pray for healing, in such

a case, would be a sign of weakness and a concession to the flesh. Consequently one could expect God to say 'No' to a prayer asking for healing.[41]

It is, of course, frank and courageous of Dr MacNutt to acknowledge the problems that have arisen for the members of the Roman Church from its departure from the Word of God and its acceptance of 'traditions' which have no basis in Scripture. Biblical Protestantism has no such difficulties.

But all this is now changed, says Dr MacNutt. Changes have been made by the Church in regard to each of the sacraments that relate particularly to healing. For example, he insists that Vatican II redefined Extreme Unction and decreed that its emphasis should be on physical healing rather than the forgiveness of sin in preparation for death, and that it should be administered to the 'seriously' rather than the 'dangerously' ill or dying. But there is little evidence that this was the real intention or that in practice there has been any real change. He says,

> Now anointing is a communal celebration involving the local caring community of the Church (including the patient's family, doctor, nurses, and others, as distinct from the former administration by the priest alone and in private).[42]

In the sacrament of Penance he sees the emphasis changed from 'confession' to 'reconciliation'; the form changed to face to face encounter between the patient and priest with no screen between; the reading of Scripture and spontaneous prayer by either priest or penitent added before or after 'absolution'. And he claims to have made the Eucharist or Mass an occasion of prayers and healing,

> I know of at least half a dozen healings that have taken place during the Mass without any prayers being said other than those in the liturgical form; and I think I can say I have seen hundreds of healings take place when I have added special prayers for healing after Communion or immediately after Mass is over.[43]

Thus it would appear that however times or viewpoints have changed within the Roman Catholic Church, there is nothing in the charismatic development which does not fit within the pattern of the Church's tradition or legend. New constructions may be put on old forms, psychological terminology and methods may replace the old theological and liturgical concepts (or appear to do so). But the new perspectives and practices of healing seem unable to cast off the old mystic paraphernalia and magic. Charismatic healing is apparently accepted in the Roman Church when practised by individuals or groups. But, as in the non-Pentecostal Protestant Churches, it takes place alongside, and is an extension, but not a part, of the normal activities of faith and worship.

IV. SUMMARY

We may sum up the doctrine and practice of healing in the Roman Catholic Church thus:

1. Faith-healing is provided for in the official doctrine and liturgy of the Church.

2. The doctrine of healing is based on the Scriptures in Mark 6:7–13 and James 5, but the practice in no way conforms to the principles or pattern of the New Testament.

3. Such healing is a sacramental process involving several of the seven sacraments of the Church.

4. The laying on of hands is appropriate to the sacrament of 'anointing of the sick'.

5. The oil used is to be consecrated by a bishop or priest and normally administered by a priest, but may be administered by others.

6. The sacrament of 'anointing of the sick' which implies (the sacrament of) penance is subordinate to and preparatory for the Viaticum in the sacrament of the Eucharist or Mass.

7. The anointing of the sick is intended primarily to effect spiritual healing and may or may not result in healing of the body according to the divine will.

8. The anointing of the sick is intended primarily as a preparation for death and judgment, hence the name Extreme Unction, but may be administered before signs of death are immediately evident.

9. The anointing of the sick may prepare the sufferer spiritually for death but it cannot deliver escape from purgatory.

10. The 'faith' element in the healing of the Church is not personal faith in Christ but confidence in the authority and power of the sacraments.

11. The healing is effected by the sacrament *ex opere operato*.

12. The healing of sickness is one aspect of the outworking of the grace of salvation.

13. Sickness may be accepted in a positive way as an aspect of taking up the cross and following Christ.

14. Healing may also be obtained by prayer in the use of relics; pilgrimage to religious shrines; or the mediation of the Virgin Mary or the 'saints'.

15. Such healing is to be attributed to the power and miraculous intervention of God.

16. Such healings may be instantaneous or gradual and may require one or more ministrations.

17. Such a ministry of healing is based on the assumption that Vatican II changed the name, form and substance of the sacrament of 'anointing of the sick'.

18. The practice of charismatic healing evidently still requires to take place as part of, or in association with, the administration of the Eucharist or Mass.

NOTES

1 Council of Trent, Sess. 14, *De Extreme Unctione* cap. 1.
2 *Ibid.,* cap. 2.
3 *Ibid.,* cap. 3.
4 *Pastoral Care of the Sick and Dying*, Study text 2, United States Catholic Conference, Washington, 1984, p. 8.
5 Prudent de Letter, 'Anointing of the Sick' in *Sacramentum Mundi Vol.1*, Burns and Oates, London, 1968, p. 38.
6 *Ibid.,* p. 38.
7 *Ibid.,* p. 38f.
8 *Pastoral Care of the Sick and Dying*, Study Text 2, United States Catholic Conference, Washington, 1984, p. 12.
9 Vatican II *Constitution on the Liturgy*, sect. 73.
10 *Pastoral Care of the Sick and Dying*, Study Text 2, United States Catholic Conference, Washington, 1984, p. 13.
11 *Ibid.,* p. 14.
12 Thomas Marsh, 'The Rite of Anointing and Pastoral care of the Sick', in *The Furrow,* Gill and Son, Dublin, 1978, pp. 89f.
13 *Ibid.,* p. 90.
14 *Ibid.,* p. 90.
15 *Ibid.,* p. 97.
16 *Ibid.,* p. 100.
17 *Ibid.,* p. 101.
18 P. de Letter, Anointing of the Sick, in *Sacramentum Mundi* Vol.1 Burns and Oates, London, 1968, pp. 39f.
19 B. B. Warfield, *Counterfeit Miracles,* Banner of Truth Trust, London, 1972, pp. 73f.
20 *Ibid.,* pp. 83, 84.
21 Georges Bertrin, *The Catholic Encyclopedia,* Vol. 9, The Encyclopedia Press, New York, 1910, pp. 390f.
22 Herbert Thurston SJ, *Encyclopedia of Religion and Ethics,* Vol. 8, p. 149.
23 B. B. Warfield, *Counterfeit Miracles*, p. 106.
24 *Ibid.,* pp. 122, 124.
25 L. D. Weatherhead, *Psychology, Religion and Healing,* Hodder and Stoughton, London, 1951, p. 149.
26 *Ibid.,* p. 153.
27 *Ibid.,* pp. 157f.
28 P. Dearmer, *Body and Soul,* Dutton, New York, 1923, pp. 327f.

29   A. Bittlinger, *The Church is Charismatic*, WCC, Geneva, 1981, p. 8.
30   *Ibid.*, pp. 56f.
31   F. MacNutt, *Healing*, Ave Maria Press, Indiana, 1975, cover.
32   *Ibid.*, p. 9.
33   *Ibid.*, p. 9.
34   *Ibid.*, p. 13.
35   *Ibid.*, p. 28.
36   *Ibid.*, p. 34.
37   *Ibid.*, p. 221.
38   *Ibid.*, p. 61.
39   *Ibid.*, p. 63.
40   *Ibid.*, p. 64.
41   *Ibid.*, pp. 65, 67.
42   *Ibid.*, p. 278.
43   *Ibid.*, p. 291.

11

THE ANGLICAN CHURCH

I. THE LAMBETH REPORTS

A Committee of the Lambeth Conference considered the subject of healing in 1908 and again in 1920 when it adopted a resolution requesting the appointment of a Committee 'to consider and report upon the use with prayer and the laying on of hands, of the Unction of the Sick, and other spiritual means of healing'. Such a Committee was appointed and its Report published in 1924 noted:

> Within the Church...the revival of systems of healing based on the redemptive work of our Lord...all spring from a belief in the fundamental principle that the power to exercise spiritual healing is taught by Christ to be the natural heritage of Christian people who are living in fellowship with God, and is part of the ministry of Christ through his body the Church.[1]

Archbishop Temple founded the 'Churches' Council for Health and Healing' in 1944. The Council was revived in 1975. In 1964 a group of priests and doctors was gathered by Archbishop Ramsey to consider the whole field of health and healing, as a result of which the 'Institute of Religion and Medicine' was formed. In 1958 a Commission on the ministry of healing set up earlier by the Archbishops of Canterbury and York reported its findings. The Report which has been long out of print stated:

> The Church as the Body of Christ and as the community through which the Holy Spirit operates is charged with a Commission to

heal the sick...many sick people are in need of an assistance which medical science by itself cannot supply. Many patients need above all else to be assured in sickness as in health God's action, wholly personal, loving and creative, is working both in their innermost being and through those who are treating them.[2] In the absence of the 1958 Report we may assume that the Report published in 1924 laid down the basic understanding of the Church regarding the 'Ministry of Healing'. The Report approached the subject under three heads: (1) the evidence of a 'ministry of healing' and its nature; (2) a comparison of the different methods of healing and their relation to Christian thought; and (3) whether such a ministry should be recognised and sanctioned. The Report identified three aspects of healing, (a) material, that is, by means of drugs, diet or surgery, (b) psychical, that is, by means of education and persuasion, suggestion or auto-suggestion including hypnosis, and (c) devotional and sacramental in which the appeal is directly to God without the use of material means. It is based on the belief that the power to heal in this way was taught by Christ to be part of the natural heritage of his people; is part of the ministry of Christ through the church, and rests upon a definite doctrine as to the nature of disease, the object of its treatment, and the results which should be expected.

It is accepted that health of body, mind and spirit is God's primary will for all his children. Disease is evil but it is permitted by God and may be overruled for good. The purpose of spiritual healing is the restoration of the whole person. It may include physical healing but this will not be the primary purpose which is spiritual strengthening (*e.g.* Paul and his 'thorn').

With regard to question (3) above—whether such a ministry should be recognised and sanctioned—the Report found:

1. Those practising this kind of healing were obtaining remarkable results.[3]

2. Readiness to co-operate with the medical profession.

3. Some claimed to possess a natural 'gift of healing'.

4. Little stress upon physical results or 'ecclesiastical technique'.

5. In the words of the Report, 'Our Committee so far found no evidence of any cases of healing which cannot be paralleled by similar cures wrought by psychotherapy without religion, and by instances of spontaneous healing'. But 'where the religious influence is of a wise and reasonable kind, greater and more permanent results may be expected than from non-religious methods'.[4]

6. A general desire for the definite authorisation of the use of anointing.

7. Considerable doubt as to the value of 'Services of Healing'.

The Committee laid down the following general principles:

1. The chief work of the Church in regard to disease is:

(a) To develop in its members a right attitude of confidence, love and understanding towards God and to approach the whole business of disease in themselves or others from this attitude.

(b) To encourage co-operation between those who care for the soul and those who care for the body.

(c) To insist on hygiene and plain living as part of the ordinance of God.

2. In practising religious healing to give full weight to the knowledge and experience of medical science.

3. Not to apply its form of healing solely for the recovery of bodily health—that is the doctor's job.

4. The primary purpose must be spiritual health whether or not physical healing ensues.

II. FORMS OF MINISTRY

The Report sets out the following forms of ministry to be used:

(a) Prayer and sacrament should be used in conjunction.

(b) While religious healing is applicable to all sickness, it is most appropriate where moral or intellectual factors are involved. These must be dealt with first and this involves knowledge of moral theology and psychology. The preliminary treatment should provide opportunity for confession and absolution if desired.

(c) Various forms of treatment may then be applied, for example, Unction (anointing with oil by a priest), laying on of hands either by a priest, layperson or both.

(d) The treatment should end with the reception of Holy Communion through which

body and soul are to be 'preserved unto everlasting life'.[5]
Other methods are: prayer in private with the patient's friends; or the exercise of a special gift of healing by particular persons.

The Committee rejected the licensing of individual healers or the official recognition of healing societies, but supported the setting up of a permanent Committee of clergy, doctors and psychologists

to advise the authorities of the Church on these matters.[6]

III. THE PRACTICE OF HEALING

Bishop Maurice Maddocks has traced the teaching and practice of healing within the Anglican Church in his account of his own ministry entitled 'The Christian Healing Ministry'. Maddocks is Co-chairman of 'The Churches' Council for Health and Healing' and President of the 'Divine Healing Mission'. In 1904 Dr. Percy Dearmer, an Anglican scholar and liturgist, and others founded the 'Guild of Health'

> to help people to experience within the fellowship of God's family the freedom and life promised by Jesus Christ.[7]

In 1905 James Moore Hickson, an Anglican layman, formed the 'Society of Emmanuel' which became the 'Divine Healing Mission' in 1933. He and his friends, Maddocks says,

> had two convictions laid upon them: the healing ministry was to be part of the preparation for the Lord's Second Coming; and that our Lord desires to use this ministry especially for the healing of his Body, the Church.[8]

The Guild of St. Raphael was founded in 1915 when the 'Guild of Health' became interdenominational. Through such men and movements the question of healing was fostered within the Church and led to the Archbishops' Commission of 1958 and the further definitive statement of 1978 when a resolution was adopted at Lambeth reaffirming:

> (1) that the healing of the sick in his Name is as much a proclamation of the Kingdom as the preaching of the good news of Jesus Christ; (2) that to neglect this aspect of ministry is to diminish our part in Christ's total redemptive activity; (3) that the ministry to the sick should be an essential element in any revision of the liturgy.[9]

Maddocks noted that the ministry of healing has been given an important role in the Irish jurisdiction of the Anglican Church as the result of the visit of J. M. Hickson in 1930. The healing ministry is now centred in St Andrew's Church in Dublin and St Anne's Cathedral in Belfast, while in the Diocese of Derry, the Bishop has allocated St Peter's Church as a focal point of the ministry.

IV. HEALING AND THE EUCHARIST

While the Anglican Church, like all other Denominations, has been affected by the rise of the Charismatic Movement with a deepened interest on the part of some in the ministry of spiritual gifts and especially in healing, the official pronouncements of the Church, as represented by the Lambeth Conference Report of 1924, appear generally to adhere to basic principles which are common to the non— Pentecostal Churches. Being a eucharistic Church, it would appear from Bishop Maddocks that the ministry of healing is to be set in a special way within the context of the Eucharist. For example, he writes,

> In any discussion of the Eucharist it must be borne in mind that participation in the ongoing, vital tradition of the Church's eucharistic worship is better than many words. It is here, in the

very centre of the Church's life, that the salvation/healing which
Christ came to bring is present in its 'timeless potency'.[10]
He even goes so far as to suggest that the Eucharist bridges the
separation of the living from the dead.

> Much of our depression and stress emanate from an
> unsatisfactory relationship with those gone before us. There is
> frequently much that is unresolved with our loved ones especially
> when they die. Why should all reconciliation and healing be left
> until the after-life? For our health it should be brought out into
> the openness of Christ and settled now; and the Eucharist is both
> the time and place for this healing to be received.[11]

None of this, of course, has any foundation or support whatever from
the Scriptures or the teaching and practice of the New Testament
Church, and indeed the latter suggestion is explicitly contrary to the
categorical prohibition of the Word of God with regard to any contact
between the living and the dead.

In referring to the practice of anointing with oil, as instructed in the
Epistle of James, Maddocks says,

> In the episcopal churches, the oil of the sick (*oleum infirmorum*)
> is usually blessed by the bishops during the Eucharist on Maundy
> Thursday. More and more is this practice being revived today
> with the beneficial result that the ministry of healing is
> increasingly and rightly taking its part within the normal,
> liturgical action of the Church.[12]

And the effects of such 'anointing' are described thus:

> Sometimes it separates the person from his disease, giving him
> freedom from pain and a consequent ability to live a normal life
> even though his body may still be ravaged by the effects of the
> disease. At other times it leads to a complete healing, for a time
> at least if not more permanently.[13]

But to suggest that it is the 'anointing' that produces such effects is
superstitious and totally foreign to the teaching of Scripture. At best
'anointing' is purely symbolical of the healing power of God
administered through his servants, at worst, it could be ritualistic magic
on the same plane as the use of relics or crucifixes for the same
purpose. Bishop Maddocks describes it thus:

> The more I ponder on my case histories, the more am I led to
> believe that the sacrament of anointing can itself be fairly
> described as a healing explosion![14]

But in his healing practice Bishop Maddocks also uses the laying on
of hands, the giving of 'absolution' after 'confession' (not to a priest
but to other Christians) especially as a means of reconciliation, and
'exorcism' though of the latter he says,

> I believe it to be a specialist ministry which needs both training

and ongoing consultation between the caring professions.... I have only been involved in one full scale exorcism in the whole of my ministry. This fact alone points to the rarity of the need for the full ministry.[15]

The Lambeth Report found

considerable doubt as to the value of 'Services of Healing'.[16]

However, as we have seen, Bishop Maddocks sees the Service of the Eucharist as central to the ministry of healing. But, in addition,

The healing service as an entity in itself and separate from the Eucharist has come into prominence in recent times. It has its critics, but the adverse criticism is far outweighed by the positive blessings of such a corporate ministry and the many 'signs following'. It also has the advantage of supplying a personal, shared, and spiritual experience in an age that is evolving from the institutional to the informal, from an emphasis on organised ritual to a more personal approach, from codified religious doctrines to an experience of faith, from academic to empirical knowledge.[17]

Thus, in Anglicanism provision is made for the healing ministry as a part of the sacramental liturgy, and, in addition, it may be practised both in a personal capacity by those who have been given a special gift of healing, or as a part of the fellowship of the congregation in Healing Services.

NOTES

1   Lambeth Conference Report 1924, *The Ministry of Healing,* SPCK, London, 1924, p. 13.
2   M. Maddocks, *The Christian Healing Ministry,* SPCK, London, 1981, p. 107.
3   Lambeth Conference Report 1924, *The Ministry of Healing,* SPCK, London, 1924, p. 16.
4   *Ibid.,* p. 16.
5   *Ibid.,* p. 20.
6   *Ibid.,* p. 21.
7   M. Maddocks, *The Christian Healing Ministry,* SPCK, London, 1981, p. 100.
8   *Ibid.,* p. 101.
9   Lambeth Conference Report 1958, p. 2.92, as cited by M. Maddocks, p. 107.
10 M. Maddocks, *The Christian Healing Ministry,* SPCK, London, 1981, p. 113.
11 *Ibid.,* p. 114.
12 *Ibid.,* p. 117.

13   *Ibid.*, p. 118.
14   *Ibid.*, p. 121.
15   *Ibid.*, p. 130.
16   Lambeth Conference Report 1958, p. 17.
17   *Ibid.*, p. 158.

12

THE METHODIST CHURCH

John Wesley, the theologian of Methodism, had a deep interest in healing and a specific view of faith-healing.

In every instance, Wesley considered prayer to be an appropriate response to illness. In some, he thought, God responded immediately to the prayer in a miracle of healing. In others, God healed the body through the 'natural' means of medicine or surgery. He thought the sick had every right to appeal for a miraculous healing, but that they should have the prudence to use medicines wisely. He often prayed with them, but he also prescribed medicines for them.[1]

I. WESLEY THE HEALER

Wesley studied medicine as a young man, actually wrote a medical guidebook *Primitive Physic: An Easy and Natural Way of Curing Most Diseases*, and established, as part of his evangelistic endeavours, dispensaries in English cities for the treatment of the sick—perhaps a forerunner of a National Health Service! But, as the American Methodist Prof. E. B. Holifield writes,

The problem of defining a continuing Methodist tradition, and of clarifying its relationship to matters of health and medicine is made more difficult by the fact that the Methodist Churches have no binding confessional statement.[2]

Wesley himself, of course, remained a 'priest' of the Anglican Church committed to the Reformed doctrines of the Thirty-nine Articles and the Book of Common Prayer.

He believed that sickness and death were not necessarily the punishment of specific sins, but were the result of man's original rebellion and fall. Since body and soul were intimately and inseparably related, physical illness might well occasion the conscience to recognise the perilous state of the soul. And the way of 'perfection' through the sanctification of the soul would also bring health to the mind and body.

When Wesley began his healing venture in 1746 it was healing by means of medicine. He believed some diseases were of demonic origin and that some cures were miraculous.

> Wesley would not have admitted to being an exorcist, and he also would never have referred to himself, in that setting, as a healer. He believed that certain persons might well be granted the extraordinary gifts of the Spirit, which included the gift of healing.... Just as there had been healing miracles in the early church, so there were healing miracles, he thought, in the eighteenth century.[3]

II. AFTER WESLEY

After Wesley's death in 1791 interest in faith-healing receded. But in the National Camp Meetings of the 1860s in America there was

> a heightened sense of expectancy about the supernatural activity of the Spirit, and a growing interest in the 'extraordinary' gifts of the Spirit, which included the gift of healing.[4]

In America in 1881 Ethan O. Allen in his *Faith Healing*,

> carried the Wesleyan doctrine of perfection to its physical extreme by arguing that purification from sin would eliminate illness.[5]

But the issue remained one of deep division and controversy so that

> proponents both of the 'second blessing' and of healing began to leave the Methodist Church and join smaller groups, some of them Wesleyan in origin, in which divine healing attracted more support. In the Pilgrim Holiness and Wesleyan Methodist and Free Methodist Churches, the advocates of healing felt more at home.[6]

English Methodists maintained their interest in healing. After the First World War Leslie Weatherhead

> concluded that the Christ church had lost its secret of spiritual healing and that the new psychology offered a way to regain it.[7]

He established a psychotherapeutic practice at the City Temple Church in London where he was minister and encouraged the training of theological students in clinical psychology, but he remained sceptical about most claims of faith-healing, though he did believe that the prayers of faithful Christians could constitute a ministry of 'spiritual healing'. In 1946 the 'Methodist Society for Medical and Pastoral Practice' was formed to promote closer association between ministers and doctors and to explore the possibilities of spiritual healing. In its publication *Religion and Medicine*,

> One New Testament scholar warned that the Bible did not 'provide us with a technique of healing which will be valid for all time' and suggested that modern faith healers might be attempting an unintelligent imitation of the New Testament grounded in a superficial interpretation of Christianity. 'Faith' he said, 'must be rescued from the faith healers'.[8]

While Leslie Weatherhead believed that intercessory prayer made little appreciable difference to the physical condition of the patient, in some instances recovery seemed effective. 'In popular English Methodism', Prof. Holifield writes, 'an interest in spiritual healing has remained an undercurrent of piety.'[9]

III. THE 1977 DECLARATION

In 1977 the Methodist Conference (the ruling body of the Methodist Church) published a pamphlet which was a statement of the Church's beliefs concerning the whole field of healing including some brief and generalised references to faith-healing. The value of the pamphlet is somewhat limited by the fact that its propositions are expressed in fairly general terms and no biblical references are supplied. By way of introduction reference is made to the

> widespread interest in the development of new medical techniques and facilities linked to confidence that disease may ultimately be curable. This interest spreads into areas on the edges of orthodox medicine, producing a fascination in all systems claiming 'healing', and often encouraging extreme and illusory expectations.[10]

It is not clear whether these 'areas' are intended to include the field of Christian faith-healing, and to indicate a concern regarding 'extreme and illusory expectations' raised by the claims of some faith-healers as well as other healing agencies. But the Statement quickly goes on to point to the importance of the Christian acceptance of the fact of death and the answer to its inevitability in the resurrection of Jesus Christ as the victory of God's triumphant plan for mankind (sec. 3).

(i) Theological affirmations

The Statement sets out a number of what it calls 'theological affirmations'. For example:

1. It is God's will that all creation should find the harmony that he has designed for it whether it be within the human person (physical, mental, spiritual), between human beings themselves, between man and the natural order, or between man and God. These intended harmonies are upset by natural disasters or by human failings such as envy, hatred, violence or greed. But there is no specific mention at this point of the disharmony between man and God or of the fall of our first parents which was the initial and universal cause of each of the areas of disharmony (secs 5, 6).

2. Jesus, whose ministry declared and demonstrated that the forces of evil were overcome and the kingdom of God released, made available supremely by his death and resurrection a new power by which the sick were healed, the lost given purpose, and sinners forgiven and restored to new life. The Statement makes no specific reference to the works of healing or casting out of demons done by Christ, nor does it explain how Christ's power to provide healing is to be applied to particular individuals or to particular disorders (sec. 7).

3. The comprehensive biblical word for the wholeness which is God's purpose ultimately for all his children is 'salvation'. Salvation, therefore, deals not only with spiritual illness but with bodily and emotional illness too. It does so as the Holy Spirit reinforces the natural forces within the human person working for wholeness, and the healing skills that man has developed. But the processes of ageing and death are natural and death itself is not essentially an enemy. While it is a manifestation of man's frailty, rebellion and estrangement from God through sin, it is also a stage on the way to life beyond (secs 8–10). Again, as a general statement of principle, all this is true. But it doesn't account for the fact that many who profess saving faith in Christ do not experience the 'wholeness' in physical, mental or emotional terms that is here suggested, nor do some ever succeed in coming to terms with the reality of death as anything other than a prospect not even to be contemplated until it cannot be escaped.

4. The grace and energy of the Holy Spirit, while necessarily experienced within the church, are not confined to the church and to Christian believers, but are active everywhere (sec. 11). Hence Christians accept that the development of scientific expertise is the fruit of the Holy Spirit's activity even though it may present such dangers as human persons being regarded as little more than superior animals, life being regarded as cheap and expendable, death regarded as the final enemy, or the spiritual dimension of life ignored or explained

away (sec. 12). But to say that the scientific method of healing is
accepted as God-given is not necessarily to say that its use is in
accordance with the purposes of God since, like every other capacity
given to the children of Adam, it is open to the misuse or perversion
of Satan, and the story of the malicious and demonic uses to which
such wisdom and skill have been put by evil men or systems of
authority, both secular and religious, is one of the darkest chapters in
the human story. Nevertheless, there can be no doubt that all healing,
by whatever means or agency, is the work of God, as is acknowledged
by the most distinguished of the healing professions.

(ii) Consequences

From these 'theological affirmations' the Statement draws a number
of consequences both for the individual and for the church.

(a) For the individual
  (i) Every person, despite his or her limitations, is intended by
  God to experience salvation as seen in Jesus Christ. There is
  therefore no place for fatalism. No person is ever 'hopeless'.[11]
Surely, however, the most we may say is 'no one need ever be without
hope', for indeed many are 'without hope' because they are 'without
Christ'. They are without hope of deliverance either from the temporal
or eternal consequences of sin, according to the Scriptures. But even
this aside, there is nowhere in the Scripture any assurance given, even
to those who have received salvation through faith in Christ, of
deliverance from the afflictions, physical or mental, to which mankind
is subject in this world as a consequence of 'the fall'. To suggest that
the gift of God's salvation in itself secures the hope of deliverance from
pain, weakness, disease or physical death is to deceive. It would,
however, have been true to say, 'No person is ever hopeless who trusts
in Christ's power to save, to heal, or to provide that grace which is
sufficient for every need or circumstance'. And this is, in fact,
acknowledged later in the Statement where it is said,
  There is then need to achieve a subtle balance between two
  hopes—that God will heal, and that he will give strength to rise
  above that condition if healing does not happen.[12]
The Statement seeks to resolve the dilemma by making a distinction
between 'healing' and 'cure'.
  In terms of wholeness and maturity there can be forms of healing
  which are not cures in the popular sense of that term. There are
  many situations in which the understanding and use of suffering
  can lead to a degree of spiritual growth which is recognisable as
  a significant achievement of healing.[13]
  (ii) Since the causes (the Statement actually says 'symptoms') of

disease are not all physical but include guilt, isolation, alienation, lack of love, despair, breakdown of relationships, or fear, that is, psychosomatic factors with physical manifestations, various forms of healing are required including,
> the skilled and compassionate help the church can offer.[14]

But the Statement goes on to make the point that,
> most suffering...results directly or indirectly from the sin and ignorance of humanity.[15]

Thus physical or psychological remedies may be totally inadequate to restore 'wholeness'. The basic need may be the spiritual healing that is to be found in the regenerating power and love of Jesus Christ. As the Statement puts it,
> Always, then, Christians should put themselves trustingly into God's care.... They live by faith in God whose love and capacity to bear suffering is shown in Jesus.[16]

The believer too can find hope and wholeness by turning in repentance and faith to Christ who said, 'Come unto me all ye that labour and are heavy laden and I will give you rest' (Matt. 11:28).

(b) For the church
(i) 'The church is called to be a community in which the constant, total healing work of the Holy Spirit is taught, sought and experienced'.[17]

And such healing, it is claimed, is present in worship, sacraments, preaching, prayer, fellowship and pastoral and social ministry of the church in which all members are to be involved. This is spelt out in the succeeding sections of the Statement.

(ii) The church must work in partnership with all healing agencies but not in
> an uncritical partnership.[18]

Presumably this is intended to mean that while the church is to recognise and support the work of medical, psychiatric and other healing agencies, such as Health and Social Services, it should also expect to be recognised and respected as having a unique and expressly spiritual dimension of healing to offer.

(iii) While some individuals
> possess special insight, knowledge, faith and power which enable them to exercise distinctive healing ministries.... Other individuals may receive a particular gift of healing from God for a specific occasion.... Every member of the church is part of a community which by its nature and activities seeks to create wholeness, health and healing.[19]

The Statement also insists that such individual healing gifts should be subject, presumably in their exercise, to the scrutiny of the church so

as to prevent
    spiritual or emotional manipulation of the sufferer.[20]
The Statement seems to be saying that the exercise of a healing gift
by any individual should be done under the discipline of the spiritual
oversight of the congregation so as to avoid abuse or harmful effect,
and this would appear to be the ideal situation. But by the very nature
of the operation, it is difficult to see how or why such a scrutiny or
discipline should be effected or required. If the person is truly
exercising a 'gift of the Spirit', what court of the church could gainsay
it, or what mischief could result from it? Besides, many faith-healers
who exercise a 'gift of the Spirit' do not do so under the discipline of
a particular congregation or church authority. In fact, it is often within
the church that opposition to, or scepticism of, the exercise of such
spiritual gifts, especially that of healing, is most evident.

    (iv) The healing ministry of the church may be concentrated in
special healing services though these should not be seen as a distinctive
or occasional activity (sec. 21). But, in fact, such services do tend to
be divorced from the normal pattern of worship and church activity.
They also tend to draw a particular clientele and to be ignored as
irrelevant or eccentric by the majority of church members until, of
course, some crisis of physical or mental health arises. To be fair,
however, the same must be said in most places with reference to the
regular prayer-meetings or other activities for the deepening of spiritual
life.

    (v) The remaining sections of the Statement (secs 22–24) deal with
social aspects of the church's life and witness such as the prevention
of illness through clean living, abstinence from alcohol or drug abuse,
moral and sexual obedience to the law of God, influence upon
economic, political, cultural, environmental and industrial attitudes and
structures in society, and training, counselling and care for the victims
of need or deprivation in society, all of which it sees as part of the
church's ministry of healing—

> Thus the Church becomes a praying, healing, caring
> community.[21]

The Statement thus presents a comprehensive overview of many of the
issues related to sickness, death and healing as understood officially
by the Methodist Church. The principles enunciated are all,
presumably, derived from Scripture, but it would have been so much
more helpful and effective if the biblical sources had been indicated.
It is a pity too that, even within such a brief and summary statement,
room had not been found to discuss in more detail some of the areas
which, since the rise of the Charismatic Movement in the 1960s, have
become matters of deep interest and concern, such as, for example, the
relevance of healing as practised in the New Testament to the present

day; the biblical principles which relate to the practice of faith-healing; the phenomenon of demon-possession and its consequences in relation to sickness and health; the importance or otherwise of 'signs and wonders' in regard to healing and the witness of the church; the nature and importance of 'spiritual gifts' in dealing with the problems of sickness.

IV. HEALING AT CHAPEL STREET

The subject is covered more specifically, though still without biblical references, in several articles in the *Health and Healing Bulletin* (January, 1991 issue) published by the Methodist Church Division of Social Responsibility. Rev. Chris Wiltsher, Director of the Wesley Study Centre in Durham, in *The Reflections of a Methodist Theologian* spells out the distinction between healing and cure which was mentioned in the Conference Statement above.

> In curing we attempt to repair, put right, or restore something damaged or impaired.... Curing involves an attempt to recreate a former state, and for that reason curing and healing are different.[22]

But he goes on to point to a further important distinction.

> Also different from healing is the process of producing wholeness. It has become common in recent years to equate health and wholeness. However, it is possible...for a person to be healthy but not whole, through, say, physical disability. Whatever wholeness is, the process of producing wholeness must involve some kind of integration of every aspect of a person's existence; however, one can be at ease with oneself and one's environment while at the same time acknowledging that not all aspects of one's existence are totally integrated.[23]

This distinction is valid. Often when people seek faith-healing all they are concerned about is the 'cure' of some particular malady or defect, and indeed, sometimes that is all that happens. Whereas in the New Testament healings, where we have sufficient information, it is evident that Jesus and the Apostles were concerned to deal with the spiritual condition of the sufferer as well, especially where the forgiveness of sin was involved.

In an article 'Healing at Chapel Street', Rev. John Horner, Superintendent of the Penzance Circuit, gives an account of the ministry of healing which has been carried on for some four years at the regular Sunday evening services in Chapel Street Methodist Church. He sets out the theology on which his practice is based in a number of propositions which include the following:

1. The local congregation, as part of the body of Christ, has the

power to heal.

2. Christ's command to 'preach and heal' has not been withdrawn.

3. Healing through prayer, laying on of hands and anointing is only one of many forms of healing whose value is to be accepted.

4. Healing is the sovereign prerogative of God which cannot be changed by prayer or fasting.

5. The effectiveness of healing is not in proportion to the faith of the healer or the healed.

6. Every church should have a trained and disciplined ministry of healing available to every Christian.

7. Members of the local church will be endowed with the necessary gifts of healing.

8. Any member of the church may exercise healing and may anoint or lay on hands in the name and the power of Jesus.

9. Some members of the church will have a permanent gift of healing and should be identified, trained and given opportunity to use it.

10. Healing should normally be at the request of the sufferer, and normally should take place in public worship or, where necessary, by visitation to the home.

11. The members of the congregation should be given regular teaching so that they may know what to expect and thus avoid disappointment or a mistaken sense of guilt.

12. The healing ministry should be part of the normal Services of Worship rather than of 'special healing services'.

There follows in the article an account of the procedure at the healing ministry in the services at Chapel Street, and the follow-up procedures including intercession and counselling, where felt appropriate or necessary, for those who have been ministered to.

Thus in Methodism there has always been an active involvement in the ministry of faith-healing though probably, as in other churches, with considerable difference of degree of interest or uniformity from place to place.

NOTES

1   E. B. Holifield, *Health and Medicine in the Methodist Tradition,* Crossroad, New York, 1986, p. 28.

2   *Ibid.,* p. 5.

3   *Ibid.,* p. 36.

4   *Ibid.,* p. 39.

5   *Ibid.,* p. 39.

6   *Ibid.,* p. 41.

7   *Ibid.,* p. 42.

8   *Ibid.*, p. 43.

9   *Ibid.*, p. 44.

10 *The Church and the Ministry of Healing,* Adopted by the Methodist Conference of 1977, (Division of Social Responsibility) London, 1977, Sec. 2.

11 *Ibid.*, Sec. 13.

12 *Ibid.*, Sec. 16.

13 *Ibid.*, Sec. 16.

14 *Ibid.*, Sec. 14.

15 *Ibid.*, Sec. 15.

16 *Ibid.*, Sec. 17.

17 *Ibid.*, Sec. 18.

18 *Ibid.*, Sec. 19.

19 *Ibid.*, Sec. 20.

20 *Ibid.*, Sec. 20.

21 *Ibid.*, Scc. 24.

22 *Health and Healing Bulletin,* Issue No. 21, (The Methodist Church Division of Social Responsibility) London, 1991, p. 6.

23 *Ibid.*, p. 6.

13

THE PENTECOSTAL CHURCHES

I. THE PENTECOSTAL MOVEMENT

The origins of Pentecostalism are said to go back to a revival amongst the negroes of North America at the beginning of the present century. The view that the baptism of the Spirit is to be recognised by the 'initial sign' of speaking in tongues, became a constituent element in the formal structure of the Pentecostal movement especially in North America.... The age of books and the newspaper as the most important means of communication is past. But what does this signify for Protestantism, the religion of the book par excellence? According to Harvey Cox (the Baptist theologian) it means the reduction of Protestantism to the ever decreasing minority of readers, unless it makes room within itself for other means of communication. The continuous spread of the Pentecostal movement in many countries must be interpreted as the discovery of new means of communication in a specific social field, which can be clearly defined for each Pentecostal group.[1] Pentecostalism has not only established its own Churches and Assemblies—The Elim Churches, the Apostolic Churches, The Assemblies of God, The Holiness Churches, The Full Gospel Businessmen's Fellowship, The Latter Rain Movement, The Charismatic Renewal Movement, *etc.*—but has affected the traditional churches both Protestant and Roman Catholic, and has become an important factor in the Ecumenical Movement. Indeed it is said to be at present the fastest growing branch of Christendom, especially in Latin America and Africa.[2]

In Britain Pentecostalism had its origin in the Welsh Revival in the early years of the present century, and largely took the form of a charismatic movement within the existing Churches. The Elim Pentecostal Church, which began as the Elim Foursquare Gospel Alliance—the 'Foursquare' relating to the four basic doctrines of the Church namely, Christ as Saviour, Baptiser, Healer, and Coming King—under the inspiration and leadership of the brothers George and Stephen Jeffreys in 1926, is the most moderate of the Pentecostal groups.

II. THE DEMAND FOR MIRACLES

Pentecostalism is based on the demand for the miraculous. This demand, in turn, is based upon the manifestation of the divine power in the life and work of the Lord Jesus Christ as the Redeemer of God's people, and the outpouring of the Holy Spirit upon the church at Pentecost with the resultant miraculous 'gifts of the Spirit' bestowed on the church and exercised by those who have been or are being sanctified by his power. George Jeffreys put it thus,

> the Christian who denies the miraculous, denies Christianity: the Christian who rejects the supernatural, rejects the religion he professes to embrace. The whole structure of the Christian religion is based upon the miraculous, as I shall proceed to shew. The man who protests against the miraculous in Christianity, undermines the whole, and is inconsistent with his profession as a Christian.[3]

And the Declaration of Faith of the British Assemblies of God states,

> We believe in...the baptism in the Holy Spirit with the initial evidence of speaking with other tongues (which) is the same in essence as the gift of tongues (1 Cor. 12:4–10, 28) but different in purpose and use.[4]

Or again, the Declaration of Faith of the Elim Pentecostal Churches declares,

> We believe that the church should claim and manifest the nine Gifts of the Holy Spirit: wisdom, knowledge, faith, healing, miracles, prophecy, discernment, tongues, interpretation.[5]

From these basic and essential elements in the doctrine of the Pentecostal Churches arises the interest and importance of the evidence of the supernatural in the life both of the individual believer and of the Church. The history of the Pentecostal Movement is dominated by this theme with special reference to the exercise of the gifts of 'tongues' and of 'healing'. This insistence upon the place and importance of the miraculous has, from the beginning of Pentecostalism led to considerable fanaticism and extreme teaching and action especially on the part of those who have become its 'healing evangelists'.

One of the forerunners of the Pentecostal Movement, the 'Restorer', 'Elias III', John Alexander Dowie, who took the title 'Doctor', believed he had been sent 'to destroy sin, to prepare the people of God, and to restore the Kingdom of the Lord'. His Zion City in Illinois, USA, its subsidiaries in Zurich, Amsterdam and South Africa, and his sermons and healings, exercised a considerable influence on the early Pentecostal movement. The American healing evangelists appealed directly to him, and many leaders of the Assemblies of God, as well as the funds for the Swiss, Dutch and South African Pentecostal movements, came from Dowie's Zion Church.[6]

Later the Jeffreys brothers, Smith Wigglesworth, Douglas Scott, William Branham, T. L. Osborne, Hermann Zaiss, the Full Gospel Businessmen's Fellowship International, Oral Roberts and other television evangelists have commanded vast audiences, though they have also created much division of opinion among Pentecostalists regarding both their teachings and their practices.

The attitude of individual Pentecostal groups to the healing of the sick by prayer in general, and to the healing evangelists in particular, varies a great deal. On the whole one can say that the more recent and more enthusiastic groups look with favour on the healing evangelists. On the other hand, the older Pentecostal groups have gone to some trouble to keep the healing evangelists at a distance, for until recently they held and taught the view of the healing evangelists which they now condemn as false: 'Anyone who believes is healed; and anyone who is not healed has not believed aright'.[7]

Accounts of raisings from the dead are also common in Pentecostalism though they are not always given credence.

For example, Lura Johnson Grubb, an evangelist of the Assemblies of God, who has risen from the dead, has described her experiences during death. She even produces her doctor's death certificate. On the other hand Paul Hug, formerly a Reformed pastor, and later a Pentecostal pastor, tried in vain to bring a dead person back to life.[8]

Rev. F. L. Wyman, one time Rector of St Paul's, York, claims that the raising of the dead is in fact an essential part of the Divine Commission to the church, and he cites a number of examples, though without apparently having had any personal experience of the phenomenon. But, on the other hand,

Kristen Heggelund says that in thirty-seven years in the ministry he has travelled in many places and has come to know many servants of the Lord with great gifts, 'but I never met one who had raised someone who was really dead'.[9]

Noel Brooks, Principal of the Bible College of the Pentecostal Holiness Church in Britain, however, insists on keeping all things in proper perspective.

The Pentecostal Revival has never been a fanatics' revival.... This shadow of fanaticism has pursued various features of Pentecostalism, not least in the matter of divine healing.... One of the most common is an antipathy to the use of 'means', whether surgical, medical or (though not always) herbal. Some preachers are quite vociferous in their denunciation of the 'physicians of Egypt', while many devout people are obsessed with a vague idea that 'faith' and 'means' are somehow incompatible, or at best 'means' is a lower thing allowed by God for those who have no 'faith'.[10]

And he goes on to show that, for example, 2 Chronicles 16:12 which might be construed by some as a pretext for regarding the use of means as being contrary to the will of God, is nothing of the kind since the censure of King Asa was not that he had sought medical help, but rather that even in his suffering he maintained his rebellion against God and refused his help. He also makes an interesting reference to Mark 5:26 where it is said of the woman with the issue of blood who sought healing from Jesus,

Extremists sometimes quote Mark 5:26 as a jibe against the medical profession. But the same words might equally sum up the case history of many who have gone the round of healing campaigns and tried the solutions propounded by various theorists. What things they have suffered mentally by crude and cruel theories! And they are 'nothing bettered', but through disappointment and frustration and agonising introspection, are frequently worse.[11]

He sets out the view of the two channels of divine healing, the natural and the supernatural, thus,

The fundamental fallacy underlying the view that to resort to 'means' is wrong is the separation of the God of nature from the God of the supernatural.... The miraculous may transcend the natural. But there is no antagonism.[12]

And he claims that George Jeffreys would endorse that view. He also makes this further important observation,

It deserves also to be put on record that an entire Pentecostal denomination has expressed a similar conviction. *The Discipline of the Pentecostal Holiness Church* contains a Doctrinal Exegesis by the late Bishop J. H. King (to this effect), which has the full

authority of the denomination behind it.... It declares, 'Natural
means, viewed as a product of the Law of Recovery, are not to
be despised. Neither are we to look upon their use as sinful on
the part of believers in Christ.'[13]
But he adds,
> The healing of Calvary's stream is the better way, and the way
> to secure complete and permanent healing of all sickness and
> diseases.[14]

III. CAUSE AND CURE

Jeffreys relates all disease to the fall of mankind in Adam and beyond
it to the work of Satan himself:
> If there was no sin there would be no suffering, no aches, no
> pains, no consumption, no cancers, no tumours, no sickness....
> But we must go further back than Adam to discover the source
> of all the trouble. The author of it all is none other than the arch-
> enemy Satan.[15]

Brooks acknowledges that disease and suffering can be a form of
punishment for personal sins or that some sins bring their own
retribution in terms of physical disease and suffering. Again, he asserts
that a disturbed heart may bring a chain of evil consequences which
affect both mind and body and can be cured not by medicine,
psychoanalysis or even physical miracle, but only by restoration to God
through the Gospel. But, in general terms, he says,
> Sickness and disease are the consequence equally with death, of
> sin and the Fall.[16]

And in reference to Job he says,
> His suffering was a trial, permitted by God and administered by
> Satan, to demonstrate Job's goodness and faithfulness.... The
> plain truth is that it is just as fallacious to say that all sickness
> is due to personal sin as it is to say that it is due to personal
> goodness.[17]

Jeffreys specifies four reasons for his belief that 'it is God's will to heal
today', namely:

1. Because the Lord who healed in the days of his flesh is
unchanging (Heb. 13:8):
> There is not a single verse in the whole of Scripture to shew that
> he has, in this age, ceased to heal the sick, to liberate the bound,
> or to uplift the oppressed. On the contrary, there is abundant
> Scriptural proof of his will to heal, and this is being confirmed
> before our wondering eyes in this the twentieth century.[18]

2. Because the Lord's commission to preach and expect signs
including healing has never been withdrawn (Mark 16:15–18);

3. Because the gift of healing and other miraculous gifts were set in the church which is still on earth (1 Cor. 12:9, 27, 28); in answer to the question 'Is it not true that the miraculous gifts, including the gift of healing, were withdrawn at the close of the Apostolic age?' he says,

> No, it is not true. There is not a single word in the whole of the Bible to prove that these miraculous gifts have been withdrawn at any time. On the contrary, there is ample Scripture to shew that these gifts, including the gifts of healing, are in the church, and the church which comprises all regenerated ones is still on earth.[19]

4. Because we are instructed how to act in the case of sickness (Jas 5:14, 15). Jeffreys explains the process of healing thus:

> The root meaning of the word 'healing' is 'a gradual recovery'. Herein seems to lie the distinction between divine healing and working of miracles. The former seems to imply that a person can through the exercise of this gift be gradually restored to health. The latter suggests an immediate divine interposition, as a result of which a person is instantaneously healed. Both were in evidence during our Lord's ministry.... It is a mistake to suppose that the person to whom the gifts of healing are given shall immediately heal everybody.... This wonderful gift, though given only to certain believers, does not preclude all believers from laying hands on the sick according to Mark 16, or elders from anointing with oil according to James 5:14. It is given in addition to those ordinary ministrations (Mark 16:17, 18; Jas 5:14, 15).[20]

But, as we have already seen, it is simply not true to say that healing effected by the Lord was ever a gradual process. Moreover, if all believers may heal by the laying on of hands, what kind of 'gift' is given to 'certain believers' to distinguish it from 'ordinary ministrations'?

IV. THE 'THREE WAYS'

Brooks also enumerates 'the three ways' in which the healing power of Christ flows to man thus: (A) through the 'gifts' of healing (1 Cor. 12:9); (B) through the anointing of the sick with oil by the elders of the church (Jas 5:14, 15); and (C) through mutual prayer (Jas 5:16). With regard to (A) he writes,

> An important question which arises in this connection...is: are they possessed by specific individuals, or are they given to the whole body of Christ, to be expressed now through one individual and now through another according to the will of the

Holy Spirit? Both views are held by Pentecostals.[21]
In regard to (B) he says,

> We take this admonition to refer to symbolic anointing of the sick
> with oil accompanying prayer for recovery. It was intended to be
> a regular feature of church life and order—as regular as the
> communion service or the ceremony of baptism. No specific 'gift
> of healing' is necessarily involved. It is the responsibility of the
> sufferer to call upon the local elders to anoint him, and it is the
> duty of the elders thus to do and to pray.[22]

And on (C) he says,

> This brings the responsibility for healing down to every
> Christian. Not only the 'gifted' person, or the elder with his
> anointing oil, but all! Healing may flow to the sick through any
> righteous man who can pray fervently, quite apart from symbolic
> oil or miraculous gifts.[23]

But again we must ask, If healing is available to any through the
fervent prayer of any believer, what need is there for the 'gifted' person
or the elder with his anointing oil? Or, if 'the prayer of faith will save
the sick', what need has the believer other than to pray for himself or
herself?

Jeffreys also distinguishes the general commission to all believers
in Mark 16:15–20 from specific gifts of healing given to particular
individuals, and relates it in a special way to evangelistic purposes:

> The command and promise of signs in Mark 16:15–20 applies
> more to evangelistic work when the message needs confirming.
> The Scripture in Mark makes manifest the love of God towards
> those who are out in the world. The evangelist is sent forth with
> the message to the outsider, and on the authority of these verses
> he lays hands on the sick, regardless of the particular person's
> faith or obedience, and the signs follow.[24]

The James 5 passage he takes to relate to the work of the local
congregation of the church. Thus,

> in the church, where the gift of healing is permanently set, the
> believer is clearly taught to comply with certain conditions if he
> expects to be healed.[25]

Moreover, healing services, he maintains, are not to be used in the
evangelistic context.

> If healing services are conducted on campaign lines outsiders
> may continually come to be prayed for and not be healed, for the
> simple reason that the gift of healing, set in the church, should
> be administered along church lines, and not expected as a sign
> which seems to be given to confirm the evangelistic message.[26]

But in the context of the fellowship of the local congregation,

> The ideal and most Scriptural way of ministry to the sick is by

adhering strictly to the pattern clearly defined in the Epistles to the Churches of the New Testament. Anointing with oil appears to be the proper method in church life (Jas 5:14, 15). Those who need healing should be given an opportunity for the ministry in the church.[27]

V. THE ISSUE OF FAITH

We have not found in Jeffreys any exposition of the place of 'faith' in faith-healing. But Brooks in dealing with the nature or necessity of 'faith' acknowledges that it is 'very confused'.

> It is our conviction that of all questions facing these groups of Bible-believing people who seek to practise the Apostolic methods of healing, this is one of the most urgent. And it is a question that needs to be faced with absolute honesty and courage. One of the charges levelled at us is just this: that we are exploiting suggestibility rather than building up faith.... Too often people are credited with 'healing faith' when they are merely highly 'suggestible', and others are condemned as 'having little faith' when, in reality, they are not easily carried along by a strong personality or a mass emotion.[28]

He also points to the problem of a distinction to be made between 'faith' and 'Christian faith'. 'Faith' he acknowledges may be nothing more than an attitude of 'positive thinking' or optimistic expectation which can be motivated by self-will or self-love with purely selfish ends:

> Sorcery, witchcraft, black magic and such like practices work on the same principle, only that they acknowledge the direct intercourse of faith with 'wicked spirits in heavenly places' and draw from them.[29]

That is why we are bidden by John to 'try the spirits whether they are of God' (1 John 4:1). 'Faith in the Christian sense', he says, 'is not a faith attitude to life. It is not a formula for health, success and prosperity. It is faith in Christ himself.... It is utter committal to him and utter trust in him, wherever the pathway of life may lead, and whatever of health or sickness, success or failure, prosperity or adversity, life may bring.'[30]

Such faith does not always result in healing, but it is able to endure and accept failure to find healing. Such faith (Heb. 11:32–37),

> endures sickness and suffering in the Spirit of Christ. It transcends the disappointment of unanswered prayer. It is uncrushed, unresentful, unembittered, though apparently unrewarded.[31]

With regard to physical healing and the atoning work of Christ (Matt.

8:16, 17) Brooks says,

> Through the power of the Holy Spirit we may have an 'earnest' and 'first fruits' of that deliverance.... But full deliverance from all the workings of death in the human body is not promised us, and cannot be expected by us, until the return of Christ in glory, who at that time 'will fashion anew the body of our humiliation, that it may be conformed to the body of his glory' (Phil. 3:21).[32]

VI. SUMMARY

From all of this we may draw some important conclusions regarding the faith and practice, particularly in regard to faith-healing, of the Elim and other Pentecostal Churches.

1. Faith-healing forms an integral part of the fellowship and function of the church. But not all who seek it are healed.

2. Healing takes place on two levels—the natural (by medical means) and the supernatural (divine healing). There is no antagonism between them.

3. Faith-healing methods are open to the same kind of abuse and failure as medical methods.

4. Some diseases which are the consequence of spiritual causes cannot be healed by medical or psychiatric means but must be dealt with by spiritual renewal.

5. God still manifests his power and purposes in faith-healing. The 'gifts of the Spirit' have never been withdrawn.

6. In faith-healing 'faith' is not mere suggestibility or 'positive thinking', but personal faith in Jesus Christ as Saviour.

7. The commission of Mark 16:15–20 extended the possibility of miracle-working to all believers.

8. The 'gift of healing' is given to individuals and especially preachers of the Word and relates particularly to the work of evangelism.

9. The gift of healing committed to the church is exercised according to the pattern of James 5:14, 15 including anointing with oil.

10. The initiative for healing in the local congregation lies with the patient who is to seek for help.

11. All believers have the responsibility of prayer for the healing of others.

12. Healing may take place as part of the normal worship of believers, but healing services are not to be used for evangelistic purposes.

NOTES

1 W. J. Hollenweger, *The Pentecostals*, SCM Press, London, 1972, p. xiii.

2 A. Bittlinger, *The Church is Charismatic*, WCC, Geneva, 1981, p. 7.

3 G. Jeffreys, *Pentecostal Rays*, Elim Publishing Co., London, 1933, pp. v, vi.

4 W. J. Hollenweger, *The Pentecostals*, SCM Press, London, 1972, p. 515.

5 *Ibid.*, p. 519.

6 *Ibid.*, pp. 353f.

7 *Ibid.*, p. 356.

8 *Ibid.*, p. 360.

9 *Ibid.*, p. 360.

10 N. Brooks, *Sickness, Health and God*, Advocate Press, USA, 1965, p. 44.

11 *Ibid.*, p. 24.

12 *Ibid.*, p. 50.

13 *Ibid.*, pp. 51, 52.

14 *Ibid.*, p. 52.

15 G. Jeffreys, *The Miraculous Foursquare Gospel—Doctrinal*, Elim Publishing Co., London, 1929, pp. 30f.

16 N. Brooks, *Sickness, Health and God*, Advocate Press, USA, 1965, p. 38.

17 *Ibid.*, p. 43.

18 G. Jeffreys, *The Miraculous Foursquare Gospel—Supernatural*, Elim Publishing Co., London, 1930 , p. 48.

19 *Ibid.*, p. 90.

20 Jeffreys, *Pentecostal Rays*, pp. 125f.

21 Brooks, *Sickness, Health and God*, p. 15.

22 *Ibid.*, p. 17.

23 *Ibid.*, p. 17.

24 Jeffreys, *Pentecostal Rays*, p. 233.

25 *Ibid.*, p. 233.

26 *Ibid.*, pp. 233f.

27 *Ibid.*, pp. 232f.

28 Brooks, *Sickness, Health and God*, pp. 27f.

29 *Ibid.*, p. 29.

30 *Ibid.*, p. 30.

31 *Ibid.*, p. 36.

32 *Ibid.*, p. 59.

14

THE PRESBYTERIAN CHURCH IN IRELAND

The Presbyterian Church in Ireland through the appropriate Committees of the General Assembly has produced two substantial reports, one in 1959 the other in 1982, setting out what that Church believes regarding the doctrine and practice of faith-healing. While these reports cover much of the same ground, they do so in quite different ways and not always with the same conclusions. For example, 2 Kings 20:7 is cited in the 1959 Report (p. 176) as evidence for the approval of the use of medicine in the Old Testament, whereas in the 1982 Report (p. 25) it is referred to as the only instance of a prescription of medical treatment in the Old Testament. Indeed the 1982 Report more than once makes the point that in the Old Testament 'no recourse to any human physician was permitted'. We propose, then, to summarise the two reports and comment upon them.

I. THE 1959 REPORT

The church's part in the Ministry of Healing
   This report is an attempt to meet the wilder assertions and the unfounded doubts and give some guidance. We shall first set forth what appears to be the intention of Scripture for the church in this matter and then examine some of the assumptions which are often made about it.[1]
The purpose of the church's Ministry of Healing
   The report suggests three reasons for Jesus' healing: (a) compassion

(Luke 7:13) though it is rarely mentioned; (b) evidence of the presence of the Kingdom of God (Luke 11:20), not proof that he was the Messiah, but the inevitable consequence of it, hence Jesus' reticence to have it made known or to take the initiative in healing; (c) his healings are 'signs' and their importance lies therefore not in themselves but in that to which they point, e.g. John 9.

His followers heal in Jesus' name and their healings are usually closely connected with the preaching of the Word, either emerging from it (Acts 8:4–8; 14:8, 9) or leading up to it (Acts 3:1ff). In the church today this pattern is continued and (a) has led to medical missions and faith-healing, (b) reveals the power of the Kingdom now in the church, (c) points to the spiritual healing of forgiveness through the redemption of Christ.

(i) Common suppositions

Four common underlying suppositions are challenged:

1. (a) *The healings of the New Testament period are to be expected today.* The missions of the Twelve and of the Seventy were limited and ended when they reported back. When Jesus gave his disciples their final commission after his resurrection he did not mention healing (Matt. 28:19f; Luke 24:45–48; Acts 1:8; probably also John 20:22, 23; 21:15–19). (Mark 16:15–18 is not part of the original Gospel.) The disciples continued to heal, however, and therefore the commission must be assumed to be operative, but the main task evidently was to bear witness to Christ and healing was subordinate to it.

(b) *All Christians should be able to exercise the gift of healing.* While Paul mentions healing as one of the gifts of the Spirit in 1 Corinthians 12:9, 28, he implies that some possessed the gift while others did not. Similarly in James 5:13–16 a particular section of the church (the 'elders' who were not necessarily equivalent to the present-day 'Kirk Session') is given the responsibility of healing by anointing with oil and prayer. Not all ministers or ministers only should be expected to do so. But all Christians should perform the duty of intercession on behalf of others.

2. *God's will is perfect health for everyone.* Sickness is only one form of suffering so the real question concerns God's will in regard to suffering. The early Christians rejoiced in suffering (Acts 16:25; 5:41; 1 Pet. 4:13; Phil. 2:17). Christ promised suffering to his followers (Matt. 5:10–12; Luke 6:22, 23). The Christian cannot avoid suffering either inflicted by others or borne voluntarily. If it is claimed that 'sickness' is different from 'suffering' it should be remembered that: (a) some sicknesses are caused by the neglect of others, and (b) the individual cannot be isolated from the universe, he will never be perfect apart from a perfect universe. This will come about in the 'new

heaven and new earth'. Evil exists in many forms; sickness, ignorance, natural catastrophe, etc. Only sin separates from God. Therefore God can and does use the suffering of the individual for his purposes. God's primary purpose is to defeat sin and reconcile mankind to himself. In doing so he may use suffering or distress. We cannot say that God wills perfect health for all men in this present time, but he does design it after the return of Christ in the new heaven and new earth.

We must also note (a) that in the New Testament some were not healed (1 Tim. 5:23; 2 Tim. 4:20; 2 Cor. 12:7), and (b) that if God wills perfect physical health for mankind on earth he must surely also will spiritual perfection. But as the Westminster Confession of Faith teaches (13:2), such perfection is not to be realised by any individual in this life.

3. *All sickness is due to sin.* This claim is never made in the sense that each sickness is the result of a particular sin (*cf.* Luke 3:1–5; John 9:3), but in the sense that since we live in a sinful world and we are sinners therefore we are subject to sickness. But if sickness is due to the fall then so are ignorance and natural catastrophe. There is no doubt that not only mankind but the world of nature also is estranged from God's purpose and will ultimately be restored to it (Isa. 11:6–9; 35:1–10; Rom. 8:19–23). Sin certainly is a contributing factor in many sicknesses and may be the main cause in some. Spiritual factors may indeed lie behind psychosomatic illness. It may be said, then, that some sickness has its roots in spiritual conditions.

4. *The cure for sickness is God's redemption of mankind through Christ.* It is claimed by some that the cross and the resurrection of Christ dealt not only with sin but with sickness as well (Matt. 8:17). Matthew 8:17 is a quotation from Isaiah 53:4. If this is a reference to the work of atonement as dealing with sickness it is unique in the New Testament and it is therefore hazardous to build a theory on one uncorroborated text. While there may be some doubt as to whether sickness in the world is the result of the fall of Adam, Paul clearly asserted that all forms of evil, represented by the 'principalities and powers', were overcome in the cross. Therefore to claim that the cross provides freedom from sickness would mean that it must also provide freedom from all other evils as well. But this is clearly not so, and it is erroneous to argue that whatever has dealt with sin must also have removed its earthly consequences. Nevertheless it is true that faith in Christ may indeed bring freedom from stress, failure, conflict, etc. and may therefore through reconciliation with God and one's neighbour bring relief from sickness which is the result of these things. One way in which sickness is overcome is the conquest of ignorance. Faith-healing appears to give too large a place to sickness as over against ignorance.

(ii) The issue of faith

'Your faith has made you whole' is a familiar saying in the New Testament (Mark 5:34; cf. 9:23; 5:36; or Matt. 9:28, 29; cf. Matt. 8:10, 13; 9:2; 21:21, 22; Luke 7:9). There are a number of different uses of the word 'faith': (a) 'confidence' in the healer; (b) faith which appears in suggestion, hypnosis, charms, witchcraft; (c) intellectual acceptance of truth (Jas 2:18ff); (d) faith in the 'invisible' things (Heb. 11:1); (e) faithfulness; (f) the principal Christian usage which speaks of salvation by faith, *i.e.* the faith by which we accept the gift of eternal life. It is based at least to some degree on knowledge of Christ and his work of redemption. Such faith may save from sin but, through lack of understanding, not from sickness.

An important text is Mark 11:22–24 (*cf.* Luke 17:6; Matt. 17:20). This would seem to imply that 'if I believe hard enough I will be cured; and if I am not cured it is because I did not believe sufficiently strongly'. But prayer is not a magical spell. It must be set within the sovereign will of God (1 John 5:14; *cf.* 3:22; John 15:7). If it is not God's will to heal then faith cannot do so. But faith must not be confused with 'suggestibility'. This is the danger in regard to particular faith-healers or healing services—'because it has worked for others it must work for me'. In psychosomatic illness the symptoms may be removed or inhibited but unless the underlying spiritual problem or sin is dealt with there can be no true healing. Healing should therefore always be conducted within the context of the Gospel.

(iii) Minister and doctor

1. The Bible assumes, accepts and commends the use of medicine and the work of medical practitioners (2 Kgs 20:7; Luke 10:34; 1 Tim. 5:23; Jas 5:14). Healing by casting out demons and the invocation of healing powers was normal medical practice in Jesus' day.

2. The use of medicines together with prayer is common to both Old and New Testaments (2 Chr. 16:12; Jas 5:14).

The close relationship between the physical and the spiritual aspects of healing therefore demands co-operation between ministers and doctors, as the Church of Scotland's Commission on Spiritual Healing insists in its report. It also demands great care in the appointment of Hospital Chaplains and in the training of theological students in regard to psychological medicine.

II. THE 1982 REPORT

There does not appear to be any uniform understanding within the church whether in relation to the biblical basis or the practice of divine healing. This perhaps is not surprising, for the interpretation of the biblical material is by no means easy.[2] Thus the report begins by identifying differing points of view with regard to the interpretation of the biblical material such as: (a) whether it is always God's will to heal; (b) the place of 'faith' in healing—does the measure of faith determine the extent or effectiveness of healing; is it a necessary condition (Mark 9:23; 6:6); does healing manifest the glory of Jesus and thus bring about faith (John 2:11; 4:54)? (c) the fact of, or need for, divine healing.

(i) Biblical teaching and practice

The Old Testament
The Old Testament 'gives the background from which we can understand something of the New Testament outlook.' Disease was seen as the result of disobedience or sin (*cf.* John 9:2), God was seen as the Healer, and the healing was an indication of divine forgiveness (Exod. 15:26). No recourse to any human physician was permitted. There is only one instance of the prescription of a poultice of figs to heal a boil (2 Kgs 20:7). Sickness is seen as a spiritual matter, hence the absence of the prescription of medical treatment except for a few folk remedies.

The New Testament
The main source of information is in the Gospels and Acts. There are only a few references in the Epistles which give some indication of the thought and practice of the church.

(a) *The Gospels.* Jesus heals and exorcises demons frequently, but that activity is directly linked with his preaching and teaching (Matt. 4:23; *cf.* Mark 1:34; 3:10). The disciples share in his ministry of healing, anointing with oil though he did not do so. His call is for 'repentance', that is, 'change', since the Kingdom of God has come to earth through him and is seen in the 'reign of God' (Matt. 11:4, 5). Jesus' priority is to proclaim salvation, the setting free from all that impairs life (Luke 19:9, 10). His healing is subordinate to and indicative of his proclamation of the Kingdom.

The early church discerned 'compassion' ('mercy') as supremely characteristic of Jesus in relation to the needy and especially the sick. Since it was part of his fulfilment of the Second Commandment—'Thou shalt love thy neighbour as thyself'—then the church is required, through the same Holy Spirit, to seek healing for others.

In the healing of Jesus, faith, whether his own or that of the patient, played a significant part (Mark 2:1–12; 9:14–29). In Mark faith is explicit or implicit in all the accounts of healing and in Luke, while it is seldom mentioned, it is assumed. Lack of faith appears to frustrate Jesus' desire to heal (Mark 6:5, 6). Possession of it makes all things possible (Mark 9:23). It is necessary for those who wish to heal as well as those who wish to be healed. It may be faith in God as God, or in Jesus as a healer, but it is not necessarily saving faith. It is not a necessary condition for healing, but in healing Jesus demands faith and prayer.

(b) *The Acts of the Apostles.* Much less space is given to healing than in the Gospels. Faith is scarcely mentioned in regard to the healings. Both believers and non-believers are healed. Some aspects of healing are missing, *e.g.* compassion, fulfilment of Scripture or the cry for healing, though it must be remembered that Luke as the author would assume his Gospel to have been known, and his outline of the progress of the church's mission could not include all the details. In any case everything, including the miracles recorded, is subordinate to the witness of the activity of the Holy Spirit in the proclamation of the Good News of salvation.

(c) *The Epistles.* There are only a few references to sickness and healing which may not have been an issue in the situations to which the Epistles were addressed. It is assumed to be the accepted practice of the church. There is no mention of exorcism, but if healing were confined to the Christian community this should not be surprising. 'Gifts of healings', not mentioned elsewhere, are listed amongst the 'gifts of the Spirit' in 1 Corinthians 12:9. They may be (1) different gifts for different diseases; (2) different members within the body of Christ with different gifts for different people. Related to these may be another gift peculiar to Paul's writings—that of 'faith' which may mean (1) a gift of faith for a specific act of healing in the service of worship at a particular time, or (2) faith for others outside the worshipping community. It is not justifying faith but possibly related to divine healing.

(ii) Sickness and sin

Having noted the fact that many were not healed, consideration is given to the problem of Paul's 'thorn in the flesh' (2 Cor. 12:7, 8). Paul accepted it as given to him by God, though described as 'a messenger of Satan' which may be either a metaphorical or traditional statement, or, as in the case of Job, fulfilling the divine intention. It gave him a fresh experience of the sufficiency of God's grace and thus indicates the effecting of the divine purpose in bringing good out of evil.

Jesus healed because he believed sickness and disease were not God's ultimate will. He looked upon the healings and exorcisms as evidence of the Holy Spirit's activity through him, and of the presence of the Kingdom of God in the world (Matt. 12:27). In Acts also those who heal assume it is part of the divine purpose (Acts 3:1ff; 9:32–43), as does Paul's experience of the unhealed 'thorn'.

The interpretation of sickness and death as the divine judgment goes back to Genesis 3:16–19. The righteous are promised freedom from disease (Exod. 16:16) while the disobedient are promised 'sudden terror, consumption and fever that waste the eyes and cause life to pine away' (Lev. 26:14–16). Job saw God as present in the midst of sickness and pain.

In view of the Jewish belief that sickness is due to evil or demonic forces over which Jesus exercises his sovereignty in expelling demons in anticipation of the final triumph of his death and resurrection, sickness may in the New Testament be seen as affording opportunity for God to manifest his redemptive power. Jesus could identify what evidently was mental illness as the work of demonic spirits (Mark 1:21–27).

But there can also be a link between sin and sickness as implied in the healing of the paralytic man where Jesus first pronounces forgiveness (Mark 2:1–12; John 5:14). Refusal to forgive others brings its own spiritual illness which can manifest itself in physical effects.

(iii) Healing methods

Various means are mentioned—word, touch, saliva, clay (which at the time was regarded as having healing properties (John 9:6)). Possibly Jesus also used oil since his disciples did so. Similarly, in Acts word and touch are used. Paul embraced dead Eutychus and even the shadow of Peter and cloths from Paul's body are mentioned.

In James healing is dealt with in the context of prayer. The sick person who is unable to attend worship is to call for those responsible for pastoral oversight. As in Jesus' case, healing and forgiveness go together (Jas 5:15). Anointing with oil was common and practised by Jewish Rabbis. The main emphasis is on the corporate prayer of the spiritual leaders of the church. It is God who does the healing through the Holy Spirit. Scientific knowledge of psycho-therapeutic methods may lead us to a better understanding of Jesus as healer, but cannot give the full truth about his unique relationship with God and people.

The Scripture says little about the relationship of medical and faith healing. In the Old Testament generally resort to a human physician is forbidden. In the New Testament, Luke is described as 'the beloved physician' (Col. 1:4), and he omits the apparent criticism of physicians in Mark 5:26. But medical science too is from God. Some doctors, unable to cure by their own skills, are happy to associate themselves with faith-healing, prayer, pastoral counselling, the laying on of hands and the total renewal, body and spirit, of the whole person.

(iv) General observations

In the Bible there is a general conviction that in the fall of Adam creation was associated with that fall and sickness along with it (*cf.* Rom. 8:22). God's ultimate plan is to recreate and restore. Thus the Bible speaks of new birth, new people, a new heaven and a new earth. In Christ God's recreative power was present in the world, but such restoration cannot be divorced from the proclamation of the good news of the kingdom or of Christ crucified.

While Jesus stressed the importance of faith, physical healing could take place without it or without being accompanied by spiritual healing. Some believers too were not healed and some outside the church could perform healings and exorcisms while some within the church could not (Mark 9:38; 9:28, 29). Whatever the link between sin and sickness, compassion rather than judgment is the main imperative for divine healing.

The church is called to the ministry of divine healing, but always with the full recognition of the expertise of medical practitioners and in full co-operation as part of the divine gift.

Addendum

How much of what is recorded in the New Testament actually took place? Equally sincere Christians differ in the extent to which they regard the records as inerrant. Nor do we depend on miracles of healing for belief in Christ as the incarnate Son of God. To reject the essential historicity of the Gospel records is to imply that the Gospel witness is false or those who supplied the information on which it was based were deluded. If we believe this, can we be sure that the teachings of Christ also as recorded are reliable? Those who doubt the historical accuracy of the healing accounts probably do so on philosophical grounds, but it is not unreasonable to hold that they are true because Jesus was, as he is represented, uniquely endowed with the Spirit of God, therefore uniquely powerful in his effects upon men.

III. ASSESSMENT OF THE REPORTS

(i) The 1959 Report

The 1959 Report takes a more practical and philosophical approach to the subject of healing and its implications than does the 1982 Report. It (the 1959 Report) faces the issues which it raises more clearly and confidently than the 1982 Report, and while its approach to Scripture appears to be more liberal, it is consistent and constructive.

To dismiss the 'commission' of Mark 16:15–18 simply as not being part of the original Gospel is hardly adequate, especially as the Report has to acknowledge that at least some of its terms were fulfilled in the later work and witness of the Apostles. As we have seen elsewhere in this study (p. 37), even if this passage were not part of the original Gospel it does reflect the conviction and experience of the early church.

While the 1959 Report fully acknowledges the miraculous nature of the work of both Christ and the Apostles in regard to healing, it appears to minimise its impact and interpret or apply it in rather mundane terms. For example, the Report demurs to see the miracles of Jesus as 'proof' or evidence of his divine Sonship but sees them rather as simply the consequence of his divine Sonship and evidence that in him the 'reign of God' in the world is to be seen, which is best represented by the spiritual benefits of forgiveness and redemption rather than by physical or material manifestations of his sovereign power and authority. Again, while it is perfectly legitimate to see modern-day medical missions as one kind of manifestation of Christian concern for the healing of the sick, it can scarcely be said to constitute a continuation of the miraculous healings of the church of the Apostles.

The 1959 Report fully acknowledges the origin of sickness to be found in the sin of the fall of mankind. It appears, however, to hesitate to attribute cosmic corruption and the other evils of this world to the same cause while acknowledging that the world of nature is estranged from God's purposes and will eventually be restored. Yet surely in the very passage (Rom. 8:19–23) to which the Report makes reference, Paul clearly identifies the 'whole creation' with the 'bondage of corruption' into which sin brought humanity and from which it has been delivered ('redeemed') by Christ and restored to 'the glorious liberty of the children of God' in prospect of the final consummation of God's establishment of his kingdom at the end of the age. Here the 1982 Report takes a different view. It says:

> What God made was good and, by insisting on this, what is not good can be attributed to other causes and, in particular, to man's sin. A general conviction is that, in the fall of Adam, creation was associated with that fall and sickness along with it (*cf.* Rom. 8:22). God has the power to create or restore. Through Jesus Christ, his ultimate plan is to set people free from all that cripples life, whether sin or sickness.[3]

On the positive side, the 1959 Report sets the whole supernatural activity of Jesus and the Apostles in the context of the proclamation and demonstration of the Good News of hope and victory over the 'principalities and powers' and all their works which has been accomplished by Christ on Calvary and ultimately will be universally displayed and shared in the 'new heaven and new earth' that are to come. That confidence enables the Report effectively to challenge any

spurious demand for continued miracle-working; the claim for perfect
health in an imperfect world or the refusal to accept that sickness or
suffering could be the will of God or part of his sovereign purpose of
testing or discipline or the demonstration of his all-sufficient grace; the
notion that the experience of saving faith in the redemption of Christ
should, in this present world, remove the physical consequences of the
work of Satan and his legions in disease or distress; the mistaken belief
that 'faith' or prayer, apart from the context of God's sovereign will
and purpose, can and must produce healing.

The logical conclusion of the argument of the Report is to advocate
a closer working relationship between the medical profession and those
who are exercising pastoral care and responsibility both for the spiritual
and general wellbeing of all in society.

(ii) The 1982 Report

The 1982 Report follows a more systematic approach to the biblical
material and exudes a more conservative theological stance than the
1959 Report, but it is more hesitant and non-committal in its
assessments of various matters and in providing specific answers to
some of the questions which it raises. For example, in regard to the
passage in James 5:15 the 1982 Report says,

> Anointing with oil for illness was common in the ancient world.
> Jewish Rabbis visited the sick and anointed them with oil to cure
> such ailments as headache. Was the oil a supplementary aid for
> awakening faith? Whatever the explanation, James shows
> remarkable confidence in bodily and spiritual healing with the
> main emphasis, in the context, on the corporate prayer of the
> leaders of the church.[4]

Here there is no real attempt (a) to explain the use of oil, the 'prayer
of faith' or the involvement of the 'elders'; (b) to consider the part to
be played by the patient; or (c) to indicate whether this practice is to
be the pattern for the church henceforward.

It is characteristic of the 1982 Report that while it takes cognisance
of many aspects of the question of faith-healing it (unlike the 1959
Report) offers little practical guidance or help in establishing principles
or patterns of practice for the church today. (a) It notes the fact of
differences of opinion regarding a number of important issues such as
whether it is always God's will to heal; what part faith has to play in
healing; whether there is need at all for the practice of divine healing
and, if so, how far it is effected by the exercise of spiritual gifts or
healing services. But it offers no guidance as to the respective merits
of the differing opinions, nor does it take up a particular position itself
leaving the reader to wonder why. (b) It in no way attempts to
pronounce upon the persistent questions in the minds of many on such

matters as the 1959 Report did, or on other important matters such as whether the 'gifts of the Spirit' are operative since the time of the Apostles.

Both the 1959 and 1982 Reports are limited in their value by their failure to make any assessment of, or even to comment upon, the increasingly widespread practice of faith-healing either in the traditionally 'Pentecostal' Churches or amongst the modern 'charismatic' elements and groups within the churches generally. Yet another common and serious defect of the two Reports is their total failure to deal with the issue of death with particular reference to the question of healing, especially of faith-healing.

Neither of the Reports offers any comment or guidance regarding the nature and conduct of healing services. Both accept the practice of healing services and note that Paul refers to healing as part of the worship in the Corinthian church, but there is no attempt to relate such services either to the exercise of a gift of healing by individual members of the church or to the implementation of the pattern set out in the Epistle of James.

(iii) Contrasts

Faith-healing as understood and practised in the Elim and other Pentecostal Churches on the one hand, and the Presbyterian Church in Ireland on the other, presents some interesting contrasts.

While the Pentecostal Churches formally acknowledge the validity of medical and psychological healing methods as being part of the 'natural' provision made by God for man's physical health and wellbeing, they are in no doubt that the 'supernatural' exercise of spiritual gifts is a superior and better way. While they are at pains not to denigrate the work of medical science and practice, they seem inevitably to be forced to the conviction that true believers will expect and choose the miraculous power of God to heal in accordance with the commission and gifts given to the Apostles and still vested in the living church. While they acknowledge that all are not to be healed, and even that sickness and suffering can be part of God's purpose and activity in the spiritual life of the sufferer, nevertheless, they seem to insist on healing both as an important (if not essential) aspect of evangelistic witness especially in the form of mass evangelism, and as an important aspect of the regular worship and life of the congregation. In conversation, however, with a Pastor of the Elim Church, the present writer was informed that only rarely does healing occur in the ministry of his congregation, and for him and his church it does not have a very high profile.

In the Presbyterian Church in Ireland the scene is different. The Westminster Confession of Faith, which is the primary Subordinate

Standard of the Church's doctrine, makes no reference at all either to faith-healing or to the 'gifts of the Spirit' as such. Nevertheless, the Church through its General Assembly has given practical recognition to the doctrine and practice of faith-healing in a number of ways:

(a) by setting up a Committee of Assembly to 'provide for the Church's ministry in divine healing' under its Board of Evangelism and Christian Training;

(b) by encouraging, through its divine healing Committee, the provision of healing services throughout the Presbyteries of the Church; and

(c) by recognising the work of a number of ministers and others who are engaged in the ministry of healing on a regular and fairly widespread basis.

Having said that, it must also be said that in most Congregations of the Church (and even in most Presbyteries) faith-healing is the concern and practice of but a few. And members of the Church at large seeking faith-healing tend to resort not to their own minister, or other ministers of the Church, but to recognised faith-healers regardless of their denominational connection. The truth of the matter is that while the biblical basis for the doctrine and practice of faith-healing is fully recognised by the Church, it takes place only in isolated instances and usually outside of the spiritual life and activity of the congregation. It is not part of the day-to-day faith and practice of the Church and usually only arises in the mind and experience of the members of the Church when some crisis arises within the family or the congregation.

IV. SUMMARY

From the two Reports the following conclusions may be drawn with regard to the Presbyterian Church:

1. Healing is available through faith and prayer with or without anointing with oil or the laying on of hands.

2. In the commission of the Lord to the church healing is subordinate to the witness of the Gospel by preaching and teaching, and is partially fulfilled in the work of medical missions.

3. Not all Christians (nor all ministers) can exercise the gift of healing, but some do. A number of ministers and other members of the Presbyterian Church in Ireland carry on a ministry of healing on a regular basis.

4. Sickness and suffering can be part of God's will for the individual. It is not always God's will to heal, nor does it always happen in response to faith or prayer.

5. While sickness (and all other evils in this present world) is the consequence of the Fall of man, and some sicknesses are the

consequence of sin and disobedience to God's Law, it is not true that all sickness is the direct result of particular sin or failure on the part of the sufferer.

6. 'Faith' in God's power to heal may be distinguished from 'saving faith'. Both or neither may be present when healing takes place. Healing can only be effected within the sovereign purpose of God and is not determined merely by the presence, absence or degree of faith manifested. Nevertheless the presence or absence of faith may assist or hinder the purposes of God to heal.

7. Medicine and faith are not alternatives in healing. The church's ministry of healing must give full recognition to and co-operate with the expertise of medical science.

8. Healing does take place in the context of healing services.

9. Christ's work of atonement on Calvary secured the ultimate deliverance of believers from both sin and sickness (and all the other works of Satan) but the deliverance cannot be fully realised in either the physical or spiritual sense until the return of the Saviour at the end of the age and in the 'new heaven and new earth'.

10. 'Gifts of healing' may be given to particular members of the church or to the whole church but to be exercised by different members at different times or for different purposes.

NOTES

1   Presbyterian Church in Ireland, *Reports,* Belfast, 1959, p. 168.
2   *Ibid.,* p. 24.
3   *Ibid.,* p. 30.
4   *Ibid.,* p. 30.

15

AS THE HEALER SEES IT

Having examined the biblical teaching and pattern of faith-healing, and having reviewed the work of healing as conceived and practised in the major churches, it is now time to look more closely at the work of individual healers and modern-day healing movements.

To do so, tape-recorded interviews were sought with five faith-healing practitioners to whom the same set of questions was submitted in advance. Three (A, B, C) agreed and gave lengthy accounts of their work and their understanding of their ministries. Two (D, E) preferred to supply rather brief written answers to the questions. The results are tabulated in Table VII and show interesting similarities and differences. The interview with A is set out and examined in some detail because it seems to represent the general approach of those who are engaged in this kind of ministry. While A had no theological training he has been exercising his ministry on a full-time basis for many years and has a very large and widely-scattered clientele many of whom are seen at his 'clinics' which are provided at churches and various centres around the country. He also ministers on request at homes, hospitals, etc. on a private basis as well as by letter and by telephone. The others are ordained ministers who practise faith-healing as one important, and they would say indispensable, aspect of their general vocation. Some hold regular 'Healing Services' or seminars in their own churches or participate in such services in other places, as well as ministering to individuals on a private basis.

I. THE INTERVIEW WITH 'A'

Q. 1. *How did you come to take up the ministry of healing?*
I was brought up as a Presbyterian and continue in the Reformed tradition. My interest in divine healing began as a result of attending Pentecostal meetings and I began to read much about the subject and to discuss it with interested friends. I was invited to attend a healing session in order to see what happened. I did so and later was invited to assist the healer. This continued for some years. Later, while I was involved in evangelistic work I felt persuaded that there was another dimension to the work. I began to minister to folk privately until the demand on my time became so great I had to give up business and devote all my time to the ministry of healing. In no sense do I claim to have a gift of healing. I would rebel against that most definitely, I am ministering the Word of God. The Word is the authority for healing. Jesus said, 'These signs shall follow them that believe'. It's a believers' ministry. It is not a matter of somebody being gifted. It is not a ministry where I have a gift of healing. It is a ministry where I am ministering to people the risen power of Christ.

Q. 2. *Do you see yourself as:* (a) *carrying on the work of Christ and the Apostles?* (b) *exercising the healing gifts of 1 Corinthians 12?* (c) *fulfilling the pattern of James 5?*
(a) Most definitely yes. I believe this is the ministry of the church, and I believe the church should have continued the way Christ and the Apostles started it off. I wouldn't be dispensational in my approach to this, that something stopped. Nothing stopped. He's 'Jesus Christ the same yesterday, today and for ever' or not. Now I have seen so many souls saved through this work that the hand of God is upon it. It is basic to the church. I often get a bit annoyed when I hear people talking about 'faith-healers' and 'faith-healing'. There is no place where Christ demanded faith. Seven times, I think, he said 'O great is your faith'. But he had 70,000 who had no faith, but he healed them because they were sick. The talk about faith-healing and faith-healers robs the church of a basic work that should be in it.
(b) Yes, inasmuch as the gifts are in the body of the church. They're not in me. I believe the gifts are given to the church and they should be manifested in the local assembly. We have here in this church (*i.e.* congregation) a very fine example of the New Testament church, because we have a tremendous teacher and preacher in the minister, we have deacons who visit, and I have this ministry here. Now this is all part of a total ministry and there's not a week in my experience in this church there hasn't been a soul saved.

(c) O yes. Very much so. Now I'm not ordained to any office in the church. I'm not a deacon. I'd refuse to be a deacon because I want to be free to come and go and be led of the Lord and his Spirit as to where I should go. So I've no ordination. I'm an ordinary pew member. But according to James 5 I am an 'elder' in the sense of being a believer. According to Mark 16:18 'These signs shall follow them that believe'. James is saying here 'Call the elder'. Now the elder is supposed to be a believer. The word 'elder' in my book is one who is ordained of God, whether he's ordained of man or not is not important. So I would say in James 5 I am an elder and I would use that as my authority for the ministry.

Q. 3. *In your ministry does healing:* (a) *take place immediately?* (b) *require further treatment?* (c) *necessitate rehabilitation?* (d) *suffer relapse?*
(a) Sometimes, very seldom. Normally I would see people three, four, five times. Very often after prayer there is a flare-up. So often when we begin to apply the Word to the person, if they're a Christian, Satan will have a real go at them to try to dispossess them of the truth of the Word of God, and there can be a very definite flare-up. Often the road to recovery is gradual, slow, gentle healing. It could be ten minutes, ten days, ten weeks, ten months. There is no limit, and I could never put a time on God's healing. Jesus said, 'these signs shall follow them that believe. They shall lay hands on the sick and they shall recover'. Now he didn't say, 'They'll recover tonight or tomorrow or next week'. Jesus on one occasion prayed twice for a man. Now Jesus didn't have to do that. He was Lord. He was totally in command. He could instantly have healed that man's eyes. But he chose to do it in two goes for the sake of you and the sake of me. (This also covers parts (b) and (c) of the question.)
(d) Yes. Sometimes they do, specially in the nervous diseases problems where there's tension, or there's a problem in the background. This can often cause a relapse and a falling back. Many of these people through their healings and through finding Christ's power in their body, find his salvation in their souls. But some don't. Now if these people are not committed and live in sin they can overcome the healing.

Q. 4. *In your work what part does 'faith' play?*
No part at all in the sick person. Totally and completely in me. I must pray 'the prayer of faith'. James 5:14 calls for the deacon, the elder, the believer, the minister 'and the prayer of faith shall save the sick'. Nothing to do with the faith of the sick person. The third category (in James 5) is 'Are any among you sick?'. Well, they're not told to pray, they're told to 'call'. They're told to go for help, or bring help, the

elder, the servant, the believer, and his prayer, or her prayer, for there
are many women in this work today, the 'prayer of faith' prayed by the
believer is the crucial thing, never the faith of the sick person. God
hates their disease because disease is evil and Satanic and Christ
rebuked it every time he saw it, and he said it wasn't of his Father, it
was of the devil. And thus it is not faith in the person (the sufferer), it
is faith in the one who ministers the Word. I rebel against those who
say that healing is only for Christians. Christ healed all who came.
Some didn't believe he was the Son of God at all. But he healed them
because they were sick. There's one criterion for healing, that's to be
sick.

Q. 5. *How do you explain failure to heal in any particular case?*
I have no quick, clear answer. I have problems here myself. I often cry
before the Lord, Why? Take cancer, I have seen many cases of cancer
healed, but I have hundreds of cases not healed. Now I would say that
if any person has to be blamed, and I don't like using the word, I would
first look at myself. Where did my prayer of faith fail? I would look
at myself first and say, 'Did I fail this person that they're not healed?'.
I would do that before I would say that I would blame them. I believe
basically it's the will of God to heal all sick. I believe it's the will of
God to save every sinner. But every sinner is not saved. At the end of
the day it's of the Lord, and I can't give you the answer.

Q. 6. (a) *Do you expect miracles to happen?* (b) *Do you encourage
patients to expect miracles to happen?*
(a) Most definitely. I set out to pray for every person believing that
they'll get a miracle. Now what is a miracle? If someone rises out of
a wheelchair, it's a miracle. Now if that person, after being prayed for
and ministered to every week for a year, rises out of the wheelchair,
that's still a miracle. It took a little longer. It took a little more work,
a little more effort, a little more faith, a little more prayer, a little more
time. It's still a miracle. I see miracles. Some instantly, some
agonisingly slowly, but they're miracles.
(b) I do. I've got to believe God's Word, and I've got to expect them
and show them that they must believe, and I would define the miracle
as a healing in God's time.

Q. 7. *To what extent do you use psychology or psychiatry in your
healing ministry?*
Not at all. In no sense do I ever ask any questions. There's another gift,
the gift of 'discernment'—the gift of 'knowledge and wisdom'—you
would have that in Corinthians. I believe that from time to time, and
maybe most of the time, I am able to discern certain things about

people's needs and problems by the work of the Holy Spirit which cuts across any need for questioning and the use of psychiatry or psychology. Now the gifts are complementary to each other. I don't think God will give any person any gift of discernment unless they need to use it. But in this ministry I believe it's important that I should get behind maybe the facade of words to find a deeper problem (in order) to minister quickly, effectively and efficiently to the person's needs. I always try to present the brighter picture, to bring encouragement to people, because so often they come here after everything else has failed and if I were looking for faith in them I wouldn't find it.

Q. 8. *How important is (a) 'anointing with oil' or (b) 'laying on of hands' in your work?*
(a) I carry a bottle of oil in my case always with me. I use it on request only. I believe that the anointing oil was really symbolic of the power of the Holy Spirit in James 5. The oil itself had no medicinal or curative power. I try to prevent the person having any faith in me or my gifts, and I don't want them also to have any faith or trust in the oil. If we use oil too openly and make too much of oil it becomes an object of faith.
(b) Now I believe that the 'laying on of hands' is essential. It is fundamental—other than in absent prayer, and this I deal with a lot in letters and in prayer-cloths, and in telephone ministry. We seek to obey the Scriptures and Jesus touched the sick and he said, 'Ye shall lay hands on the sick', and James required anointing with oil, and you can't anoint with oil without touching. I would not minister to a person that was with me without the laying on of hands. Often when I lay hands on a person, not always, and it's not important, but from time to time there's a very definite awareness of heat. The heat is not in my hands. The heat is generated in the ministry, in the obedience. It is not hot hands. It is simply the power of God. It is answered prayer, if you like, in the sense of heat. So much of medical healing comes through heat. Now God has his own heat treatment.

Q. 9. *Do you believe in public Services of Divine Healing?*
Yes and No. I feel that so many services for public healing tend to be non-events because it's a very general service. It's an open service and the person ministering is not getting down to the needs of the individual. I see this work as essentially in the modern age a very private and personal thing. I'm not opposed to services of healing, I think they only touch the fringe of the problem. I would question the larger healing services. I have seen healings take place at one of these, and I myself was gloriously healed at one. So I can't just cut them out.

But in the modern problems of today to me they don't offer the right answer.

Q. 10. *Do you think all ministers of the Gospel should be exercising a healing ministry as distinct from the other aspects of their ministry?*
I do within limits. I believe that all ministers (who are believers) from time to time should be prepared to minister, to lay hands on the sick in a very clear-cut and definite way for healing, not just pray a general prayer. They should get down to the fundamentals of carrying out their anointed and appointed jobs as ministers of the full gospel to bring salvation and healing to all who need it. I would differentiate the work of the minister from my own work in that this is for me a very specialised and a very single-minded work that I am doing. I know that the minister as such today, in the rather unscriptural way that the church is constituted, can't properly do the work, and cannot always minister as he should. But I feel that if the minister is worthwhile in his work, since I don't think this is a gift or calling, it is his responsibility to look after the souls of his flock, to reveal Christ to them and to point them to Christ. It is his responsibility also to minister to their bodies from time to time. Now I know that this would be on a lesser basis because of the time-consuming work. I'm not saying that everybody should do what I'm doing. God, I believe, has called me to a very unique and special ministry. But I feel that men like yourself would probably have a greater opportunity of getting through to people when you're able to bring them the help they need physically, because it brings a new relationship between you and them, and between them and the Lord, and sinners are so much easier saved and brought face to face with Christ when you have demonstrated the reality of the living Lord and his power to heal first and then ultimately to save.

II. ASSESSMENT OF THE INTERVIEW

In attempting to evaluate the meaning and import of his presentation there are two immediate difficulties—(1) his looseness in handling the text of Scripture, and (2) the confusion of thought and inference in his application of biblical statements. He of course makes no claim to theological training or expertise, though he does not hesitate to present his understanding of these matters with confidence and dogmatism. This seems to be somewhat characteristic of statements of those who practise faith-healing, even when they are not evidently confirmed by subsequent experience or events.

(i) Dealing with the 'Word'

It is clear throughout the healer's statement that he is concerned to act only upon the authority of Scripture, and that he believes he is doing so. He is 'ministering the Word of God' (Q. 1.), and he claims no authority or power in his work other than that of the Scripture and the Holy Spirit, and it is evident that he has no intention other than to comply with the express instruction and content of the Word.

But when he comes to quote the Word, or to interpret it, he does so with little regard to accuracy or consistency. For example, he says, 'Jesus on one occasion prayed twice for a man' in reference to the healing of a blind man (Q. 3.). But the Scripture makes no reference to Jesus' having prayed at any time for anyone's healing. Jesus, the Scripture says, 'touched' the man twice. Furthermore, in his reference to James 5 he repeatedly misquotes the Scripture (Q. 2, (c)). For example, he says, 'James 5:14 calls for the deacon, the elder, the believer, the minister'. Now leaving aside for the moment his interpretation of 'elder' in this chapter, it is noteworthy that James actually said, 'Let him call for the elders (plural) of the Church'. Or again, in dealing with the James passage he says, 'I would use that as my authority for the ministry'. But when we examine his treatment of the matter of 'anointing with oil' and 'laying on of hands', he dismisses the 'anointing with oil' which James requires (Q. 8 (a)) as being optional or of indifferent account to such an extent that in his practice he omits it altogether except on request, while he regards as 'fundamental' and essential the 'laying on of hands' which James does not even mention (Q. 8 (b)).

Now there is no desire to quibble about words, but it would seem to be a basic requirement of any doctrine or practice said to be founded on the Word of God, that the Scripture should be dealt with accurately and consistently. Yet we find him frequently making sweeping generalisations or absolute statements which are not borne out consistently in Scripture, or which may even be directly contrary to the Word in other places. For example, in his answer concerning the 'laying on of hands' he makes reference to 'absent healing' and to the use of 'prayer-cloths' (Q. 8 (b)) which we presume to be a reference to the 'special miracles' associated with Paul's ministry in Ephesus (Acts 19:11, 12). But in the Scriptural account of this event there is no reference to prayer or 'prayer-cloths'. What is referred to is the 'sweat-cloths and aprons' which Paul used in the course of his daily work at his trade. And again, perhaps one of the most unfortunate examples of this looseness in regard to the precise text of Scripture is his statement in the answer to Q. 2 (a) where he says 'There is no place where Christ demanded faith'. This statement is simply not true (Matt. 9:29; Mark 4:40; 11:22). Again he says (Q. 5.), 'I believe it's basically the will of God to heal all sick'. But the Scripture shows clearly that not only is this not so, even in the case of the Apostle Paul, but that, in fact, God actually inflicted sickness from time to time for his own purposes. Nor did Jesus heal all the sick who were around him, for example at the Pool of Bethesda (John 5:1–9).

As we shall see later, this is not just a matter of words. It involves sometimes a subtle change of concept seemingly for the purpose of creating apparent Scriptural warrant for something other than the original intent of Scripture. It is important also that due regard should be paid to the general teaching of Scripture and that particular texts and passages should not be unrelated to each other nor interpretation or application inconsistent.

(ii) Which is it?

The second problem is really an extension of the first and arises from confusion in the interpretation and application of Scripture teaching. At first glance it might appear that the questions put to the healer had received direct and decisive answers, as the healer himself doubtless intended. But further examination of the answers given leaves many things unresolved. For example:

(a) *Gift or no gift?* He says in answer to Question 1, 'In no sense do I claim to have a gift of healing. I would rebel against that most definitely.... It's a believers' ministry. It is not a matter of somebody being gifted. It is not a ministry where I have a gift of healing'. But in Q. 2 (b) when asked if he sees himself as 'exercising the healing gifts of 1 Corinthians 12', he replies, 'Yes, inasmuch as the gifts are in the body of the church'. Presumably by being 'in the body of the church' he means they are entrusted to individual members or groups of members within the church. For he goes on to explain that the gifts of the Spirit are severally distributed among, and exercised by, individuals in his own congregation—the minister in his preaching and teaching; the deacons in visitation; and himself in the healing ministry. Furthermore in Question 7 he refers to the 'gift of discernment' which he claims to possess and use, and goes on to say, 'Now the gifts are complementary to each other'. In the context of his answer this would appear to mean that the gift of discernment is complementary to the gift of healing (and this is thoroughly good Scripture, of course). But it implies that he has the gift of healing!

(b) *Calling or no calling?* In answer to Question 10, speaking of the responsibility of the minister for the physical as well as the spiritual needs of his flock, he says, 'I feel that if the minister is worthwhile in his work, since I don't think this is a gift or calling...'. But a few sentences later, in justification of his own 'unique and special ministry' he asserts, 'God, I believe, has called me'. The point at issue here is whether any or every believer is to be involved in the ministry of healing, as the healer would seem to imply when he says, 'It's a believers' ministry', or whether a particular gift or calling is required. Is it a 'unique and special ministry' reserved to those who are specifically called to it by God, or is it the kind of operation in which believers generally are to be engaged?

(c) *Elder or no elder?* In answer to Question 2 (c) 'Do you see yourself as fulfilling the pattern of James 5?' he said, 'O yes. Very much so'. But immediately he goes on to assert that he was not an ordained office-bearer in the church, nor indeed would he undertake such office. Now there can be little dispute as to what James meant by the phrase 'Let him call for the elders of the church'. They were those duly elected and ordained according to the requirements laid down and explained at some length in the Pauline Epistles, and appointed to the spiritual oversight of each of the churches (congregations) (Acts 14:23). But, says the healer, 'the word 'elder' in my book is one ordained by God. Whether he's ordained of man is not important'. As a personal opinion this may be respected, but it can scarcely be accepted as a fulfilment of the pattern of Scripture in James 5 where the instruction is clearly for the sick person to seek the help of 'the elders' as a body, and not the ministrations of an individual healer.

(d) *Following Christ and the Apostles or not?* Asked in Question 2 (a) 'Do you see yourself as carrying on the work of Christ and the Apostles?' he says, 'Most definitely yes'. But when the answer to Question 3 is examined, it is evident that the healings effected in his ministry fail to conform in scarcely any respect to those effected by Christ and the Apostles. For example, they are not usually immediate, they require repeated treatment and rehabilitation, and they are subject to relapse.

(e) *Faith in the sufferer or not?* Asked in Q. 4 'In your work what part does faith play?' he says, 'No part at all in the sick person. Totally and completely in me'. If this be true there can be no real analogy between the work of preaching the Gospel and that of the healer, as he insists there is, because souls can never be saved by the faith of the preacher. There must be the exercise of personal saving faith in Christ on the part of the sinner himself if he is to be saved. Whereas the healer's statement here implies that no exercise of faith is required on the part of the sufferer in order to obtain healing, but rather on the part of the healer. Nor can there be any analogy, such as the healer suggests in answer to Question 5, between the failure of some to be saved as the result of the preaching of the Word, and the failure of some to be healed as the result of the ministration of the healer, since in the one case faith is required on the part of the recipient, and in the other case, in his view, it is not.

The effectiveness of the healing depends, he says, upon 'the prayer of faith prayed by the believer' which, he adds, is 'the crucial thing, never the faith of the sick person'. Now these are pretty dogmatic statements. They would seem to imply that the healing of the sufferer is totally dependent on the faith of the healer and works '*ex opere operato*'. But when asked in Question 5 'How do you explain failure to heal in any particular case?' he says, 'I would first look at myself, where did my prayer of faith fail? I would look at myself first and say "did I fail this person that they're not healed?". I would do that before I would say that I would blame them'. Now if in no circumstances faith is to be required of the sufferer, and if responsibility for faith rests 'totally and completely' with the healer, on what grounds, or in what circumstances could the sufferer possibly be blamed? Or, for that matter, in what circumstances could the 'prayer of faith' fail, since the promise is 'the prayer of faith shall save the sick'? So that failure to heal must be the result of failure, on the part of the healer, to pray the 'prayer of faith'. Yet in his answer to Question 6 (b) 'Do you encourage patients to expect miracles to happen?' he says 'I do. I've got to believe God's Word, and I've got to expect them and show them that they must believe'! But which is it? Must they believe or not?

(f) *Miracle or no miracle?* He defines a miracle as 'healing in God's time' regardless of the length of the time or what has taken place during that period. The sufferer may have been receiving repeated treatment by his visits to the healer through which he has been comforted, sustained, encouraged, or sympathised with, and given counsel concerning not only the particular malady which is to be healed, but also relating to other personal problems, anxieties, difficulties and surrounding circumstances, personal, domestic, social, or spiritual which may have direct or indirect bearing upon his physical condition. All of this, of course, is accepted as perfectly legitimate and Scriptural activity in fulfilment of the multiplicity and variety of the 'gifts' to be exercised. He may also be receiving medical treatment. If at the end of this period he is healed, this, according to the healer, is to be regarded as a miracle. But surely in these terms all healing is 'miracle'. And in the sense of its being the evidence of the power of God working through human instrumentality, it is indeed 'miracle'. But this can scarcely be said to be 'miracle' as effected in the healings of Christ and the Apostles where the effect is immediate and without the use of medical skills or 'medicine' either physical or psychiatric.

(g) *Psychiatry or no psychiatry?* The answer to Question 7 'To what extent do you use psychology or psychiatry in your healing ministry?' was again uncompromising—'Not at all. In no sense do I ever ask questions'. Now if the healer here intended to say that he did not make a practice of protracted questioning or psycho-analytical procedures this might be understood. But to say 'In no sense do I ever ask any questions' is difficult to comprehend simply because it is not true. What he was really trying to say would appear to be that whereas the doctor or psychiatrist in making his diagnosis obtains information by means of question and answer, he, the healer, obtains the information he requires by means of the spiritual gift of 'discernment'. This is borne out by the instance with which he illustrated the point. 'I had a case where a woman came in with a little boy covered in psoriasis, and I asked him just to come and stand beside me and I put my hands on him.... I put my hands just round him and I sat here and talked to the mother and grandmother who was also present, and immediately I sensed—there's trouble around this child, there's struggle, there's stress, there's trouble; there's nothing wrong with the child, there's a problem in the home. So I said to the mother, "Now look, this child has psoriasis but it's caused by tension in the home, there's something wrong". And she looked at her mother, and the mother looked at her, and the granny said, "You'd better tell the man everything". Now it turned out that this woman's husband had become almost an alcoholic. He had hit her. The child was terribly devoted to both parents, and he was split between father and mother. He didn't sleep. He was missing out at school. And he broke out in psoriasis. They had tried every cream and treatment. Now right away I put my finger on it—*discernment*! Now this cuts through knowledge, human or anything else, and you get right to the core of the person's need'.

Here we have a perfectly normal example of diagnostic procedure—the healer first 'talked to the mother and grandmother'. It is difficult to imagine that the conversation did not concern the background of the child's condition—whether he had symptoms of any other illness, how long he had been affected, when or how the trouble started or was first noticed, what treatment had already been used, whether the doctor had been consulted and what his opinion was, *etc*. It would appear, moreover, from the interjection of the granny 'You'd better tell the man everything' that, in fact, the mother had already told a good deal, but had hidden the embarrassing domestic problem. From this the healer had concluded that 'there's nothing wrong with the child', that is, there was no evident physical cause for the child's condition. It did not therefore require anything more than natural 'discernment' to conclude that there must be another cause. Besides, a person dealing with many cases of eczema, dermatitis, psoriasis, etc., would be well aware that these are often psychosomatic in origin, and would therefore at once look for underlying 'stress' or 'struggle' or just 'trouble'. This is not in the least to discount the reality of the gift of 'discernment', but simply to make the point that all diagnosis—medical, psychiatric or spiritual—is based on right and wise discernment. When the doctor or the psychiatrist diagnoses a difficult or uncommon cause of suffering or distress he may well be consciously or unconsciously exercising the 'gift of discernment' given by God. Indeed, this may well be so in any case of true diagnosis. But that does not make the procedure less medical or psychiatric.

(h) *Anointing or no anointing?* The answer to Question 8 (a) raises interesting issues. Here the healer says he anoints with oil 'on request only'. It is not his normal practice. In summing up parts (a) and (b) of the question he said, 'So it is very much the laying on of hands always, and the anointing with oil when requested. This (request) often would be by very knowledgeable people who know the Word, and who believe the Word, and who feel they should totally obey it, in which case I go along with them'. What a strange business! He does not normally anoint with oil, though this is expressly required in James 5:14, as indeed in part (b) of the answer he fully acknowledges— 'James required anointing with oil'. He does, however, insist on the laying on of hands in every case although this practice is not even mentioned by James. But, perhaps strangest of all, when he received requests from people 'who know the Word, and who believe the Word, and who feel they should totally obey it' he 'goes along with them'. This would appear to be an acknowledgement of specific disobedience to the Word on his part in those instances when anointing with oil does not take place, that is, in his normal practice. But in regard to the laying on of hands he says, 'We seek to obey the Scriptures and Jesus touched the sick and he said, "Ye shall lay hands on the sick"'. The reason given for the healer's failure as a normal practice to anoint with oil is the fear of superstitious association on the part of the sufferer of the power of healing with the oil. But why should there not equally be the possibility of superstitious association of the power of healing with the laying on of hands? Or does he mean to suggest that it is, in fact, the laying on of hands that heals? This might appear indeed to be suggested by his reference to God having 'his own heat treatment' (effected through the healer's hands?).

III. COMMON GROUND

From the foregoing analysis of the answers given by one healer it would be easy to conclude that he was unable to give a coherent or consistent account of his ministry. But an examination of Table VII shows that, in fact, his account is largely corroborated by the four others to whom the same questions were put. All the divergences in the answers of A are reflected in the general picture presented by the five healers.

Thus, from Table VII we may conclude that two of the five took up the ministry of healing directly as the result of having received such healing for themselves, while two were challenged by the suffering of others to put the teaching of the Scriptures, as they understood them, to the test, and one was convinced of the necessity and validity of the healing ministry by the study and observance of Pentecostal teaching and practice. From this it would appear that their involvement in the healing ministry was based, in the first place, upon personal or practical considerations rather than upon any clearly defined or understood command or requirement of Scripture. Having become involved in the practice, however, they would then appear to have gathered from Scripture to support their particular practices.

On five matters there appears to be complete unanimity by all five. (1) They all claim to be carrying on the work of Christ and the Apostles, even though none of them claims to produce the same results. (2) They all deny that they are simply praying for the sick with fruitful results, though they do not all agree that they are exercising a special gift of healing. (3) They all expect miracles to happen when they minister, although all but one acknowledge the possibility of complete failure. (4) They all encourage their patients to believe that miracles will happen, although none appears to lay the onus of 'faith' on the patient, and again, while they encourage patients to believe that it is the sovereign purpose of God to heal, when healing does not appear to take place two of them attribute the result to divine sovereignty while the others explain it as the result of some deficiency in the administration or the extent or degree of progress of the disease. (5) They all claim to be fulfilling the instruction of James 5, yet, contrary to the direction of James, they all deny the necessity or importance of anointing with oil while insisting on the necessity and importance of laying on of hands.

On the other matters dealt with in the questions there is a variety of opinion and practice without much consistency. Asked whether they are exercising a specific 'gift' of healing, three claim they are, one categorically denies any claim to such a gift, and the other denies having such a gift himself though he appears, in fact, to be exercising it along with other gifts of the Spirit. Again, asked if in their ministry healing takes place immediately, three say it does but not usually, and two say it doesn't. With regard to the necessity of repeated treatment, two say it is normal, and three say it is required sometimes. None claims to have witnessed spectacular and immediate healing, which was invariably the case in the ministry of Christ and the Apostles. Four acknowledge that some patients do suffer relapse, and one fails to comment on the question. In the case of complete failure to heal, three acknowledge that it does happen, one denies that it ever happens, and one does not comment.

In regard to the nature of 'faith' all seem to believe that faith is required, but there is little attempt to specify what the nature of such faith must be. It seems to be agreed by three that the faith required is not 'saving faith in Christ', and two at least would require the faith not of the patient but of the healer or of others involved in the event. Asked about the use of psychological or psychiatric methods, one acknowledges their use, one categorically denies their use, and the others obviously use such techniques to a greater or lesser degree but are rather reluctant to say so and minimise their importance. With regard to healing services, three positively participate in such while two do so only occasionally and with considerable reservation. One of the healers believes that all ordained ministers should be practising faith-healing as a necessary part of their ministry. Two assert that only those who have received a 'gift' of the Spirit should do so. And two would seem to imply that failure to do so may be indicative not merely of disobedience but of deficiency of spiritual experience.

From the interview with A and the comparison with the replies of the other four healers, there would appear to be no very consistent pattern either in their understanding or practice of their ministry. Each would seem to be acting upon a personal conviction that he is being obedient to what he believes the Word of God to teach. But there is no doubt that healing by means of prayer and spiritual counsel is being offered to, and received by, many who are being ministered to.

16

AS THE DOCTOR SEES IT

I. ESTABLISHING THE FACTS

When we attempt to investigate the phenomenon of faith-healing from a purely medical point of view, we at once encounter a number of basic problems. First, there is the problem of knowing all the relevant facts. Reliable scientific conclusions can only be derived from adequate and scientifically authenticated evidence which, in many cases, is either simply not available, or is bedevilled by such complex aspects as mistaken diagnosis, mistaken prognosis, temporary or prolonged remissions, or spontaneous cures.

> It is seldom easy to ascertain all the relevant facts concerning any reported case of miraculous healing and...the overwhelming majority of recorded cases of healing are insufficiently documented to enable exact diagnosis to be made.[1]

Second, there is the problem of the degree to which even modern medical knowledge is able to explain the nature and history of disease. For example,

> Some consideration must be given to what is known of disease and especially of its unusual outcome. In dealing with malignant conditions the medical man feels himself to be on safe ground; he is able to give a tentative prognosis and therefore better able to test a 'cure'. Nevertheless, even here we must be wary in accepting claims too readily. We are still ignorant of much of the 'natural history' of disease. From time to time reports have

appeared in medical literature of the spontaneous regression of almost every known form of new growth. In fact, histological appearance can no longer be accepted as the sole criterion of malignancy; biological behaviour must also be taken into account.[2]

Third, there is the problem on the one hand of failure or unwillingness to take into account the factor of divine intervention, and on the other hand of confusing or equating such divine intervention with the psychological power of 'suggestion'.

Thus, it would appear, from our point of view at least, any investigation to be satisfactory would require to be undertaken by Christian doctors or those at least who were prepared to be open-minded regarding the reality and implications of the divine dimension. But even then, as doctors Edmunds and Scorer put it in their revised report of a study group of Christian doctors,

> On the one side are some Christians who, in their anxiety to preserve the divine reputation, think it praiseworthy to exaggerate or to minimise some of the evidence; on the other side are certain scientific interpreters who imagine that objectivity demands of them that the explanation of any given phenomena, however fully and accurately accredited, should never in any circumstances be attributed to the supernatural.[3]

With these considerations in mind, then, we turn to the investigation of faith-healing 'As the doctor sees it'.

II. MIRACLES DO HAPPEN

Rex Gardner is a consultant gynaecologist and former missionary doctor turned ordained minister who has written a valuable volume on *Healing Miracles*. His book is different, and for that reason specially interesting, because in it he sets out to investigate the subject not merely on the basis of 'popular descriptions' of instances of faith-healing, but on the basis of medical records showing

> the true nature of a diagnosis before the claimed healing, and, if possible, Case Papers or some certainty from medical observers that the change was lasting.[4]

It is also interesting (though not unusual) that he chooses to begin not from clear and definitive statements from Scripture, since, he believes, biblical interpreters are often in conflict or cancel one another out, but from recorded and authenticated experience. And this he does with considerable effect, though not always with first-hand evidence or entirely convincing conclusions.

He defines healing miracles as

> those cures for which, apart from the intervention of God, there

is no logical explanation[5]
and gives much space to proving or illustrating such miracles. He
carefully examines with examples six categories of alternative
explanations to that of 'miracle': (1) physiological process; (2)
spontaneous remission; (3) therapeutic response; (4) incorrect
diagnosis; (5) psychosomatic origin; (6) natural history of the disease
where

> sudden improvements, such as periods of amelioration in the
> chronic stress diseases, or the reduction of a hernia[6]

may take place. Having acknowledged the possibility of such
'alternative' explanations, he nevertheless rightly insists that even
where they might appear to be established on medical grounds, there
is still the possibility that they could be associated with, or the result
of, united, believing, persevering prayer (p. 40).

Gardner acknowledges that,

> Much of the contemporary concern (regarding healing miracles)
> seems to be inspired directly (or sometimes indirectly) by the
> movement for charismatic renewal, and arises out of a fresh
> discovery in the 1960s of the possibility of this ministry.[7] With
> this experience and knowledge...a whole new area of co-
> operation between Spirit-filled doctors and Christians:
> congregations, fellowships, prayer-groups, is rapidly developing.
> There are general practices which operate on church premises,
> and an increasing number of young doctors work only part-time
> in order to devote energies to the local fellowship and
> community. At last we are beginning to see something of true
> holistic medicine: body, mind and spirit all being renewed by
> God the Holy Spirit.[8]

III. SPIRITUAL GIFTS CONTINUE

He writes, of course, as one who rigorously accepts the continuance
of the 'gifts of the Spirit' from New Testament times till the present
without any interruption, and in his book he traces the history of the
Spirit's operation in and through the church, whether in 'the
Northumbrian saints' in whom he had a special interest, or in the great
'Revivals of Religion'.

This leads eventually to a discussion of the assertion

> If the gifts of God the Holy Spirit—including miraculous
> healings—are still being poured out in the late twentieth century,
> then surely healing is ours of right.[9]

He cites Kenneth Hagin (of the Kenneth Hagin Evangelistic
Association 1975) for the view that on the basis of Galatians 3:13,
'Christ hath redeemed us from the curse of the law', taken in

conjunction with Deuteronomy 28:61 which says every sickness is a
curse of the law,
    You can Scripturally claim healing from any sickness.[10]
Colin Urquhart, 'who is one of the most respected leaders in the
charismatic movement', is quoted as reaching a similar conclusion, but
including the involvement of the medical profession; 'You have every
right to pray; to ask, believing his promise; to seek the good offices of
the medical profession. To believe God not only to alleviate the pain,
but remove the disease, whether it is physical, mental or emotional; and
to give you the healing you seek in the way he chooses.'[11]
Others, he says,
    can see no reason to involve medicine.[12]
But, he asks,
    If that is how it can always be done, then are we not negligent
    if we allow any sick to remain in our congregations?[13]
From this it would appear Gardner does not in fact endorse the claim
of 'healing by right'. Indeed he does not accept that even the evidence
of faith guarantees healing. And he summarily dismisses the dictum
proclaimed by some that 'You are healed although the symptoms have
not disappeared; disregard them' (p. 172)—
    Diseases are diagnosed principally on symptoms: if they persist
    the disease persists. It is as easy as that. Let us stop calling black
    white, ostensibly to protect the good name of the Lord, but in
    reality to get ourselves out of an embarrassing situation, and—
    even worse—from having to rethink our dicta. This view is not
    only worrying because it is dishonest but, worse, because it can
    be highly dangerous.[14]
He cites twenty-four Case Records covering a wide variety of
maladies. In eleven instances healing took place immediately upon the
ministry of prayer, or prayer and the laying on of hands, or (rarely)
anointing with oil. In the remaining instances healing was revealed
soon after the event by medical examination, or took place in stages
or gradually over a short period.

IV. STARK EVIDENCE

Included are two instances of people having been raised from the dead.
In the first (7.1) Gardner acknowledges that there was no medical
evidence to prove that the person was dead. It happened in a
missionary situation in Northern Thailand. A fifty year old woman who
had renounced her animistic religion and become a Christian believer
had disposed of the objects of her heathen faith and worship only to
be assured by her friends and neighbours that ill-fate would befall her.
It did! She became ill. And while the missionaries prayed for her

recovery and the local animist priest jeered at the evident judgment that had befallen her and their apparent inability to help, she died. The missionaries felt themselves to be in a corner, rather like Elijah on Mount Carmel (1 Kgs 18:19–39), and that all they could do was hand over the situation to God in prayer. After ten minutes the woman was heard to be speaking quietly and calmly. Her eighteen year old son asked her to whom she was talking and where she was. What they heard was evidently her part of a conversation with Jesus who was walking along with her. At one stage she got frightened and agitated when near to a pit demons tried to grab hold of her, but Jesus took her hand. She sat up, called out to the villagers individually by name and revealed some of their previously unknown secrets.

So accurate and devastating were these that the village priest's son fled, to return half an hour later and announce that he wished to become a Christian. (He is now an elder of the Church).[15] The second instance (7.2) took place in Chile, South America. A girl of thirteen or fourteen years of age had died. In this case there was a greater lapse of time and the corpse was already stiffening when the native Christian evangelist came on the scene. After he had prayed once, and again the second time, nothing happened. But when he prayed the third time the girl coughed, moved and was able to take food. Gardner uses these two instances as the most convincing proof that the miraculous gifts of the Spirit were not withdrawn after the first two generations of Christians.

The two most bizarre instances recorded by Gardner relate to cases of the filling or replacement of decayed teeth in answer to prayer during a Service of Worship and in circumstances where any kind of dental treatment was totally unavailable. In the first instance (9.1), as reported by a missionary, a small church was crowded with 150 villagers most of whom suffered great pain and discomfort from badly decayed teeth due to deficiencies in their diet. The evangelist and pastor of the church after prayer laid hands on as many as they could reach, and the others were asked to put their own hands on the place where healing was needed—their mouths. As the result the pain ceased and the decayed teeth were filled. The missionary was invited to inspect the mouths of those who had been healed and she testified,

these teeth have been filled. And the filling has the form of a silver cross set in each tooth. One little boy...can show me a tooth into which is set, delicately but quite distinctly, a golden cross.[16]

In the second instance (9.2), an eleven year old girl was in severe pain. After having been prayed for in the course of an evangelistic service,

We sensed a tremendous warmth and presence of the Lord and she said her mouth was burning, then we looked in and saw that where there had been dark decay and in some places no teeth at all, the decayed areas had been filled with beautiful stoppings with little silver crosses on, and in areas where there were no teeth at all she was sensing pain as well. (We subsequently found that new teeth had grown and she had completely, as it were, a new set).[17]

Gardner suggests three reasons by way of explanation. (1) Compassion for suffering, as in the Gospels. (2) As a witness to God's power in circumstances where there could be no other explanation. (3) As a demonstration of God's blessing on man's healing skills and techniques, as, he suggests, Jesus did on those occasions when he used clay or saliva. His purpose in using these instances is to demonstrate the intellectual integrity which he believes is necessary by taking account of, and being willing to give credibility to, God's work which might easily be dismissed as an embarrassment to, or contradiction of, our 'rational' view of the world.

Gardner takes serious issue with B. B. Warfield whom he regards as typifying the position of those who would explain away the church's failure in these days to manifest or exercise the power of God in spiritual gifts and miracles as in other days by asserting that God has withdrawn the gifts. But, he says,

He (Warfield) has misunderstood the function of the Holy Spirit's gifts[18]

when he asserted that their purpose was only

temporary support for the infant church[19]

which became unnecessary when the canon of Scripture was complete. In reply to Warfield's rejection of the healings at Lourdes as

not the direct acts of God,[20]

he cites the instance of a diabetic who suffered three strokes which brought him to the point of death. After receiving the Eucharist from a priest he was able to get out of bed and walk to the window. Shortly after this at the end of a Service of Ordination to the priesthood of a friend, the new priest laid his hands on the patient's head, and his ability to walk increased to the extent that he was now able to walk upstairs though he had still to use a wheelchair. Later, after a reluctant visit to Lourdes, he was able to abandon his wheelchair altogether and resume a full-time job. Here Gardner comments: (1) While the major problem—his heart condition—was completely cured, the diabetes remained. (2) The healing was not instantaneous but in stages. (3) The final step occurred in circumstances uncongenial both to the patient and his wife. And his conclusion is that

God does not work according to a template.... We must not try to stereotype God's work, least of all make acceptance of it conditional on its falling within the bounds of *our* presuppositions and *our* historic bulwarks.[21]

V. GARDNER'S CONCLUSIONS

His formal conclusions to his whole investigation are (1) Intellectual honesty demands that after all other possible medical explanations have been taken into account there are some cures beyond medical explanation. (2) In these cases the association of prayer cannot be discounted or regarded as mere psychological boost. (3) Such healings which occurred in the ministry of Christ and the church did not cease at the end of the Apostolic age. (4) Although Christ on the cross purchased physical health as well as spiritual redemption and adoption as God's children, the benefits of none of these can be fully realised during present life on earth. (5) Healing is not an automatic response to sufficient faith. It is in the sovereign will of God. (6) The Christian is entitled to ask for healing but subject to the condition 'If it is thy will'. (7) Intellectual honesty requires acknowledgment that only a small percentage of those for whom physical healing is sought by prayer actually obtain it. (8) A belief in the occurrence of miraculous healing today is intellectually acceptable (pp. 205, 206).

All of these conclusions are totally in line with the picture that emerged from our own survey of the Bible teaching and practice of healing. The significance of them is that they are endorsed by a qualified medical authority on the basis of personal, well-researched and scientific evidence.

VI. DOCTORS DIFFER

The conclusions reached by doctors Edmunds and Scorer (pp. 51–55) are not contrary to those of Gardner, but their emphases are different. They may be summarised thus:

1. While all processes of repair in the body are ultimately attributable to a divine source, and while God can and does sovereignly intervene as and when he wills, he normally works by 'natural' means.

2. In both the Old Testament and the New Testament miraculous events were 'signs' given to authenticate his special messenger at particular times, in particular circumstances, and for particular purposes. This is specially true in regard to Jesus as Messiah as shown by his reply to John the Baptist's question (Matt. 11:2–6).

3. There is no New Testament evidence that the power of miraculous healing given to the Apostles was intended to be permanent in the church. Moreover, the gifts listed by Paul in 1 Corinthians 12 consisted of miraculous and non-miraculous, but the Apostle's special commendation to the church was to seek the non-miraculous (1 Cor.

12:31).

4. The James 5 passage emphasises the fact that through faith we may and should bring all our needs to God in prayer, including physical sickness (Heb. 4:14–16).

5. In view of the covenant-relationship of God to his people should the 'prayer of faith' be regarded as applicable to any others than those who are 'of the household of faith'? If so, are 'healing missions', to which all and sundry are invited, in keeping with the biblical promise 'the prayer of faith shall save the sick'?

6. The Christian doctor must not be averse to abnormal intervention by God in response to the prayer of his people, nor, on the other hand, must he regard God as little more than an extra 'remedy' in the pharmacopoeia.

7. The general impression gained from the examination of the results of the work of faith-healers is that

> little which can be honestly said to be truly miraculous occurs today.[22]

Doctors Edmunds and Scorer add a number of significant considerations from their findings:

1. There appears to be no significant difference between the longevity of members of healing movements or Christian Scientists as compared with people in general.

2. While statistics are hard to come by, the number of 'spontaneous cures' and those attributed to faith-healing are significantly similar.

3. The vast majority of cures claimed by healing movements relate to functional conditions common in neurological and psychiatric departments of hospitals and being successfully treated by ordinary medical means.

4. It is often difficult for faith-healers, due to lack of medical training or experience, to distinguish between the effect of the mind on the body and what is truly inexplicable and therefore possibly miraculous.

VII. NO PRESCRIPTION

The problem remains, however, that beyond confirmation of what has already been accepted as the 'facts' of biblical revelation and experience, the conclusions of the doctors can provide no prescription as to the form or requirements of any 'ministry of healing' that may or should be practised today. Indeed, the formulation of any pattern of such ministry Gardner himself finds impossible:

> When I first met cases of miraculous healing…and became interested in what God is doing in this field, I decided that one day I would sit down with all the case histories I could collect

and identify the patterns. I would aim to elucidate God's criteria, find out the methods Christians should use and get some systematic guide-lines worked out. That is the standard method of medical investigation. However from the case records presented one thing is clear—there is no pattern.[23]

He then proceeds to catalogue all the anomalies or apparent contradictions that we have already encountered in the faith-healers' accounts and explanations of their procedures and results. His conclusion to this catalogue is,

Not only is there no pattern of method, there is no pattern for knowing who will be healed by God, or how it will happen.[24]

NOTES

1   V. Edmunds and C. G. Scorer, *Some Thoughts on Faith Healing,* Tyndale Press, London, 1956, p. 40.

2   *Ibid.,* p. 46

3   *Ibid.,* p. 8.

4   R. Gardner, *Healing Miracles,* Dartman, Longman and Todd, London, 1986, p. 3.

5   *Ibid.,* p. 15.

6   *Ibid.,* p. 37.

7   *Ibid.,* p. 59.

8   *Ibid.,* p. 64.

9   *Ibid.,* p. 155.

10   *Ibid.,* p. 156.

11   *Ibid.,* p. 157.

12   *Ibid.,* p. 157.

13   *Ibid.,* p. 158.

14   *Ibid.,* p. 172.

15   *Ibid.,* p. 138.

16   *Ibid.,* p. 178.

17   *Ibid.,* p. 181.

18   *Ibid.,* p. 133.

19   *Ibid.,* p. 104.

20   *Ibid.,* p. 104.

21   *Ibid.,* p. 108.

22   V. Edmunds and C. G. Scorer, *Some Thoughts on Faith Healing,* Tyndale Press, London, 1956, p. 54.

23   Gardner, p. 199.

24   *Ibid.,* p. 200.

17

THE HEALING MINISTRY CONGREGATION

Having examined the beliefs and practices of individual healers we now look at the teaching and work of modern healing movements. Of these there is a wide variety so it is necessary to be selective. It could be said that the whole Charismatic Movement is a healing movement because of its particular emphasis on the gift and work of healing. For this reason we have chosen three movements which would appear to be representative of different approaches to the matter—one which is carried on within the life and witness of a traditional Anglican congregation, the second which is the largest ministry of faith-healing being carried on within the Roman Catholic Church on an international basis throughout the American Continent, and the third which is centred in a thoroughly charismatic situation apparently with all the sophistication and financial resources of an American religious corporation.

I. THE HEALING MINISTRY

Canon A. J. Glennon developed his healing ministry over a period of seventeen years (1961–78) on the staff of St Andrew's Cathedral in Sydney, Australia. The work was centred in the Cathedral through what he calls the 'Healing Ministry congregation' which was a group consisting of members of the church who had a special interest in and concern about healing and which met weekly. His account of the healing ministry in his book *Your Healing is Within You* is in two parts.

The first is largely anecdotal and the second is
a scriptural exposition of the healing ministry.[1]
The substance of the latter part originally formed a paper submitted by
Canon Glennon as a member to a Synodical Committee of the Diocese
of Sydney which enquired into 'the neo-pentecostal movement and the
healing ministry'. The Canon claims,

As far as I know, this is the first time that both a pastoral and
scriptural presentation of this ministry has been offered in the one
book.[2]

The healing work of Canon Glennon is centred on what he calls the
'Healing Ministry congregation' which apparently is a particular group
of people within the Cathedral membership which he describes as

a team, a family, a community—one in which each person has
played his or her part in ministry.[3]

This 'congregation' meets each Wednesday evening for a Healing
Service. It would appear to be a 'congregation' within a congregation,
and therefore raises interesting questions as to what he means by 'the
church' when he declares:

The elders of the church represent the whole body of believers,
and so it is the faith of everyone that is drawn upon and
used...the person who is sick must have faith to come and ask;
and the faith of the church must be added to his faith that he may
receive the healing he needs.[4]

His reference to 'elders' obviously relates to James 5:14, but it offers
no explanation as to how elders are to be constituted in his Anglican
system. Furthermore, the responsibility of the elders is emphatically
stated:

In these circumstances (Jas 5) the elders of the church are to be
the channels of healing for the person who has called them; yet
there is no suggestion that they have a gift of healing.[5]

But then he seems to cast real doubt on the reality of his recognition
of the standing and responsibility of the elders when they appear to
have no place in his own personal practice of healing, and are
explained away by the device,

I, representing the elders of the church, have prayed the prayer
of faith.[6]

So that insisting on the necessity of the involvement of the faith of the
church in the work of healing, he claims that,

the elders of the church represent the whole body of believers.[7]

But even this is not the end, for, he goes on,

I represent the elders,[8]

so that 'the faith of the church' becomes 'the faith of the elders'
(representing the church), and then 'the faith of me' (representing the
elders), which can scarcely be said to be treating the Word of God with

real integrity.

Again, in Canon Glennon's account of his ministry, as in our previous interviews (Chapter 15), there is considerable divergence from the healing methods and effects of our Lord's ministry.

> There is one thing that needs to be said about divine healing generally before we look at it in more detail.... It is this: only a minority of people are healed at once. The majority of those who are healed find that this healing is progressive.[9]

Yet on the following page we read,

> Christ heals today in the same way as he healed in the days of his earthly ministry, because he is the same today as he was yesterday.[10]

Here surely is the same kind of dichotomy which we found in our interviews. Things are set down side by side and equated with others which appear to be quite different, and this makes it difficult to reach logical and clear conclusions. For example, speaking of the Gospel record of our Lord's healings, he says,

> These stories differ from one another, but each one makes a distinctive contribution to our understanding. They add up to this: Jesus healed, he always healed, he never failed to heal, and he healed them all.[11]

The latter assertion just does not square with the biblical facts. There were places where 'he could do no mighty work', that is, he could not and did not heal. There were occasions when he selected individuals for healing while he left others unhealed, for example, at the Pool of Bethesda where out of the 'multitudes' of those requiring and waiting for healing only one man was healed without so much as the question of faith even being mentioned!

In his account of his own experience the Canon does not claim to have a 'gift of healing'. He recounts how under the influence and instruction of Mrs. Agnes Sandford he received the 'fullness of the Spirit' ten years after his ordination to the ministry.

> I shall not go into details about her ministry to me, except to say that Agnes prayed deeply for me on three occasions. The end result was that I felt I was being *immersed* in the Holy Spirit. It was as though something like a dye had gone all the way through my being, in contrast to a stain or colouring that was previously only skin deep. I certainly knew that something wonderful had happened to me.... Following this wonderful experience I was quite different, and so was my ministry.... I found, too, that I could lay hands on people and pray that they be healed and they were healed; if not immediately, then in a progressive way.[12]

He believes that God gives a gift of healing to some:

> God has given such people a special endowment of spiritual

power by which they are able, in Christ's name, to lay hands on others to heal.[13]

In keeping with the plural form 'gifts of healings' (1 Cor. 12:9) in Paul's list of spiritual gifts, he believes

there can be different gifts of healing for various kinds of physical and mental disorders.[14]

And for himself this means

if I myself have any gift of healing, it is to do with fear. Because I understand that type of problem, I am able to relate to those who are sick with fear, and to pray for them effectively.[15]

But a 'gift of healing' is not necessary in all cases. For example, as we saw in reference to the ministry of the 'elders' in James 5, he says,

there is no suggestion that they have a gift of healing. True, they will have a gift of ministry of some kind, and with one or more it may be that of healing. But that would be incidental. The particular qualification they have in this situation is that they are the representatives of the church. And because they represent the body of Christ, God administers divine healing through them.[16]

In fact he goes farther,

Every Christian can share in the healing ministry, but some Christians will have a special calling to that work.[17]

II. BASIC PRINCIPLES

We now look at some of the particular emphases of Canon Glennon's theory and practice.

(i) The reasons for Christ's healing work and the commission to heal

The Canon observes a number of reasons for Christ's healing ministry. Some of these present no difficulty, for example, as

a sign of compassion...to draw attention to his work of redemption...to glorify God[18]

(though this must be said of all that he was and did),

to stimulate faith[19]

(though there is some question as to what constituted the nature of that faith, as we shall see). There can be no objection to Christ's healing being seen as means to a number of ends. It is when it is seen as an end in itself that difficulties arise. For example, it is equated with the 'work' which the Father sent him to do (John 4:34). But this 'work' is usually understood to mean the whole work of redemption. Again, it is equated with 'a fulfilment of prophecy' (p. 136), the prophecy being that of Isaiah as quoted in Matthew 8:16, 17. Here he asserts that Isaiah 53

in the view of some can only mean that healing is included in the atonement
though without attempting to enlarge upon or explain what this means. When people came to Christ for healing he responded, more often than not, without any comment about spiritual things. He never said, 'I am willing to heal you, but you must realise there is something more important'.[20]
But this scarcely does justice to the fact that on a number of occasions he did say to those healed, 'Go and sin no more', and in the case of the man brought by his four friends, Jesus drew particular attention to the fact that the physical healing was 'easier' and less important than the fact that the man's sins were forgiven.

But the Canon also sees Christ's healing work as in some special sense part of his purpose 'to destroy the works of the devil' since 'so far as Jesus was concerned, sickness was the work of Satan'[21], and, 'The positive corollary of destroying the works of the devil is extending the Kingdom of God'[22] which was 'The ultimate reason why Christ healed'.[23]

In asserting that by the mere fact of effecting physical healing Christ was 'extending the Kingdom of God', the Canon seems to have become the victim of his own circuitous reasoning.

> The ultimate reason why Christ healed was to extend the kingdom of God. Healing was only part of that work, but it *was* part and it was an *essential* part.... These reasons for Christ's healings were not personal to him alone but were, he said, to be the ministry that he and his disciples would have in common.[24]

But would it not be more correct to say that the purpose of Christ's healing, and that of his disciples, was not so much 'to extend the kingdom of God' as to reveal the glory and power of God as it was personified in the name and person of Jesus the Christ? 'It is obvious', he says, 'that our Lord did not look upon the healing ministry as being unique to himself because he committed the same ministry to his followers'.[25]

This commission he refers to the sending out of the Twelve (Matt. 10:1–16; Mark 6:7) and the Seventy (Luke 10:1–12) and from it he concludes,

> Evangelism and healing were to go hand in hand; healing was to be as normal a ministry as preaching the Word; they were spoken of and practised together. The followers of Christ were never sent out to preach but that they were also sent out to heal.[26]

On the other hand, from a general review of the recorded healings in the Acts of the Apostles, he concludes,

> it could be said that no specific commission to preach and heal was regarded as necessary in the early church. Its members were

all witnesses and they all had a ministry, and healing was an essential part of their witness and ministry.[27]

So that now the assertion is that every member of the church, that is, every Christian, was equally commissioned by the Lord to witness by both preaching and healing. Yet Paul roundly asserts that while there are a variety of gifts distributed among believers, 'not all have the same gift' (1 Cor. 12:4), and, in fact, he specifically asked the rhetorical question 'Have all the gifts of healing?' (1 Cor. 12:30) with the implication that the answer was 'No'. No more are all Christians, then, to be healers than are all to be 'apostles, prophets, teachers, workers of miracles, speakers with tongues, or interpreters' (1 Cor. 12:29, 30). So that it would appear that Paul was not aware of a 'general commission' to all believers to practise healing, and he is in direct conflict with the Canon's assertion that

the commission to the seventy disciples, with its ongoing authority could have been understood as a general commission to all disciples.[28]

On the contrary, it would appear both in the experience of the Lord himself and of the Apostles that the commission to heal was not general but rather given to particular people at particular times and probably for particular purposes. There is certainly no evidence in the New Testament that all believers exercised, or were capable of exercising, the power of healing.

Because of the difficulty which he himself has created by the assertion of a 'general commission' to heal, the Canon is obliged to treat the James 5 passage in a summary and altogether unsatisfactory way. It must be looked at in its New Testament context, he says, and he then proceeds to do so by asserting, without the slightest evidence from other Scriptures, in regard to the Lord's commission first to the Twelve and then to the Seventy that,

The equivalent of that today would be the elders and the general members of the congregation.[29]

But in the James passage it is not 'the congregation' which is called upon to exercise the healing ministry, it is specifically 'the elders'. So that far from being, on the Canon's analogy, 'a logical development of all that has gone before', and, 'a natural conclusion'[30], the James passage is a complete departure from the principle of the individual healer, and sets the healing ministry in a totally new context.

As was noted earlier, the Canon in fact makes no attempt whatever to deal in a realistic and credible way with the position of 'the elders'. Rather, like the other faith-healers in our interviews, he simply glosses over the office of the eldership set forth in the New Testament simply attaching to it whatever meaning and significance suits his purpose at the time.

(ii) The issue of 'faith'

In a chapter entitled 'Only believe', the Canon seeks to deal with the whole issue of 'faith' in the healing process. First, there is the 'prayer of faith', and here we have the startling assertion,

> to conclude a prayer with the proviso 'if it be thy will' expresses doubt right away.[31]

But, of course, it may express nothing of the kind, as is divinely manifested in our Lord's own prayer in the Garden of Gethsemane. The proviso, 'if it be thy will', far from expressing any doubt regarding either God's power to heal or his willingness to do so may, in fact, be, and usually is, a humble acknowledgement of our human incapacity fully to understand God's purposes; a sincere confidence in his sovereign wisdom and love; and a faithful submission to his 'good and acceptable and perfect will'.

It is indeed true that in his sovereignty God may grant a request that is pursued contrary to his will. The appointment of the first King of Israel, Saul, is a case in point. But the consequences of such an event usually prove to be, as one would expect, disastrous. More than once in the ministry of the author of this document there have been known those who learned this lesson in a particularly distressing way. For example, a mother whose child was sick and likely to die was rebellious against God's apparent will to take away her child, persisted in prayer that her desire that the child should be spared should overrule all other considerations. Only after many years of pain and distress for the child, for herself, for her home and family, was she convinced that God's merciful will, which seemed so cruel at the time, would indeed have been better, and that if only she had been willing, like Christ, to say 'nevertheless not my will but thine be done' the whole sad story might have been so different.

> Healing in the New Testament was always prayed for with complete assurance that it was going to eventuate, however serious the sickness or incapacity. It was never associated in thought or word with the proviso 'if it be thy will'.[32]

But, of course, as a matter of fact in one of the earliest cases of a leper seeking (*i.e.* 'praying') for healing by Jesus, he says 'Lord, if thou wilt, thou canst make me whole' (Mark 1:40). The father, too, who brought his convulsing boy to Jesus said, 'If thou canst do anything, have compassion on us and help us' (Matt. 9:22). But the Canon goes on,

> Our Lord's utterance 'not my will but thine be done' is, with respect, irrelevant, because it concerns suffering, not sickness.[33]

But surely this is a distinction without a difference, but necessary to sustain the unproven assertion in the next sentence,

> In any case, as far as healing is concerned, there is an express

promise which reveals God's will on this matter[34]
which presumably refers to the assumption that it is always God's will
to heal the sick. But even the Canon has to admit,

> If, on the other hand, it is reverently believed that the sick person
> has come to the end of his life span (and presumably this is
> reflected in the medical treatment), one no longer prays for
> healing. Rather does prayer accept the blessing of God
> appropriate to the circumstances.[35]

But you can't have it both ways, Canon! According to your earlier
assertion the *only* 'blessing of God appropriate to the circumstances'
is healing, since 'as far as healing is concerned there is an express
promise which reveals God's will on this matter'[36], that is, to heal. In
any case, at what point or by what means are we to determine,
according to the Canon's scheme, whether the sick person has come
to the end of his life span? At seventy years or seven months? Other
faith-healers would claim that it would be revealed to them by a 'word
of knowledge' (one of the 'gifts of the Spirit') rather than by
observation of the medical treatment. But however the situation may
be assessed, perhaps the Canon would agree that the distraught mother
should 'no longer have prayed for healing' for her child, in which case
the whole of his thesis dismissing the validity of the qualification 'if
it be thy will' would be demolished. His concluding words on the
matter are significant,

> When one acts in faith (*i.e.* in praying the 'prayer of faith' for
> healing) God guides and overrules.[37]

We would heartily agree, but what does this mean in face of a specific
promise always and in every circumstance to heal, as the Canon
asserts?

Turning to the question as to whose responsibility it is to exercise
faith the Canon concludes,

> There is no general rule.... Vicarious faith is effective when it
> complements the faith of the sick person. Conversely, unbelief
> in those being ministered to can render impotent even perfect
> faith in those who pray from the 'outside'.[38]

So that 'vicarious faith' is only complementary to the faith of the sick
person and can be undone by the unbelief of the patient. But we have
noted already that Jesus often healed without even the mention of faith
on the part of the patient, and, in fact, in at least two recorded instances
the person healed, far from exhibiting any faith whatever in the Healer,
was not even aware at the time of his identity. All intercessory prayer
implies faith on the part of one who prays on behalf of another. There
is nothing exceptional or dramatically extraordinary about such faith
in the case of healing. By its very nature the exercise of faith must be
personal. It is a foolish and unnecessary confusion of terms to speak

of 'vicarious faith' on the part of one person for another. The person
praying is exercising faith 'in the interests of' but not 'in the place of'
another. No more can I exercise 'vicarious faith' for another's healing
than I can do so for the salvation of his soul. According to the notion
of Canon Glennon it would seem justifiable to ask, Why didn't the
'vicarious faith' of Abraham, that outstanding exemplar of faith, save
Sodom and Gomorrah? The fact is, of course, that Abraham was
exercising real faith in his prayer for those doomed cities, but it was
not, nor could it be, 'vicarious faith'. The very idea is completely
foreign to Scripture.

Yet another doubtful assertion made by the Canon is this:
> In principle, the provision of God is there as soon as we believe
> and in proportion to our belief.[39]

But, according to the Lord Jesus Christ, faith as small 'as a grain of
mustard seed' may 'remove mountains'. And this hardly seems like a
pro rata proportion. When the distraught father brought his convulsing
boy to Jesus and prayed for healing, he said, 'Lord I believe, help thou
my unbelief' thus indicating that he himself was aware and ready to
acknowledge the smallness of his faith. Indeed, he was not even
convinced as yet that Jesus could help at all, for he said, 'if thou canst
do anything, have compassion and help us'. But Jesus did not say, 'I
can help you only to the extent and proportion of your belief', rather,
he said, 'If thou canst believe (at all?) all things are possible to him
that believeth' and he healed the boy at once (Matt. 9:22ff).

(iii) The analogy of preaching and healing

Perhaps one of the most perplexing aspects of the Canon's thesis is the
attempt (common apparently to many faith-healers) to make an
analogy between a universal commission to all believers to preach the
Gospel, and a similar universal commission to heal the sick. The
argument generally runs thus: the commission of Christ to preach the
Gospel was given to all believers. As the Gospel is preached the lost
are challenged to 'believe' for salvation. Some do believe and are
saved, many do not believe and, to all outward appearances at least,
are lost. Furthermore, the experience of salvation is for some a sudden
and permanent experience, while for others it is the end of a more
gradual process—'first the blade, then the ear' to use the words of the
Canon (p. 171). There is also a 'growth in grace and in the knowledge
of Christ', to use the words of Paul. The effectiveness of the whole
process is dependent upon the initial 'prayer of faith'—'God be
merciful to me a sinner'—followed by an ever deepening experience
of God's grace through the indwelling presence of the Holy Spirit
received at the 'new birth', and a continuing practice of prayer and
fellowship with God's people. Now, argues the faith-healer, the

situation in regard to the practice of healing is precisely parallel. But is it? No indeed, far from it!

To begin with, there is no general commission in Scripture to all believers to preach the Gospel. There is a general commission to all believers to be 'witnesses' to Christ by word of mouth and example of life. But such witness is to take a variety of forms according to the believer's particular abilities (Matt. 25:15); gifts (1 Cor. 12:4); opportunities (Eph. 5:15, 16); responsibilities (Eph. 5:22–6:9), etc. The commission to 'preach the Word' is a particular commission based on particular gifts (Eph. 4:11; 1 Cor. 12:28 N.B. 'some') which all do not share. This is the specific Scriptural authority for the preaching and teaching elder (1 Tim. 5:17) as distinct from the ruling elder (1 Tim. 5:17), though some share both responsibilities. Furthermore, it is clear that in the New Testament church certain individuals were 'called', 'appointed' and 'ordained' by prayer and the laying on of hands of the Presbytery (1 Tim. 4:14) to this particular office. This is indeed in keeping with the Lord's commission and appointment of the Twelve and the Seventy, and totally contrary to a general commission to all believers. Moreover, it was to those commissioned to preach the Word that the commission to heal was given in the first place (as indeed the Canon agrees), and in confirmation of this intent, it was 'the elders' to whom the sick members of the church were to appeal in the James 5 passage. Nowhere in the New Testament is there a single instance either of someone being commissioned to heal apart from the commission to preach the Word, or to be a ruling elder; nor is there a single instance of anyone doing so. Thus, it may be concluded that there is no general commission to all believers to heal the sick any more than there is such a commission to all believers to preach the Word. All indeed will by the use of the 'gifts' God has given them witness to his love and power, and in some cases this will be by the exercise of the 'gifts of healings'. If any are commissioned to heal the sick, it is only those who are commissioned to preach the Word, but the difficulty is that in the New Testament there is no such commission to any others than the original disciples.

The second point of analogy claimed by the Canon and other faith-healers is that as not all are saved to whom the Gospel is preached and the Word of life spoken, so it is not surprising that not all are healed for whom the 'prayer of faith' is offered. But of course again we have here fallacious reasoning. The Scriptures make plain in every place and in every instance that the absolute condition of salvation is the faith of the sinner who seeks it. There are no exceptions. 'He that believeth on the Son is not condemned; but he that believeth not is condemned already, because he hath not believed in the name of the only begotten Son of God' (John 3:18). It is absolute and final. Saving faith is the inescapable condition of salvation. But not so, as has been pointed out so often already, in the case of healing. Thus it is quite untrue to say that healing works on the same principle as salvation in terms of the response on the part of the recipient. If it did work on the same principle then all who believe would be healed. But in fact it is admitted by all faith-healers that not all who exercise faith are healed. The analogy therefore simply cannot be sustained.

On the question of the 'growth' process, as the Canon calls it, the analogy again fails hopelessly. It represents, in the first place, a complete failure to understand the distinction between 'justification' and 'sanctification'. Of course it is true that the process of 'being made holy' is one of growth and development. But the 'act' of justification is immediate and final—'He that heareth my word, and believeth on him that sent me, hath everlasting life, and shall not come into judgment but is passed from death unto life' (John 5:24). Now in the case of each of those who 'passed from death unto life' in the physical sense at the word of Jesus (Jairus' daughter, the widow of Nain's son, Lazarus) the effect was immediate, as indeed, in every case of the healing practised both by the Lord and the Apostles. To use the process of sanctification therefore as the basis for 'gradual' healing is neither logical nor Scriptural. And to suggest that conversion may be gradual is nothing short of heresy. The process leading up to the experience of salvation (conversion) is usually gradual often spread over many years, but conversion itself is 'an act of God's free grace'. There may indeed be a process of rehabilitation after, or as part of, healing by medical means, but there is no evidence of such a necessity in the case of any of the New Testament healings. For example, some who had never in their lives walked before were immediately, and without any rehabilitation whatever, 'loosed' and able to walk and leap without difficulty (Acts 3:8).

There is therefore no analogy whatever between the ministry of the Word and the ministry of healing in the New Testament. Any apparent analogy is based upon a superficial and inaccurate understanding or observation of such work.

III. OBJECTIONS TO HEALING

The Canon deals specifically with what he calls 'Four Common Objections' to the practice of healing: (i) the value of suffering, (ii) Paul's thorn, (iii) the cases of Trophimus, Timothy and Epaphroditus, and (iv) the will of God.

(i) The value of suffering

Here he distinguishes categorically between 'sickness' and 'suffering'.

The meaning of 'suffering' in the New Testament, as far as the Christian is concerned, is the persecution that comes from being a Christian. This is the broad and consistent theme and there are no exceptions.... As with the suffering of Christ, the use of the word in relation to the Christian is not in any way a reference to sickness.... Sickness is always sickness; it is never described as suffering. And we are to react to it quite differently.... Suffering is to be redemptive; sickness is to be healed.[40]

But is this distinction real? There can be no doubt that 'suffering' is a more comprehensive term than 'sickness'. Physical sickness is certainly a form of suffering, but suffering takes a variety of other forms as well, and both are seen in the Scriptures.

Whether it speaks of the suffering of bodily sickness (Matt. 17:15; Jas 5:13) or of moral temptation (Heb. 2:18; Jas 1:12), or, as often, of persecution (2 Tim. 3:10f), the New Testament proclaims that suffering has been overcome by Christ but not yet done away: through the life of faith it becomes a state of grace in which the believer can rejoice here and now, for it is the pledge of future glory (Acts 5:41; Rom. 8:17ff; Phil. 3:10; 1 Pet. 4:13).[41]

The point in seeking to make a clear distinction between 'sickness' and 'suffering' is, of course, to make possible the conclusion that 'suffering' may be the will of God for the Christian, but not sickness.

Suffering for the Christian is intended to be a redemptive experience by which we learn the obedience of trusting not in ourselves, but in God. This is the value of suffering, and its importance cannot be overstressed. Nowhere does the New Testament speak of 'sickness' in the same way.[42]

But, of course, precisely the same could be said of sickness in the life of the Christian, as has been demonstrated again and again in Christian experience both within and beyond the New Testament. The Canon declares,

Jesus suffered but he was not sick.[43]

But such a statement seems extraordinary in the light of the fact that it is one of the cardinal arguments of the Canon, as of many other faith-healers, that Isaiah 53:4, as quoted in Matthew 8:17, asserts that our Lord in his atoning work bore not only our sins but also 'our sicknesses'.

This prophecy comes from the Suffering Servant passage in Isaiah 53 and in the view of some can only mean that healing is included in the atonement.[44]

But it must then also mean that 'sickness' is part of the 'suffering' process. Indeed when dealing with this passage it is claimed categorically by some that the reference is to physical sickness and hence to the fact that healing of the whole man in redemption requires healing of bodily sickness. And again it might be asked, if Christ could only deal with the physical consequences of our sin—physical death—by experiencing death 'for every man', could he not only deal with the physical effects of sin—sickness—by experiencing sickness too?

But it is neither necessary nor desirable to press the point so far. The Scripture says, 'He was touched with the feeling of our infirmities and tempted and tried *in all points* as we are yet without sin' (Heb. 4:15), and if words mean anything it is plain that the Lord Jesus did suffer all the frailties of our human existence—hunger, weariness, pain, and distress—so that while there is no specific reference to his being 'sick' in body, there can be little doubt that 'the things which he suffered' included many of the afflictions which in human life are either the cause or the consequence of bodily sickness. To limit the meaning of 'suffering', therefore, in the New Testament to 'persecution' is unwarrantable.

Nor is the Canon consistent on the matter. When he illustrates Paul's assertion that suffering has a redemptive purpose, he uses the Apostle's reference to his 'trouble' in Asia in which he says, 'we were pressed out of measure, above strength, insomuch that we despaired even of life' (2 Cor. 1:8, 9). The commentators would seem almost universally to agree that the strength and sentiment of the words used by the Apostle could simply not be in reference to the riot in Ephesus where, it would appear, his own life was not in danger, but rather to

> grievous bodily sickness, which brought the Apostle to the gates of death...and it would be necessary to contemplate its recurrence (v.10).[45]

Indeed the whole tenor of the passage is that of a man ill to the point of dying who was restored in answer to the prayers of God's people. Such an interpretation of the passage would seem to be strongly supported by Paul's reference to his being 'troubled on every side' in 2 Corinthians 4:8, and his explanation in 4:10 as 'always bearing about in the body the dying of the Lord Jesus', and his further reference in 12:9 to his readiness in regard to his 'thorn' to 'glory in (his) infirmities'. From this particular example, chosen by the Canon himself, we can only conclude that the artificial distinction made between 'suffering' and 'sickness' is wrong and misleading. If, as he claims,

> suffering is to be redemptive and sickness is to be healed[46]

there are many Christians who are getting the worst of both worlds. Of course the saving truth of the matter is that 'whom the Lord loveth he chasteneth' and many a Christian tested in the fire of physical weakness, pain and distress has proved to be 'pure gold'.

(ii) Paul's 'thorn'

The Canon agrees that the incident of Paul's thorn is either the one exception which sets aside what is otherwise the rule in regard to

> our Lord's teaching and practice that only faith was needed for healing[47]

and this he rejects on the ground that 'the exception proves the rule', or else it had reference not to physical sickness at all but rather, from the analogy of Paul's understanding of the Old Testament Scriptures, to people: 'The inhabitants of the land...shall be as pricks in your eyes and thorns in your sides...'(Num. 33:55). This he believes is confirmed by Paul's statement 'A thorn was given me in the flesh, a messenger of Satan' (2 Cor. 12:7). The word 'messenger', he says,

> is always translated as a person, never an object, and it has no connection with sickness.[48]

Now this again seems a strange argument from one whose basic premise is,

> as far as Jesus is concerned, sickness was the work of Satan.[49]

Thus, the Canon quite illogically concludes,

> as there is no reason to think the 'thorn' was a sickness, this further identifies it with the 'suffering' syndrome,[50]

and hence

> it was a redemptive experience (p.160) in which the circumstances which led to the thorn and which prevented its removal were obviously unique to Paul and therefore cannot be applied generally to others.[51]

Having said all this, however, the Canon feels obliged to add,

> Notwithstanding what has been argued...we would accept that it is possible for a 'messenger of Satan' in the shape of sickness, not to be removed by God[52]

thus demolishing his own previous objections, but then adding,

> This means that if the person is not to be healed, this fact will be revealed by God (and thus) the sick person will 'all the more gladly boast of (his or her) weaknesses', as did St Paul, and will not continue to seek their removal.[53]

By all of which it would appear to be accepted, in direct contradiction to the former assertion of the Canon,

> Nowhere in the New Testament is sickness shown to be suffering which is beneficial[54]

that sickness may indeed be 'the messenger of Satan' used by God for the discipline and development of his faithful servant.

(iii) Trophimus, Timothy and Epaphroditus

The Canon argues that Epaphroditus (Phil. 2:25–30) was in fact healed

and therefore there is no case to answer. But, of course, the question
is not whether he was healed, but rather, why Paul or no one else
exercised the power of healing. With regard to Trophimus and Timothy,
the Canon comments

> There is nothing to say that Trophimus and Timothy had been
> prayed for, and there is nothing to say they were not subsequently
> healed.[55]

But this will just not do. For one thing, Paul actually recommended
medicine to Timothy for what appears to have been a recurring
complaint ('frequent ailments' 1 Tim. 5:23). Such advice seems
eminently sensible, but it clearly shows that, for whatever reason, the
Apostle made no attempt to heal his 'own son' nor did he suggest any
way by which effective faith-healing might have been obtained. Such
a situation seems nothing short of incredible if, as the Canon and others
contend, the practice of faith-healing was common in the church and
essential to the commission of the Apostle. Secondly, to suggest, as he
does, that these friends of Paul were not even 'prayed for' is so
outrageous as to be absurd, especially in view of Paul's statement in
2 Timothy 1:3 'without ceasing I have remembrance of thee in my
prayers night and day'.

Surely it would be much more simple and honest to say that
Epaphroditus, Trophimus, Timothy and Gaius represent the position of
many fine Christian folk who, in the good providences of God, are
called upon to endure all the hazards of normal life in terms of sickness
and its consequences, to seek whatever medicinal help may be
available for its relief, and with grace to accept and 'turn to account'
spiritually the experience so that God may be glorified, their own faith
and courage reinforced, and others challenged by their sincere and
convincing witness to the sustaining and triumphant power of the Holy
Spirit.

(iv) The will of God

This matter has already been dealt with so that it is only necessary to
note that the only attempt the Canon makes to answer the 'objection'
to faith-healing posed by the problem of God's will in the matter is to
make a number of generalised and unsubstantiated statements
regarding prayer and God's promises concerning it. He says, for
example,

> The view that 'there are magnificent promises in the scriptures
> to do with prayer', but that it may not be God's will for us to
> have them in reality, is a contradiction in terms[56]

But it may not be so. It is true that there are great, unconditional and
absolute promises in the Scriptures concerning God's loving and
eternal purposes. But it is also true that many of his promises,

especially in regard to matters of daily life and experience, are conditional or are related to more than one factor in the situation. The Canon himself admits this when for example, in a desperate attempt to account for the failure of some of God's promises to be fulfilled in particular cases, he attributes the cause to such factors as

the quantitative aspect of faith[57]

And, more importantly, as he had to admit in another place,

it is possible for a 'messenger of Satan' in the shape of sickness, not to be removed by God[58]

in order that his loving purposes of good might be effected towards his servant.

The conclusion which the Canon has drawn from consideration of the 'Four Common Objections' is,

It is clear that none of these four common objections can be sustained.[59]

But alas, it is often his answers to them which are neither agreeable to Scripture, reason, nor fact and therefore unsustainable.

IV. CONCLUSION

Canon Glennon in his account of the work of the 'Healing Ministry congregation' certainly attempts to face the issues commonly raised in regard to faith-healing with honesty and integrity. But, like the individual healers whom we have already considered, while he can provide a wealth of anecdote from his own and others' experience, his explanations lack cogency and consistency when he endeavours to interpret and apply the patterns and perspectives of the biblical scene. The problem lies not in the truth or validity of the events described, or of his description of them, but rather in his efforts to explain them in terms of biblical precedence and authority.

NOTES

Unless otherwise indicated quotations are taken from:
A. J. Glennon, *Your Healing is Within You*, Hodder and Stoughton, London, 1979.

1   p. 14.
2   p. 14.
3   p. 15.
4   pp. 31f.
5   p. 113.
6   p. 44.
7   p. 31.
8   p. 44.

9   p. 33.
10 p. 34.
11 p. 28.
12 pp. 100f.
13 p. 112.
14 p. 112.
15 p. 112.
16 p. 113.
17 p. 151.
18 p. 136.
19 p. 137.
20 p. 137.
21 p. 138.
22 p. 139.
23 p. 142.
24 p. 142.
25 p. 144.
26 p. 146.
27 p. 149.
28 p. 149.
29 p. 153.
30 p. 153.
31 p. 166.
32 p. 167.
33 p. 167.
34 p. 167.
35 p. 168.
36 p. 167.
37 p. 171.
38 p. 170.
39 p. 171.
40 p. 156.
41 S. Amsler, *Vocabulary of the Bible,* Ed. J. J. Von Allmen, Lutterworth Press, London, 1958, p. 414.
42 p. 156.
43 p. 155.
44 p. 136.
45 J. H. Bernard, *Expositors Greek Testament Vol. 3,* Hodder and Stoughton, London, 1903, p. 40.
46 p. 156.
47 p. 157.
48 p. 159.
49 p. 138.
50 p. 159.

51 p. 161.
52 p. 161.
53 p. 161.
54 p. 156.
55 p. 163.
56 p. 164
57 pp. 38, 163.
58 p. 161.
59 p. 165.

18

PRIESTLY HEALING

Dr Francis MacNutt, O. P. had wanted to become a doctor but his call-up for military service in 1944 prevented his entering University, though he worked in the Medical Department of the Army as a surgical technician. He later entered the Dominican Order and in 1956 was asked by a Protestant friend to heal his son's partial blindness which he felt unable to do. But some time later when he was teaching homiletics at the Aquinas Institute of Theology, he felt something was missing from his ministry. After much enquiry and attendance at various conventions and conferences, he met Mrs Agnes Sandford and the Rev. Tommy Tyson who in a five-day 'workshop' convinced him that the healing ministry should be part of the normal work of any minister.

> I was the first Roman Catholic priest to attend one of these schools of Pastoral Care and immediately saw that the basic teachings on healing were very much in line with the Roman Catholic tradition.[1]

He sees praying for healing in no way in conflict with the need for doctors, nurses, counsellors, psychiatrists or pharmacists. He acknowledges too that

> some prayer can have a psychological effect through the power of suggestion.[2]

Nevertheless, he is convinced that prayer for healing brings into play forces far beyond anything human factors can contribute. We base this summary of his teaching and practice on his first volume entitled *Healing*.

I. DIFFICULTIES ABOUT HEALING

Dr MacNutt sees the loss ('unbelief', as he puts it) of the practice of healing in the church as the result of five prejudices against it, namely: (1) Scepticism or revulsion—because of bad impressions made by faith-healers (p. 39), (2) Acceptance of suffering as a 'cross' to be borne as God's chastening or discipline (p. 41), (3) The mistaken belief that only 'saints' could exercise the power to heal (p. 43), (4) The emphasis on faith based on doctrinal belief regarded signs and wonders as no longer necessary to prove the truth of God's Word (p. 44), (5) Miracles became associated with 'primitive' thinking; they didn't really happen or could be explained by science or reason (p. 45).

But the reality and significance of miracles and healing is confirmed by Jesus in his own description of his ministry in Luke 4:16–22 as a fulfilment of Isaiah 61:1, 2, and by his message to John the Baptist when from his prison John sought confirmation of the Messiahship of Jesus, and when Jesus pointed to his healings and miracles as the evidence which John required (Luke 7:20–33). Besides, Dr MacNutt argues, the miracles are no longer regarded as intended to be 'proofs' of Christ's divinity and Person, but rather as manifestations of the character and actions of God (p. 53). Christ commissioned the Twelve and the Seventy to preach, teach, heal and cast out demons as he himself did. The Acts of the Apostles shows that the early church exercised the same gifts and powers (p. 55) and the ending of the Gospel of Mark showed that the commission was extended to all 'believers' (Mark 16:17, 18) (p. 8). 'The test of orthodoxy is not doctrine alone', he says, 'for doctrine remains incomplete unless it is accompanied by the power to make the doctrine come true in our lives' (John 14:12).[3]

II. THE CHURCH AND SUFFERING

He traces the changes in the church's view of healing from the second century when the early Fathers

> moved gradually from a wholehearted belief in healing...to a view that the body's suffering is preferable for the sake of the soul (St. Gregory in the fifth century).[4]

The Platonic, Stoic and Manichean philosophies regarded the body as a prison of the soul which hinders spiritual growth.

> An exaggerated model of the flesh warring against the spirit, the Spiritual Combat, tends to put the body in the category of an

enemy to be subdued through punishment rather than an ally to
be healed (p. 64). (But) Today...we find that psychology has
effected a return to the Hebrew view of man: man as a person
who is not separated into body and soul, but is a whole individual
whose emotions and body very much affect his mind and spirit.[5]
This attitude is reflected in the Roman Church's attitude to the physical
aspects of marriage as being primarily for the procreation of children;
and to the changes which have taken place regarding the sacrament of
the Anointing of the Sick which originally was regarded as a sacrament
of healing based on James 5 but became Extreme Unction or Last
Anointing and was regarded as a preparation for death, while in recent
times (since Vatican II) it has been restored (officially) to its healing
role.

Since praying for healing was no longer performed by the living
representatives of the Church, the priests, the people turned to the
saints to pray for their ailments. Mary, the Mother of God, in
particular was sought for healing at Lourdes and her other
shrines, which were really centres of healing.[6]

III. THE MEANING OF SUFFERING

Dr MacNutt deals with the 'apparent contradiction' in the Bible
teaching regarding suffering and our reaction to it.

Jesus tells his followers to bear their cross; yet, whenever he
meets people who are sick, he reaches out and cures them. Was
he inconsistent, or have his words been misunderstood?[7]

The problem is how to reconcile the merit of carrying one's cross with
the apparent cowardice of seeking healing. But he endeavours to solve
it by making the distinction between 'suffering' and 'sickness' which
we have already encountered in Glennon and Wimber.

The kind of cross that Jesus carried was the cross of *persecution*,
the kind of suffering that comes from outside a man because of
the wickedness of other men who are evil.... The suffering that
Jesus did not himself endure, and which he took away from those
who approached him in faith was that of *sickness*, the suffering
that tears men apart from *within*, whether it be physical,
emotional or moral.[8]

He sums up his view of suffering thus:

1. In general it is God's desire that we be healthy. Hence 'he will
respond to prayer for healing unless there is some obstacle, or unless
sickness is sent or permitted for some greater reason.'[9]

2. Sickness is in itself an evil, although good may result from it.

3. There comes a time for a person to die.

We should pray for light as to when to ask God to take away the sickness and when to pray for happy death—which is passing to a deeper life with God and not a tragedy at all.[10]

4. Some sickness may have a higher purpose. He mentions such examples as Paul's blindness at Damascus which brought Ananias to heal him by his receiving the gift of the Holy Spirit, and Paul's illness in Galatia which resulted in the Gospel being preached in that area as it might not otherwise have been.

It is interesting to note his readiness, unlike other faith-healers, while distinguishing between 'suffering' and 'sickness' to accept that sickness can serve a positive and constructive purpose in God's will.

IV. BASIC ATTITUDES TO HEALING (P. 115)

Here he reflects on a number of differing attitudes to healing.

1. Healing is simply man's responsibility and he has the resources to do so. This is faith in man.

2. Healing is possible but extraordinary. Here is faith in God's power to heal, but doubt as to his desire as a matter of course to do so. This is the view of many Christians.

3. Healing (through prayer) is ordinary and normative, but does not always take place when sought. This is the view of Dr MacNutt:

> Usually a man glorifies God more mightily in every way when he is healthy than when he is sick. Therefore, a man can and should pray to God with confidence for healing. Yet there are exceptions: sometimes sickness is directed toward a higher good, for the kingdom of God...consequently, healing does not always take place, even where there is faith.[11]

4. Healing always takes place where there is faith.

But these basic attitudes raise questions regarding the nature of the 'faith' that is entailed in faith-healing. Dr MacNutt provides the following principles: (1) My faith is in God—not in my faith. It may not be perfect or complete faith and there may be doubts or problems— 'Lord, I believe, help thou mine unbelief' (Mark 9:24), (2) The 'gift of faith' is not the same as the virtue of faith.

> The 'gift of faith' (1 Cor. 12:8, 9), or fullness of faith, is given to some but not all, Christians.... The 'gift of faith' is a ministry-gift which God imparts to help us pray with confidence...for a given intention.... The gift of 'the word of knowledge' is closely connected with the 'gift of faith'. Through the word of knowledge, God intimates to the person(s) praying that his will is to heal a particular person at a particular time.[12]

(3) The faith needed for healing can be in anyone—or no one. The faith can be in the person praying, the sick person or

> Sometimes it just seems that God wants to manifest his goodness

when *no one in particular* seems to have faith.[13]

V. TYPES OF HEALING AND OF PRAYER

There are four kinds of healing relating to the different types of sickness and their basic causes:

1. Sickness of spirit which is caused by personal sin.
2. Emotional sickness and problems caused by past emotional hurts.
3. Physical sickness in our bodies caused by disease or accidents.
4. Any of the above three can be caused by, or related to, demonic oppression.

Healing requires four related prayer methods thus:

1. Prayer for repentance (for personal sin).
2. Prayer for inner healing, for example, healing of memories (for emotional problems).
3. Prayer for physical healing (for physical sickness).
4. Prayer for deliverance (for demonic oppression).

In some instances any or all four of these may be required.

The last of the four categories requires fuller attention. Dr MacNutt distinguishes between 'exorcism' which he defines as *formal* ecclesiastical prayer to free a person *possessed by* evil spirits (which is rarely used), and 'deliverance' which is a process, mainly through prayer, of freeing a person who is *oppressed by* evil spirits. He is convinced, he says, of the reality of 'demonic oppression' by the tradition of the Roman Catholic Church's doctrine concerning the Devil as a

> living spiritual being, perverted and perverting[14]

and by his own experience. Whereas formerly he assumed the only way to treat psychosis was to refer the patient to a psychiatric or mental hospital, now he believes many such people can be helped through the 'prayer for deliverance' if the cause of the psychosis is demonic. This kind of prayer, he believes, should ideally be undertaken in conjunction with a psychiatrist if possible.

> I find that possession is rare, but people who are demonized, who are attacked or oppressed by demonic forces, are a relatively common occurrence.[15]

He specifies a number of signs which may indicate the need for 'Prayer for deliverance': compulsion, as in alcoholism, drug addiction, or self-destruction; the patient might feel the problem is demonic, though this could be part of the psychosis; the failure of prayer for inner healing to be effective might also indicate the need for 'deliverance'. However, the problem is such that the gift of 'discernment' is clearly necessary to determine the proper diagnosis and indicate the proper response. And the condition is such that only those who have been specifically called or gifted by God should attempt to deal with it since it may require special discernment, prayerful preparation, and unlimited time; it should be done in private rather than in public because of unhealthy curiosity on the part of spectators; and ideally it should be undertaken not by an individual on his own but by a team who would share a diversity of 'gifts' in dealing with the situation. In addition, it is important that after deliverance the patient should be filled with the Holy Spirit and with God's love; should be encouraged to break behavioural habits; should regularly participate in the study of the Word of God, prayer and the sacraments; and should become personally and actively involved in a Christian church or fellowship. Dr MacNutt makes a strong plea,

> For those who have had no experience in any kind of deliverance ministry.... I would only ask that you put it all on the back burner, as it were, until such time as you have a chance to see for yourself.[16]

VI. REASONS FOR FAILURE

Dr MacNutt lists eleven reasons as to why people are not healed as follows:

1. Lack of faith. General scepticism regards healing as no more than psychological process. Even those who do believe in it need their faith constantly deepened.

2. Redemptive suffering. At times God uses sickness for a higher purpose.

3. A false value attached to suffering. Most sickness is not redemptive.

4. Sin. No healing can take place until associated sin (if there be such) is dealt with.

5. Not praying specifically. The root cause must be discovered and prayed for, otherwise even healing obtained may be lost.

6. Faulty diagnosis. If the healer lacks discernment he is bound to fail. The cause must be properly discerned or we cannot know how to pray properly.

7. Refusal to see medicine as a way God heals. Physicians and medicines are the instruments God normally uses. To set healing by prayer in opposition to that by medicine is to create unnecessary suffering and mutual suspicion.

8. Not using the natural means of preserving health. Neglect to care for the health of the body, or to live a good life may make healing by prayer less likely.

9. Now is not the time. There is often a right time. But God may require us to wait.

10. A different person is to be the instrument. The wrong healer may have been approached.

11. The social environment prevents healing from taking place. Wrongful relationships must be put right first.

This list of reasons as to why healing does not take place in response to prayer raises a number of further questions especially in reference to some of the principles already enunciated by Dr MacNutt. For example:

1. It is understandable that modern philosophies and scientific scepticism might result in fewer people seeking faith-healing than might otherwise do so. But that could not explain failure to heal since, in fact, healing would not be sought. On the other hand, if it is implied that the degree of success is related to the degree of faith exerted either by the healer or the healed, this is contrary to the principle already stated that

the faith needed for healing can be in anyone or no one.[17]

2. As we have noted already, he does not seem to be quite sure about the distinction between 'suffering' and 'sickness'. This would also apply to reason 3.

4. Having already laid down the procedure for dealing with sin in his four types of prayer, and the responsibility of the healer through the gift of discernment to use the appropriate type of prayer in the right order, any failure must surely be occasioned not by the sin of the patient but by the ineffectiveness of the method used by the healer to deal with it. This would also apply to reasons 5, 6 and 11.

7. Here is a particularly difficult problem. In view of the fact that by definition faith-healing is healing that comes about in response to prayer apart from the use of medical, psychiatric or other treatments; and that in the New Testament healings no question of medical or other treatments arose either as part of the cure or as a follow-up requirement; it is difficult to understand how failure to be healed by prayer can be explained by failure at the same time to put confidence in, or persist in, medical treatment. Of course there need be no 'opposition' between healing by prayer and healing by medical treatment. As Dr MacNutt puts it:

> Medicine and prayer are not opposed, but the doctor, the nurse and the person with the gift of healing prayer all together form God's healing team (p. 265).... Sometimes God cures directly through prayer; at other times through nature, assisted by doctors who have learned how the body can be assisted to throw off the sickness that oppresses it (p. 267).... A similar relationship should exist between prayer for inner healing and counselling, psychology and psychiatry.[18]

But it can scarcely be satisfactory to explain the failure of one by the failure to use the other. Unless, of course, the healing process is understood to be a partnership between them. But this is not the accepted pattern or principle of faith-healing.

8. Here is a piece of extraordinary reasoning surely. The neglect by the patient to take the normal means of preserving bodily health may be a sound reason for laying the responsibility for his condition on the patient, and may therefore rightly demand of him repentance and a change of heart. But it can hardly be said to explain the failure of faith-healing to be effective. Did our Lord not say to the man at the Pool of Bethesda when he met him later in the temple after he had been successfully healed, 'Sin no more, lest a worse thing come unto thee' (John 5:14), which might seem at least to lay some blame on the patient for his condition. But it did not hinder his being completely healed.

9. This would seem to be the ultimate fall-back position of the faith-healer when the process appears to have been ineffective—God's sovereignty in the matter. And indeed it may be so. But the faith-healer cannot have it both ways. He cannot claim to have the gifts of discernment and knowledge to direct him infallibly as to what the divine will and purpose is, and then claim that failure to effect it is due to a misunderstanding or misapplication of the sovereign purpose of God. This would also apply to reason 10.

VII. PRACTICAL QUESTIONS

Dr MacNutt concludes his survey of 'Healing' by addressing a number of practical questions. We may summarise his answers to these 'Questions often asked' thus:

1. Every Christian may be used in faith-healing, but for ministers and priests it is an essential part of their calling, and some Christians are specially 'gifted' by the Holy Spirit for a ministry of healing. The proof of such a calling is the effectiveness of its exercise.

2. Physical phenomena such as heat, trembling or surge of power may and often do accompany the exercise of the healing gift.

3. Healing can be dispensed either by the individual or 'in community'. There is no fixed rule.

4. Praying for a patient 'at a distance' is difficult in respect of physical sickness, but less so in respect of 'inner healing' and of 'deliverance' from demonic oppression.

5. Other 'gifts' involved in healing are the 'discerning of spirits', the 'gift of faith', the 'word of knowledge' and 'miracle-working'.

6. The patient may be, and often requires to be, prayed for more than once, as taught by the Lord in the parables of the Importunate Friend and the Importunate Widow.

7. Leg-lengthening does happen, but what happens is not really leg-lengthening but changes taking place in the spine or hips which result in the equalising of leg-length.

8. Some faith-healing may be the result of 'suggestion' but most is due to a power vastly greater than any human powers.

9. In regard to 'psychic' healers, apart from divine power, there are natural powers of healing and 'life energy' which can be transmitted by the laying on of hands, and there are demonic powers, but to seek healing from anyone whose powers are connected with the demonic is likely ultimately to result in greater evil.

VIII. HEALING AND THE SACRAMENTS

Dr MacNutt, as one would expect, has a section on the relation of the sacraments of the Roman Catholic Church to healing. Reference has already been made to the developments in respect of the sacrament of Anointing with Oil (Extreme Unction), and in the section on 'The Churches Healing' we discussed the place of the sacraments with reference to healing in the Roman Catholic Church (see 'Sacramental Healing' pp. 150ff), and with reference to Dr MacNutt in the section 'Charismatic Healing' (pp. 159ff). It will suffice here, therefore, to recall his conclusion to his section on the sacraments thus:

> I think that the churches at large are undergoing the same kind of renewal and change of attitude that St Augustine underwent. In his early writings he held that healing was meant for the beginnings of Christianity but that Christians were not to look for a continuance of healing. Then his attitude changed and he frankly admitted in his book of 'retractions' that he had been wrong.... Wonderful things will happen through the sacraments as we learn to believe more in their potential.[19]

IX. CONCLUSION

We conclude in Dr MacNutt's own words from his second volume, *The Power to Heal*:

> Many of the things I have seen are so wonderful as to sound incredible to those who have not themselves experienced them. These saving actions of God include spiritual healings (such as being freed instantly from long-standing alcoholism), emotional healings (such as schizophrenia and deep mental depression), and physical healings (such as growths disappearing in a matter of minutes). For some these healings are immediate; for some they are gradual and take months, and for still others nothing at all seems to happen. But I would estimate that about 75

percent...are either healed completely or experience a noticeable improvement. Almost everyone regards prayer as a real blessing and experiences the presence of Christ in a very direct way.[20]

NOTES

Unless otherwise indicated quotations are taken from:
F. MacNutt, *Healing,* Ave Maria Press, Notre Dame, Indiana 46556, 1975.

 1   p. 13.
 2   p. 14.
 3   p. 60.
 4   p. 64.
 5   p. 73.
 6   p. 71.
 7   p. 78.
 8   p. 78.
 9   p. 84.
10   p. 85.
11   p. 117.
12   p. 126.
13   p. 131.
14   p. 212.
15   p. 216.
16   p. 230.
17   p. 131.
18   p. 269.
19   p. 298f.
20   F. MacNutt, *The Power to Heal,* Ave Maria Press, Notre Dame, Indiana 46556, 1977, p. 22.

19

'SIGNS AND WONDERS'

John Wimber, after many years of resistance to the work of faith-healers, joined the staff of Yorba Linda Friends Church in 1970. In 1974 he became founding Director of the Department of Church Growth at the Charles E. Fuller Institute of Evangelism and Church Growth. In 1977 he became the instrument of his wife's healing and was finally convinced that God's healing power is operative today. In May of the same year he became the founding Pastor of the Vineyard Christian Fellowship at Anaheim, but continued as a 'full-time Church Growth Consultant'. In 1984 he moved with 600 of the 4,000 members of the Anaheim Church back to Yorba Linda to open a new Vineyard Fellowship Church there from which his healing ministry and Conference lectureship has grown to international proportions.

I. THE WORK OF WIMBER

When we turn to the writings and the work of John Wimber and the Vineyard Christian Fellowship Church, we are in a somewhat different world from anything encountered so far in our survey of the ministry of healing. Here we are dealing with a highly organised and complex system of healing ministry which embraces the total range of human personality—body, mind and spirit; the total field of medical application to disease; and the total scope of human affliction whether from the natural effects of the fall of mankind or the invasion of demons from the spirit world.

He sets out the whole field of his healing ministry under five categories thus: (1) 'healing of the spirit', that is, healing spiritual sickness caused by sin; (2) 'healing of the effects of past hurts'—inner healing—that is, healing of hurtful memories and damaged emotions; (3) 'healing of the demonised and mental illnesses', that is, the external influence of evil spirits and the internal emotional disturbances they may create; (4) 'healing of the body', that is, the healing of illnesses (a) in which the structure or tissue of the body is damaged through accident or virulent and bacterial infection, or (b) which are the result of malfunction of organs as in certain heart diseases, ulcers or psychosomatic problems; and (5) 'healing of the dying and the dead', that is, comforting the dying or raising the dead (pp. 77, 78).

(i) Biblical principles and patterns

The system is based on principles and patterns of practice derived from both the Old and New Testaments, and especially from the practice and example of Christ and the Apostles. It assumes:

1. That miracles are as possible today as in Bible times. It rejects the view that miraculous gifts ceased after the time of the Apostles.

> There is a long tradition of theological thinking that believes miracles no longer happen. Most of them propose that scripture teaches the cessation of healing in the early church.... Dispensationalists...are the most ardent defenders of the cessation position.... Many Reformed and Lutheran Christians also teach the cessation theory of the gifts. Both Calvin and Luther (the latter changing his position in later life) thought the charismatic gifts ceased after the first century.... In contrast with many Protestant theologies, Roman Catholic theology asserts the possibility of modern miracles.[1]

2. That while suffering through sickness may play a part in spiritual growth, divine healing and the discipline of suffering are not mutually exclusive.

> Jesus understood sickness as an enemy of men and women. Its source was evil and from Satan's kingdom. The deepest sickness is sin, and all other consequences of sin, including physical sickness and poverty, are subordinated to that. This does not mean that every sick person who is prayed for will be healed in this life; but it does mean that forgiveness of sin is available to all, and for many there will be physical healing. In the age to come there will be complete healing of all who turn to Christ: the eradication of all disease and poverty, hatred and sin.[2]

It is noted that when the New Testament writers use the term 'suffering' they are usually referring not to sickness but to persecution and its consequences, whereas in this century the two are equated.

3. That God guides Christians not only through the four traditionally accepted means—a 'burden' or concern to do something, Scripture illuminated by the Holy Spirit, the counsel of others, and circumstances—but as in the Old and New Testaments through dreams, visions, prophecies and messenger angels.[3]

4. That in the New Testament healing is associated with repentance from sin and conflict with Satan and that it aids evangelism.

> It is a 'gospel advancer'.... The Third World students at Fuller (Theological Seminary) claimed it is easier to pray for people's healing than to tell them about Christ. In fact, they said, it is very easy to tell people about Christ after they have been healed. Scripture verifies this; notice how Christ frequently first healed the sick then proclaimed the gospel of the kingdom of God.[4]

5. That all Christians have been given authority to heal the sick just as they have been given authority to preach the gospel of forgiveness of sins (Matt. 9).

> In the Matthew passage the crowd was in awe that Jesus would heal the paralytic and forgive his sins. In response they praised God 'who had given such authority to men'. The implications of this passage seemed clear to me: Christians are commissioned by God to heal the sick. *I* am commissioned to heal the sick.[5]

(ii) Aspects of healing

Wimber deals at length with each of the five categories of healing already indicated above. Much of what he says relates to ground which has already been covered in our own survey but with interesting emphases.

> 1. 'The healing of our spirit, in which our relationship with God is renewed and restored, is the most fundamental area of healing'.[6]

Since, as Martin Lloyd-Jones put it,

> All the varied and complicated problems of the human race today, as they have always been throughout the running centuries, all emanate from just one thing, that man is in the wrong relationship to God. He is alienated from God. There is a state of warfare between man and God. That is the cause of all our troubles,[7]

the renewal and restoration of our relationship with God through repentance and redemption makes 'all things new' (2 Cor. 5:17). It does not remove all struggle, conflict or adversity, but the power of the Holy Spirit makes victory and endurance realisable.

> 2. 'I define inner healing as a process in which the Holy Spirit brings forgiveness of sins and emotional renewal to people suffering from damaged minds, wills and emotions'[8]

whether as the result of being born into a sinful world, wounded by others—parents, family members, friends, acquaintances, even strangers whether intentionally or not—or personal sin or failure. The essential elements in dealing with memories and associated hurts which hold back from true freedom in Christ, are repentance and forgiveness both in relation to ourselves and others, and learning to see past experience in the perspective of God's mercy and forgiveness—what he calls 'conversion therapy'.

4. On 'healing the body' he says,

Of the different types of human healing, physical healing is the most difficult for most people in Western civilisation to believe in; it appears far easier to pray effectively for spiritual or psychological hurts than for physical hurts caused by sickness or accident. Surely the influence of modern materialism and rationalism contribute to most people's scepticism about physical healings.[9]

Most of Jesus' healings, he says, related to organic disease, but

it is possible that many functional disorders were healed when Jesus ministered to big crowds (p. 145). Mental illness, in which personality and emotional disturbances result from brain disease, emotional factors or demonisation[10]

Jesus also regularly healed. It is important to note that Wimber encourages

most of the people whom I pray for to seek medical help, especially if they have a life-threatening disease.[11]

He does not regard physical healing necessarily as an immediate event since it may be complicated by emotional, psychological or demonic factors. Nor does he expect healing always to be accomplished by prayer on only one occasion. It may require several periods of prayer. Moreover, having commented on the four cases in the New Testament of those who were not healed, he says,

What makes those four instances of God not healing even more remarkable is that they involved men who were highly esteemed, gifted and mature Christian leaders. Explanations such as personal sin, defective faith or ignorance in those who were sick or those who prayed over them for healing are not plausible for these men.[12]

The explanation is, he believes, that God is selective about whom he heals.

5. With regard to ministering to the terminally ill or dying, he says,

For these people offering a false hope for healing brings unnecessary pain and deflects their attention from trusting in God for eternal life.... Telling the truth in the face of death is one of the most helpful things we can do for a terminally ill person. That way he or she can talk about it and work through their relationship with God.[13]

This raises immense problems, however. Indeed in his own practice it would appear that in the case of Rev. David Watson Wimber did precisely 'offer a false hope', though in the Introduction to his book he goes out of his way to deny it (see p. 171). Certainly according to Watson's account, he (the patient) believed he had been given a categorical assurance by Wimber that his cancer had been healed or would be healed. In any case, how is one to determine at what point the hope of recovery is false if, in fact, the prayer of faith is always to expect a positive result? With regard to 'raising the dead' he has little to say.

> In sum, raising of the dead was a dramatic and infrequent event in the New Testament, something that I believe is still possible today.[14]

But he records no instance of it in his own experience.

(iii) Healing of demonisation

It will have been noted that no reference has yet been made to the third category of healing. This is because Wimber's treatment of the matter of 'healing the demonised' is so explicit and different from anything that we have encountered in our investigation of the practice of faith-healing so far as to require examination in some greater depth. His section dealing with 'healing the demonised' is actually the largest single section of Wimber's book, and, as we shall see, dealing with demonic activity is a prevalent part of his healing ministry.

1. While at one time people attributed all kinds of things to the direct intervention of the devil, in the modern scientific age the activity, or even the existence, of the devil is treated generally with cynicism and disbelief. 'Yet I believe', Wimber says, 'that the understanding Jesus and the apostles had about the significance of Satan and evil spirits is so much a part of the New Testament that we cannot ignore their existence and influence'.[15]

On the other hand, Wimber says, belief in the supernatural and the occult is increasing. But

> Modern belief in the supernatural is losing its Christian roots; movements like Scientology.... Transcendental Meditation, Silva Mind Control, and parapsychology all claim to be based on a mixture of science and metaphysics. I believe these so-called New Age movements are conduits into Western culture for Eastern religions, the occult and direct demonic attack. They introduce people to supernatural experience while denying the source of great spiritual harm: evil spirits. Thus though many men and women are more open to supernatural encounters, often

they are unaware of the danger of encountering Satan and demons.[16]

The belief in Satan and demons was maintained throughout the history of the early church and of the Reformers. It was the purpose of Christ in coming into the world to destroy the kingdom of Satan and its evil works and to establish the kingdom of God. Jesus taught:

(1) God's reign came into the world in the person of Jesus (Matt. 12:28). (2) By repenting of personal sin and believing in Jesus Christ, men and women are redeemed from the world, the flesh and the devil, and they come under the reign of God's kingdom (John 3:5). (3) The kingdom of God is destroying the kingdom of Satan (1 John 3:8). (4) At the return of Christ, when he ushers in the fulness of the kingdom of God, Satan will be eternally destroyed (Matt. 13:36–43).[17]

The ministry of Jesus had two elements: *proclamation* of the good news of the kingdom and *demonstration* of its power through casting out demons, healing the sick and raising the dead. He commissioned the Twelve and the Seventy to do the same (Matt. 10:5–8; Luke 10:1–20), and by implication this commission extends to every believer (John 20:21–23).

2. Wimber concludes from the New Testament that there are two groups of demons: first, those 'reserved (*i.e.* 'bound') in everlasting chains under darkness unto the great day of judgment' (Jude 6); and second, those who are free to roam the earth (Eph. 6:12). He identifies from the Scriptures many characteristics of these demons: they have intelligence, they are spirits, they manifest themselves in different forms, they are malevolent, they know their own doom, they have supernatural strength, and they must bow to the authority of the name of Jesus. He believes that many of the problems—spiritual, psychological, physical from which people suffer and cannot find healing through medicine, psychiatry or even prayer—are caused by these demons. Satan attacks in three ways: by temptation through our 'flesh' or 'sinful nature'; by opposition through accidents, counterfeit supernatural gifts or other diversions; and by demonisation in which demons use physical affliction, moral weakness, or emotional problems to attempt to gain control of a person. Wimber says the Greek word means not 'demon-possessed' but 'to have a demon' or be 'demonised', that is, influenced, afflicted or tormented by demonic power but not 'possessed' or absolutely controlled by it. Demonisation may vary from mild to severe.

In mild demonisation, evil spirits exert power over people. This influence varies from harassment to more extreme forms of bondage[18]

which may result in blindness, hardness of heart towards the Gospel, apostasy and doctrinal corruption, indulging in sinful, defiling behaviour. Severe demonisation, represented by the Gadarene demoniac, produces much more serious results such as: epileptic-like seizures with convulsions or self-destructive behaviour; taking over almost complete control of the person invaded; unusual physical strength; a changed personality; strong resistance to the name or presence of Jesus; the ability to convey abnormal knowledge; causing the person to speak in voices or languages not their own; or moral depravity.

> Immediate deliverance from the evil spirit is possible for the demonised. For those whose mental illness is caused purely by demons, health is immediate. For those whose mental illness is more complex, they must go through a long and costly process of psychological healing.[19]

Christians can be affected or even controlled by evil spirits if they live in unconfessed or serious sin. Demons may gain a foothold in people's lives through such means as unrighteous anger, hatred of others or of self, revenge, unforgiveness, lust, pornography, sexual wrongdoing or perversion, drug or alcohol abuse or involvement with the occult, and may thereby open the door to the lives of others such as children, relatives or friends.

3. Demonisation may be resisted or deliverance from it gained by the use of the 'spiritual weapons' described by the Apostle Paul in Ephesians 6:10–18.

> We have been given total authority over demons. But this does not mean that we should be surprised when we encounter demons. God has equipped us for battle, and he expects us to use all the armour to advance the kingdom of God.[20]

This leaves the question as to how 'demonisation' is to be recognised or diagnosed. Wimber provides what he describes as

> an incomplete list of symptoms[21]

but the list would appear to cover almost every conceivable circumstance of mental, physical or psychosomatic disorder and to apply would demand a lengthy and exhaustive process of inquiry and investigation which is not evident in those instances which he describes in his own experience of dealing with demons. For example, his account of his dealing with a demonised Christian believer is as follows:

> At our first meeting a demon manifested itself through Bill, which was the first time something like this had happened to him. Bill's voice and personality changed, his face became contorted, and the spirit challenged my authority for being there...I said, 'Identify yourselves'. They said they influenced Bill towards using pornography, rage, self-hatred and practising masturbation.

I said, 'In the name of Jesus, leave Bill right now' (see Luke 10:17). At first the demons resisted my commands, so I prayed further and again told them to leave. After about thirty minutes of prayer, they were gone. Bill told me that for the first time in years he felt free from compulsions to sin sexually.[22]

He concludes his discussion of 'healing demonisation' by indicating three forms of deliverance apart from self-deliverance through commitment of every area of life to the Lordship of Christ, confessing and renouncing the particular area of sin or temptation in question, commanding the spirit in the name of Jesus to leave, and destroying all objects associated with the area of sin or temptation, *e.g.* books or occult material.

> Some people are too severely demonised for self-deliverance to be effective. This calls for other types of deliverance. Fraternal deliverance is when Christian brothers and sisters help cast out demons. Pastoral deliverance, ministry from pastors is helpful in more extreme cases of demonisation.... The last type of deliverance comes from people to whom God has given 'special gifts of discernment, revelation and authority to overcome Satan and evil spirits at their most profound levels of activity'.[23]

4. Wimber's description and analysis of 'demons' as exhibited in the Gospel accounts of the ministry of Christ are quite correct. Moreover, that Christ himself cast them out of human lives and gave his disciples power to do so effectively is equally clear. But a number of other important things are also clear:

Firstly, while demons could cause sickness and other physical disorders such as blindness, deafness, dumbness, fits, nervous disorders and even mental derangement, there was a clear distinction in the Gospels between sickness or disease and demon-possession or 'demonisation' (Matt. 4:24)! It is therefore highly dangerous and wrong easily or readily to identify physical or mental disorder with demon-possession unless there is other clear evidence.

Secondly, there is but one reference in the Acts of the Apostles to the casting out of an evil spirit (Acts 16:18). It was done by the Apostle Paul. Otherwise there is not a single reference to the casting out of demons by any other Apostle or anyone else.

Thirdly, the only references to demons in the New Testament, apart from those already referred to, occur in 1 Corinthians 10:20; James 2:19 and Revelation 9:20, but in none of these is there any connection either with demon-possession or with the casting out of demons. So that apart from the Gospels and one place in the Acts of the Apostles, nowhere else in the New Testament is there any reference whatever to demon-possession or to procedures for dealing with the phenomenon.

Fourthly, there is in the New Testament Epistles frequent reference to the conflict between Satan and the Christian believer. The believer is exhorted to 'resist the devil' (Jas 4:7; 1 Pet. 5:9), and to 'withstand' him (Eph. 4:27). But the answer to the power of Satan and his demons is not 'exorcism' (which belongs to the world of magic and the occult), but the disciplined and persistent use of 'the whole armour of God' described by Paul (Eph. 6:11–18).

Fifthly, there is not a single word of command or instruction to believers in the New Testament with regard to the necessity of (a) recognising, by means of spiritual gifts or otherwise, instances of demon-possession; or (b) using words of command or other forms of 'exorcism' (see pp. 19–23).

It would appear, therefore, that while the activity of Satan and his legions is persistent in the world and will continue to be so, with increasing vehemence as the age draws to a close, the phenomenon of 'demon-possession' was peculiarly associated with the ministry of the divine Christ on earth. It was a particular manifestation of the strength of Satan's reaction to Christ's work which, contrary to Satan's intention, furnished Christ with a particular opportunity to demonstrate his divine power and Lordship over the powers of evil as one evidence of his divine Sonship. That same power was extended to the Apostles through his personal commission to them and to Paul. This would appear to be the reason why there is no account of the need or use of this power ever having arisen in the New Testament apart from the ministry of Christ and the Apostles. It would therefore also appear that Wimber's approach to the phenomenon of demon-possession and its removal would require to be handled with the utmost caution.

The approach of modern psychiatrists too, even some of Christian conviction, seems a far cry from the biblical pattern. For example, Dr M. Scott Peck, Medical Director of the New Milford Hospital Mental Health Clinic, Connecticut, who has dealt with the whole subject of human evil in his publications, describes 'exorcism' as a psycho-therapeutic technique in which,

> the healer calls upon every power that is legitimately, lovingly available in the battle against the patient's sickness. First of all, exorcism, as far as I know, is always conducted by a team of at least three or more. In a sense the team 'gangs up' on the patient. Unlike traditional therapy, in which it is one 'against' one, in exorcism the patient is outnumbered.[24]

Exorcism sessions, he says, may last three, five, even ten or twelve hours. It is seen by exorcists as spiritual warfare which summons not only human resources but the power of God,

> as far as the Christian exorcist is concerned, it is not he or she who successfully completes the process; it is God who does the healing. The whole purpose of the prayer and ritual is to bring

the power of God into the fray.[25]
But having said this he acknowledges that

exorcism is indeed a form of brainwashing.... What prevents exorcism from being true rape is that, as with surgery, the individual consents to the procedure.[26]

He insists that exorcism is not a magical procedure.

As in psychotherapy, it makes use of analysis, of careful discernment, of interpretation, of encouragement, and of loving confrontation. It differs from traditional psychotherapy only as open-heart surgery differs from a tonsillectomy. Exorcism is psychotherapy by massive assault.[27]

Interestingly he too, like Wimber, distinguishes between 'deliverance' and 'exorcism'.

Deliverance is a sort of 'mini-exorcism' frequently conducted over the past two decades by charismatic Christians to treat people suffering from 'oppression' (defined as a sort of halfway state between demonic temptation—which charismatics would say we all undergo—and frank possession).[28]

In a footnote in which he discusses 'oppression' and 'deliverance' he says,

The charismatics generally are not dealing with true demons, but occasionally they catch a real fish![29]

In the struggle with the demonic, Peck says, many skills are required,

analytic detachment, compassionate involvement, intellectual formulation, intuitive insight, spiritual discernment, deep understanding of theology, thorough knowledge of psychiatry, great experience with prayer, and others.[30]

Since no one person can possess all these skills the involvement of a 'team' is 'absolutely necessary'. But it is inconceivable that even the 'two-man' teams which Jesus sent out could have exhibited such capabilities. Perhaps most strangely of all, Peck asserts

Ultimately it is the patient herself or himself who is the exorcist.[31]

With reference to two patients whom he witnessed being exorcised, he says,

Human free will is basic. It takes precedence over healing. Even God cannot heal a person who does not want to be healed. At the moment of expulsion both these patients voluntarily took the crucifix, held it to their chests and prayed for deliverance. Both chose that moment to cast their lots with God.[32]

But all this surely bears little or no relation whatever to what happened when Jesus dealt with the poor man from Gadara or when Paul set free the demon-possessed girl in Philippi!

(iv) Integrated model of healing

Over the years, and out of his own experience of the ministry of healing, Wimber has developed what he describes as 'an integrated model of healing'. The model is built upon six principles: (1) God wants to heal the sick, (2) the importance of corporate ministry, (3) our trust in God is demonstrated by action, (4) we are empowered by the Holy Spirit, (5) the importance of loving relationships within the Christian fellowship, (6) God wants to heal the whole person not just specific conditions.

A vibrant healing ministry is dependent upon: (1) a healing environment, that is,

> When the Holy Spirit is present and when people are full of faith in God for healing.[33]

Such an environment which increases faith for healing can be created particularly by worship which includes praise and prayer. (2) Time for ministry, that is, opportunity for people to learn how to pray for the sick by instruction and practice. (3) Training of others by those who are already experienced. (4) Lifestyle healing, that is, the ministry of healing as a lifestyle (or full-time occupation?) in which every event or circumstance may become an occasion for the exercise of the ministry.

Effective healing ministry involves: (1) Hearing, that is, being open to the Holy Spirit's leading and power. (2) Seeing, that is, observing the signs that the Holy Spirit is at work (or the absence of such signs). (3) Speaking, that is, words of love and encouragement to the afflicted, words of authority and command to the disease or its cause, words of prayerful petition, or words of counsel and direction. (4) Touching, that is, laying hands on the sufferer.

(v) The Ministry of healing in the congregation

In his Church Wimber has trained healing teams available at almost any time. They are trained at healing seminars. The folk who are trained must themselves 'have faith for healing' by which we take him to mean they must believe both that God has commissioned them and will be pleased to heal through them. This does not necessarily imply a spiritual maturity; nor is the gift of healing to be confused with

> a natural talent for healing.[34]

It means they are open and ready through the gifts of the Spirit to minister the power and grace of God in healing. It does not necessarily imply a permanent 'gift of healing' either, but that

> All may at different times experience any of the gifts.[35]

But, in fact, he says,

> Few Christians will be called or drawn by God to the ministry

and office of healing' (p. 202). But for those who do not have an on-going ministry of healing there are occasional anointings.[36] These anointings, or 'gracelets' (lit. *charismata*) as he prefers to call them, include a 'word of wisdom' or godly insight into a specific situation; a 'word of knowledge' or godly revelation regarding the facts about a situation of which a person had no previous knowledge, for example,

exact details of a person's life, to reveal sin, warn and provide safety, reveal thoughts, provide healing or provide instructions;[37]

the ability to discern spirits, that is,

the supernatural capacity to judge whether the motivating factor in a person is human, divine or demonic. It is supernatural insight into the source of spiritual activity;[38]

and the gift of faith, that is,

a mysterious surge of confidence in God that arises within a person faced with an insurmountable situation or need.[39]

In setting out a Biblical pattern of praying for the sick, on the basis of the 'gracelets' described, he delineates five steps to healing power: (1) The interview. This is not the taking of a medical case history, but an assessment of the situation in natural and spiritual terms. (2) The diagnostic decision, which determines the type of prayer needed to bring healing. (3) The prayer selection. For example, 'prayer directed towards God' (*i.e.* praying in 'tongues'), or 'words from God' (*i.e.* words of command either to evil spirits or to the condition itself, prophetic pronouncements, prayer of rebuke, prayers of agreement that comply with what the Father is perceived to be doing). (4) The prayer of engagement, in which people may respond with 'manifestations' physical, emotional or even demonic, that is, such manifestations as occur in religious revivals—apparent drunkenness, bodily writhing and distortions, prolonged and exuberant expressions of praise. The prayer of engagement may also involve helping the sufferer to experience forgiveness; to extend forgiveness to others for hurts received; to announce, by the authority of Christ, guilt or innocence; speaking to the condition (*e.g.* bidding twisted bones to straighten; conversing with demons and rebuking or expelling them). (5) Post-prayer directions, that is, counsel and instruction to the healed. He concludes the whole matter thus:

I believe that if the Old and New Testaments are going to be a source of constant reforming power in the church, the doctrine and practice of divine healing must be brought into contact with them. That was a fundamental presupposition in this book.[40]

II. COMMON GROUND

There is a good deal of common ground in the experience of the three healing movements which we have examined. For example,

1. Each is based on the exercise of the gifts of the Spirit by those who are engaged in the ministry of healing. That is to say, while each of the writers insists that the work of healing is not effected by them, but by the Holy Spirit, nevertheless, they are the agents of healing through the endowment of spiritual gifts on the basis of Paul's catalogue of gifts in 1 Corinthians 12 (Glennon p. 4; MacNutt p. 5; Wimber p. 10).

2. Each acknowledges that not all who are prayed for, or ministered to, are healed although each insists that the ministry is a continuance of the work of Christ and the Apostles (Glennon p. 3; MacNutt p. 5; Wimber p. 4).

3. Each claims that all believers are commissioned to preach and heal even though Paul insists that not all believers have the same gifts (Glennon p. 6; MacNutt p. 2; Wimber p. 3).

4. Each insists on the necessity of the exercise of faith in 'the prayer of faith' for healing though they distinguish between the normal exercise of faith (personal or vicarious) by others and the 'gift of faith' required by the healer (Glennon pp. 8, 11; MacNutt p. 5; Wimber p. 9).

5. Each wrongly makes an analogy between the commission to preach the Gospel and to heal the sick (Glennon p. 11; MacNutt p. 2; Wimber p. 3).

6. Each unsuccessfully attempts to make a distinction between 'suffering' and 'sickness' for the purpose of concluding that 'suffering' may be the will of God, but not 'sickness' (Glennon pp. 15ff; MacNutt pp. 3f; Wimber p. 2).

7. Each divides sickness into the same four or five categories (Glennon p. 5; MacNutt p. 5; Wimber p. 1).

III. WIMBER DISTINCTIVES

Each, of course, has distinctive features which in the case of the other two have already been discussed. Now we must look more closely at the ministry of Wimber whose teaching and practices have created or brought to light some of the most serious questions in regard to the charismatic approach to healing.

(i) Healing and evangelism

The first problem surely arises out of his use of healing primarily as a means—perhaps *the* means—of evangelism. Hence his term 'Power

Evangelism'. Power Evangelism is evangelism effected not by the preaching or *proclamation* of the Word of God alone, although it is an essential element, but rather by the *demonstration* of the power of God which becomes the opportunity to present the Word to the one who has been healed, and creates the readiness and ability for the right response to be made by the healed. 'Power Evangelism', he says, 'was one of the most effective means in the early church.... [It] is that evangelism which is preceded and undergirded by supernatural demonstration of God's presence.'[41]

Wimber's approach to the whole matter of healing is determined by what he would call his 'worldview'. That worldview stands in deep contrast to the twentieth century materialistic or secular worldview of Western society.

> The assumption of secular minds is that we live in a universe closed off from divine intervention, in which truth is arrived at through empirical means and rational thought. Inherent in the modern Western worldview is a desire to control everything—people, things, events, even future events.[42]

By contrast

> The Christian worldview makes room for mystery in the relationship between the spiritual and material worlds. For example, [it] sees some illness as caused directly by demons and other illness having physical causes. Instead of being forced to the extremes of empiricism or animism, Christians see *the possibility though not the necessity* for supernatural intervention in all earthly experience.[43]

That 'supernatural intervention' is manifested in two directions—the activity of God, and the activity of Satan.

> Satan's captivity of men and women has many facets, denial of final salvation being his primary goal. But there are other types of dominion: bondage to sin, physical and emotional problems, social disruption, demonic affliction. Our mission is to restore those who have been taken captive as a result of Adam's fall.[44]

On the other hand, God is sovereign and intervenes in the affairs of the universe, and of mankind, according to 'the pleasure of his own will', as the Reformers would have said. He did so most significantly of all in the death and resurrection of Christ.

> Two fronts, two kingdoms, two economies had hit head on. And in the resurrection and ascension, Christ came out the Victor, Satan the loser. It was in this, the ultimate power encounter, that salvation was secured for all men and women who place their faith in Christ.[45]

That ultimate power-encounter of Christ with Satan is to be reproduced in the daily conflict with Satan in the life of the Christian believer.

Many Christians do not adequately recognise that though Christ's victory is irreversible, its application to everyday events is ongoing. Satan is still alive and well, even though his time on earth is limited.... There is a war yet to be fought, an enemy still capable of inflicting great harm—if we allow him to.[46]
Part of that 'harm' is done through 'demonisation' of individual lives. And the remedy lies in the power of
the Holy Spirit, the go-between God, who holds the key to power encounters.[47]
That the remedy fails to happen so often may be due to the fact that the Christian's worldview may be undermined by the Western worldview as the result of which he consciously or unconsciously denies the possibility of the supernatural, for example, in supernaturally inspired dreams, visions, or revelations, or the reality of 'signs and wonders' in the present time. Or his worldview may be so affected by Western rationalism that while he acknowledges that signs and wonders may happen, he consigns them to the irrational. But,
Clearly Jesus envisioned a group of people—his disciples—who would perform not only the same but even greater miracles than he did. The only limitation for receiving this power is lack of faith: '*Anyone* who has faith in me.... '(John 14:11,12). It was Christ's intention that the kingdom of God be spread in the same way that he spread it—through power evangelism.[48]
As a pertinent illustration he notes that having failed to accomplish his mission in Athens by his preaching and disputation—'a *few* men became followers of Paul and believed' (Acts 17:34)—the Apostle changed his tactics in Corinth—'When I came to you, brothers, I did not come with eloquence or superior wisdom.... My message and my preaching were not with wise and persuasive words, but with a demonstration of the Spirit's power, so that your faith might not rest on man's wisdom, but on God's power' (1 Cor. 2:1, 5). And as the result of *demonstration* being added to, or substituted for, *proclamation* '*many* people in this city' believed (Acts 18:10).
Wimber claims that while Western evangelicals acknowledge the necessity of signs and wonders to authenticate the divinity of Christ and the authority of the Apostles, they generally refuse to accept the continuance of them beyond the first century.
This diminishes the effectiveness of Christ's example for us, discounting much of what Christ intended that we do. What Christians—including evangelicals—are often left to follow is a good moral example, not a dynamic, Satan-conquering Lord. This results in overly intellectual disciples—certainly not a people who cause demons to tremble.[49]
But Wimber goes even further. He suggests that with the development

of early twentieth century Pentecostalism
> The conservative evangelicals claimed that the gifts ceased in the early church, that Pentecostalism was a serious error, perhaps even demonic.[50]

Thus, he believes, conservative evangelicalism has largely lost out both on the benefits of the healing ministry and on the effective evangelism which are both the product of the manifestation and exercise of God's power in signs and wonders.

Now there can be no doubt that people were brought to faith in Christ by the demonstration of his divine power, and why not? But there is no evidence in the New Testament that Jesus used such 'signs and wonders' as an evangelistic method, and certainly not that he used them as his primary method of evangelism. Nor is there any evidence that the Apostles or evangelists of the New Testament church did so either. His explanation of Paul's change of method at Corinth, in contrast to that in Athens, is a misinterpretation of the Scripture. For the contrast that Paul himself made was not between preaching the Gospel, on the one hand, and working wonders, on the other, but rather between the weakness of human knowledge or philosophy and the power of the simple 'word of the cross'—'Jesus Christ and him crucified'. As G. G. Findlay put it,

> All through, he opposes the practical to the speculative, the reality of God's work to the speciousness of men's talk.[51]

Or again,

> Right from the beginning Paul had wished to ground his converts in the divine power and to make them independent of human wisdom. That was why he had made no attempt to employ rhetorical arts, but had contented himself with the simplest approach. That was the reason for his concentration on that message which was so unpalatable to natural men, the message of the cross.[52]

But Wimber's problem arises from the fact that he and his Movement have redefined the 'Gospel'. In the New Testament the good news of the Gospel is that 'whosoever believeth in him (Christ) should not perish but have everlasting life' (John 3:16). The answer of Paul and Silas to the Philippian jailer's question 'What must I do to be saved?' was 'Believe on the Lord Jesus Christ' (Acts 16:31). The Good News was that men could be saved by faith in Christ alone—'By grace are ye saved through faith' (Eph. 2:8). And this was the great liberating truth restored at the Reformation, that faith in Christ alone was both necessary and sufficient for salvation. But the Wimber Movement would appear to require something more. For example, in the account by Graham Banister of a personal interview at a Conference in Sydney, Australia, in 1990 with Dr Jack Deere, one of the Wimber team, and

the leading theologian of the Movement, we find the following:
> Jack Deere then commented, 'I used to be just like you'.... Then
> he added, 'Thinking the gospel was simply justification by faith'.
> I responded, 'Are you saying that the gospel is more than
> justification by faith?' 'Yes', he said. 'What would you add to it?'
> I asked. 'Deliverance', he said. Then I asked, 'What do you mean
> by Deliverance?' He explained, 'Things like demons and healing
> and.... 'Pausing for a deep breath, I said, 'So let me get this
> straight. You would add as an essential part of the gospel things
> like the exorcising of demons and healing?' He nodded. I
> continued, 'Sort of like what John Wimber was saying last night
> at the evangelistic rally that it's the 'complete package'—the
> word and the works of Jesus'. 'Yes', he said. 'But you're not sure
> exactly what should be included?' I asked. 'No', he said, 'not
> yet.'.... After this we chattered on about a few other things but
> I remained stunned that one of the leading minds, if not the
> leading theological mind in the Signs and Wonders Movement
> did not know what was the gospel.[53]

'Signs and Wonders', it would appear, is not only the method of
evangelism, it is 'the Gospel'!

(ii) Healing and 'prophecy'

A second problem in the Wimber system is his theory of the 'word of
knowledge'. Other faith-healers speak of the 'gift of discernment', by
which they mean a God-given capacity in a particular situation to
discern what may not otherwise be evident to reason or observation.
With Wimber it is a much more complex matter. In fact it is not so
much an enhanced ability to understand or interpret the circumstances
or symptoms of the case, but really falls within the sphere of the 'gift
of prophecy'.

> A word of knowledge is God revealing facts about a situation
> concerning which a person had no previous knowledge. An
> example of this is God giving someone exact details of a person's
> life, to reveal sin, warn and provide safety, reveal thoughts,
> provide healing or provide instructions. The discerning of spirits
> is the supernatural capacity to judge whether the motivating
> factor in a person is human, divine or demonic. It is supernatural
> insight into the source of spiritual activity.[54]

This discernment he explains comes through 'inspirations', dreams and
visions, impressions ('a deep knowing in one's spirit'), Scripture
verses, or pains in the body (corresponding to the pains of the person
to be healed). In an appendix to Power Healing he gives an analysis
by a Social Anthropologist (Dr David C. Lewis) of the phenomena of
'words of knowledge' as exhibited at a Wimber training conference at

Sheffield in 1985.

Dr Lewis notes the similarity of some of the 'words of knowledge' to those derived by spiritualistic mediums from telepathy or clairvoyance, though he believes the Wimber form to be more specific. He also sees the Wimber phenomenon as less open to the possibility of fraud, and not using objects or 'inductors' as mediums do. He believes Wimber's (or his associates') words of knowledge are not attributable to 'statistic probability'. While it may be of a different kind from that which takes place between close friends or relatives, he says, it may still be open to explanation in telepathic terms. As people are identified as those whom God wants to heal, and are prayed for, physical manifestations of the Holy Spirit's presence are observed, such as shaking, laughing, crying or stiffening of the body, which are reminiscent of the times of the Wesleyan and other 'revivals' (or even the 'apparent drunkenness' of the disciples on the Day of Pentecost). Lewis comments,

> In subsequent sessions there may have been more expectancy of seeing such behaviour and so the element of psychological suggestion cannot be ruled out for later meetings even if it is difficult to account for phenomena at the first 'clinic' by such theory.[55]

Nor does he accept that while emotions are obviously involved, such behaviour can be explained by 'emotionalism'. Again, while some of the physical phenomena manifested closely resemble trancelike or hypnotic states, such a theory cannot account for the whole range of phenomena exhibited, nor can it account for the accuracy of some of the words of knowledge spoken, or the behaviour of those referred to. Nevertheless,

> It is clear from scripture that real signs and wonders can be done by 'false Christs' and 'prophets of falsehood' (*e.g.* Matt. 7:22; Mark 13:22; Acts 8:9; Rev. 13:13), and also the name of Jesus can be invoked improperly but effectively by non-believers (Acts 19:13–16). Subsequent history confirms that healings and wonders can be brought about in the names of other gods and of demonic powers.[56]

Doris Collins, for example, is a necromancer and clairvoyant who has been exercising psychic powers publicly for over forty years. As an entertainer she has exhibited her skills on theatre platforms before huge audiences in many countries. She has worked through radio phone-in programmes. She has participated in experiments conducted in conjunction with the *Sun* newspaper. And she has been investigated by Polly Toynbee of the *Guardian*. Although she says,

> I was born a Christian, and I still acknowledge my Christian faith, but I have learnt that there is no exclusive path to

knowledge. I am also a spiritualist[57]
the Bible categorically forbids her activities. 'Let no one be found
among you...who practises divination or sorcery, interprets omens,
engages in witchcraft, or casts spells, or who is a medium or spiritist
or who consults the dead. Anyone who does these things is detestable
to the Lord' (Deut. 18:10–12 NIV). Yet her latest book teems with
instances of her having received and imparted 'facts about a situation
concerning which (she could have) had no previous knowledge',
which, of course, is precisely Wimber's definition of 'words of
knowledge', together with some of the same sources of such
knowledge as he describes, and acts of healing which are
indistinguishable from many of those described by Wimber as
instances of 'power healing'. She says,

> The techniques of clairvoyance and healing are altogether
> different, but in my case I know that I often use my clairvoyant
> ability to help me with my healing. Sometimes a patient will tell
> me he has something wrong with one part of his body, when I
> know that his pain emanates from a different part.[58]

Apparently it is often by her clairvoyant powers that she identifies
those who are in need of healing, and the specific nature of the
complaint. As the late Roger Cowley, a former member of staff at Oak
Hill College, London, put it,

> if we take seriously the scriptural statements about false prophets,
> sorcerers and the like, we cannot simply say, 'So-and-so was
> healed, so it must have been the Holy Spirit'.[59]

(iii) Other problems

But there are other serious questions too. For example, in a three-hour
interview, an account of which has been published, with 'three leading
evangelicals' in Sydney, Australia prior to a 'Spiritual Warfare
Conference' held there in 1990 by John Wimber and a team of his
'Signs and Wonders Ministry', the following results came to light:

1. Of the two hundred Downs-syndrome children for whose healing
Wimber had prayed only one showed signs of partial healing, that is
0.5%. Wimber confessed to have no idea as to why this malady should
be so resistant. Moreover, failure to provide Christian doctors with
cases to verify which had been healed during the Conference raised
doubts as to the genuineness of the miracles claimed.

2. Whereas in his books Wimber claims to be carrying on the work
of Christ and the Apostles, when faced with the obvious differences
between the results obtained by him and them, he replied that through
Jack Deere he had come to understand that his miracles fit into the New
Testament pattern not at the point of Christ and the Apostles, but in 1
Corinthians 12–14, the gifts of healing (of which, of course, there are

no examples with which to compare).

3. When challenged about the distinction he makes in his book between 'natural' evangelism and 'power' evangelism, he acknowledged that the book was imbalanced and that it was not written by himself but compiled by Kevin Springer from his lecture-notes and tapes and had not been read by himself before publication.

4. While claiming to accept the infallible and sufficient authority of Scripture in all matters of the Christian life, he also admitted that the ministry of gifts (especially the 'words of knowledge') added significantly to the Scripture as the authoritative voice of God.

5. Questioned about the references in his books to charismatic conversions and healings effected by Roman Catholics or opponents of evangelical faith, he accepted that healing in the name of the Virgin Mary was wrong, but pleaded ignorance of some of the examples given in his books.

6. Although he acknowledges the centrality of the cross in theory as the moment of crisis in the battle between God and Satan, in fact victory over Satan is to be seen in the display of God's power in fresh revelations and miracles of healing which are therefore an essential part of the Gospel. To receive redemption through faith in Christ entails not only belief in Christ's finished work, but in his continuing work through the miraculous exercise of the 'gifts of the Spirit'.

7. Although he declares his belief in the authority and power of the Scriptures, he gives an apparently more important and essential place to new revelations received on the personal level by means of dreams, visions, voices or intuitions. In this regard Jack Deere was most specific:

> Satan understands the strategic importance of Christians hearing God's voice so he has launched various attacks against us in this area. One of his most successful attacks has been to develop a doctrine that teaches that God no longer speaks to us except through the written word. Ultimately, this doctrine is demonic even (though) Christian theologians have been used to perfect it.[60]

8. During the conference there was little evangelism in the sense of proclaiming the great truths of the Gospel, rather people were invited to believe on the evidence of what they had seen in the miracles performed, thus confirming the contrast between 'proclamation' and 'demonstration', that is, between 'natural' and 'power' evangelism.

9. While claiming that it is God's desire to heal all who are sick, Wimber at this conference (apparently in contrast to other conferences) indicated that not all would be healed, nor would all be healed instantly.

10. The so-called 'third wave of the Holy Spirit' (the first was

Pentecost and the second the charismatic movement of the 1960s), which is predicted to come in this century, and which C. Peter Wagner, Professor of Church Growth at Fuller, would identify with the 'signs and wonders' ministry, Wimber believes will unite conservative evangelicals and charismatics, not on the basis of theology but of 'power evangelism'.

> Perhaps the next stage of the Holy Spirit, one affecting conservative evangelicals, will come with different models of how the charismatic gifts should function, such as in power evangelism.[61]

The unity thus achieved, since it will be based not on theology but on charismatic experience, he would see, presumably, as embracing both 'reformed' and 'non-reformed' Christians.

(iv) Gunstone's questions

John Gunstone is an Anglican parish minister with personal experience of the Wimber ministry. He has written a sympathetic and supportive but serious and searching assessment of what he calls 'The Wimber Phenomenon'. Gunstone writes of Wimber with affection and appreciation expressing his conviction that through Wimber and his ministry, (1) we are being given a new vision of what it means to be an evangelistic church; (2) we are being shown that congregations can grow and plant new churches if they are open to God; (3) we are being confronted afresh with the challenge of charismatic renewal, and (4) we are encountering the Pentecostal spirituality of the growing churches of the Third World. But he nevertheless poses real questions to which he seeks for real answers.

1. *Should we expect signs and wonders to follow the preaching of the Gospel today as in the New Testament?* Pentecostal teaching, he says, insisted on the association of healing with the preaching and acceptance of the Gospel. The 'signs and wonders' ministry is a development of this teaching. But while in the sovereign grace of God signs may follow the preaching of the Word,

> Power Evangelism cannot be programmed[62]

that is, it cannot be guaranteed, and indeed, it could easily become a distraction from the real purpose which has to do with sin, guilt, grace, forgiveness and salvation by faith in Christ rather than physical or psychological healing.

2. *Does the 'signs and wonders' ministry have a theology for those who are not healed?* Gunstone acknowledges that in his early visits to this country Wimber may have given the impression that he did not give sufficient weight to the possibility or, even the necessity, of receiving God's grace through sharing in the sufferings of Christ. But this he believes Wimber has corrected in a later booklet entitled

Kingdom Suffering (1988) where he says,

> We have no right to presume that unless God heals in every instance there is something wrong with our faith or his faithfulness.[63]

3. *Is the use of 'words of knowledge' in the Wimber-Vineyard meetings justified scripturally?* While Gunstone accepts that 'words of knowledge' are one of the gifts listed in 1 Corinthians 12:8, he expresses serious reservations about its use especially in large audiences, and he is persuaded that

> Only Wimber himself and one or two of his team seem to be gifted with real words of knowledge in open sessions[64]

whereas, in practice all the members taking part in his 'clinics' are encouraged to exercise the gift.

4. *Do we have to abandon our Western worldview if we are going to see signs and wonders?* Again, while Gunstone acknowledges the difficulties that arise from our scientific and cultural Western worldview in accepting the reality of divine intervention and demonic activity, nevertheless, he admits, 'I believe that God is sovereign over all that happens, and that he can and does intervene in our world when it is necessary for his will to be fulfilled.' But, 'I do not believe we should be trying to force on contemporary western Christians a worldview which is contrary to what they know is true in other ways'.[65]

And with regard to dealing with demonic activity he says,

> Certainly he [Christ] treated many illnesses as if they were caused by demonic agencies, because that was what they were to him. He would not have been a man of his age if his diagnosis had been based on modern medicine. But that does not mean that he would have treated them all in the same manner if he had been born in the twentieth century instead of the first.[66]

5. *Does the Wimber-Vineyard ministry imply a demonology that goes beyond what our understanding of the New Testament texts requires?* While Gunstone acknowledges that people do find release from serious problems, including illnesses both physical and mental from the 'authentic' exercise of 'deliverance', his answer to the question seems to be 'yes'. He notes that charismatics tend to blame all sorts of troubles on the devil rather than on themselves or those concerned. He recalls that while Jesus did cast out demons, this was not the general pattern of his healing ministry. He points out that many illnesses which are often identified with demonic attacks have strong psychosomatic associations. By a strange irony, he says,

> The fascination of the occult, masonry, spiritualism, and so on, has brought the need for deliverance even to technological man.... But we should remember that those who have turned to Christ, repented, been baptised and filled with the Spirit have

already stepped outside the realm of darkness. Satan can do little more than occasionally disturb them.[67]

NOTES

Unless indicated quotations are taken from:
J. Wimber, *Power Healing,* Hodder and Stoughton, London, 1986.
1   pp. 30f.
2   p. 35.
3   p. 43.
4   pp. 60f.
5   p. 66.
6   p. 82.
7   p. 84.
8   p. 95.
9   p. 139.
10   p. 147.
11   p. 151.
12   p. 163.
13   p. 175.
14   p. 177.
15   p. 113.
16   p. 286.
17   pp. 114f.
18   p. 123.
19   p. 125.
20   p. 136.
21   p. 136.
22   p. 128.
23   p. 138.
24   M. S. Peck, *People of the Lie,* Rider, London, 1988, p. 186.
25   *Ibid.,* p. 186.
26   *Ibid.,* p. 187.
27   *Ibid.,* p. 188.
28   *Ibid.,* p. 193.
29   *Ibid.,* p. 193.
30   *Ibid.,* p. 199.
31   *Ibid.,* p. 197.
32   *Ibid.,* p. 197.
33   J. Wimber, *Power Healing,* Hodder and Stoughton, London, 1986, p. 185.
34   p. 200.
35   p. 201.
36   p. 203.

37 p. 204.

38 p. 204.

39 p. 204.

40 p. 245.

41 J. Wimber, *Power Evangelism,* Hodder and Stoughton, London, 1977, p. 16.

42 *Ibid.,* p. 77.

43 *Ibid.,* p. 87.

44 *Ibid.,* p. 27.

45 *Ibid.,* p. 33.

46 *Ibid.,* p. 33.

47 *Ibid.,* p. 43.

48 *Ibid.,* p. 60.

49 *Ibid.,* pp. 108f.

50 *Ibid.,* p. 138.

51 G. G. Findlay, *Expositor's Greek Testament Vol. II,* Hodder and Stoughton, London, 1901, p. 777.

52 L. Morris, *Tyndale New Testament Commentaries, 1 Corinthians,* Tyndale Press, London, 1958, p. 53.

53 G. Banister, *John Wimber, Friend or Foe?,* St. Matthias Press, London, 1990, p. 24f.

54 J. Wimber, *Power Healing,* Hodder and Stoughton, London, 1986, p. 204.

55 *Ibid.,* p. 264.

56 R. Cowley, *Signs, Wonders and Healing,* Inter-Varsity Press, Leicester, 1989, p. 93.

57 D. Collins, *Positive Forces,* Grafton Books, London, 1991, p. 23.

58 *Ibid.,* p. 168.

59 R. Cowley, *Signs, Wonders and Healing,* Inter-Varsity Press, Leicester, 1989 p. 93.

60 M. Thompson, *John Wimber, Friend or Foe?,* St. Matthias Press, London, 1990 , p. 18.

61 J. Wimber, *Power Evangelism,* Hodder and Stoughton, London, 1977, p. 130.

62 J. Gunstone, *Signs and Wonders,* Darton, Longman and Todd, London, 1989, p. 96.

63 *Ibid.,* p. 100.

64 *Ibid.,* p. 103.

65 *Ibid.,* p. 106.

66 *Ibid.,* p. 106.

67 *Ibid.,* p. 111.

20

PASTORAL PRINCIPLES

We must now seek to formulate the biblical principles on which the pastoral practice of faith-healing is to be based. Some general principles may first be recognised:

1. God's original purpose for mankind was perfect health and wholeness, but the 'fall' into sin changed the condition of mankind physically, mentally, morally and spiritually, and also that of his environment, both of which will be fully restored by the redemption of Christ, but only at the end of the age and the return of the Lord.

2. All sickness is the consequence of mankind's fall and sinfulness.

3. Some disease is the direct result of sinful living or of abuse or neglect of the body, mind or spirit.

4. Generally sickness is not to be attributed to personal or particular sins.

5. There are at work in the created world evil powers or 'spirits', under the control of Satan, which may affect the natural processes of the environment and attack human beings by means of the physical, mental or emotional aspects of human personality or circumstance.

6. God is sovereign in his authority and power over all things and will ultimately restore the whole of creation to his perfect plan. Meantime, he may intervene at any time and in any situation to accomplish his purposes of grace and judgment, but normally he operates through 'natural' means, that is, so far as healing is concerned, through human means enlightened and enabled by medical science and

its progressively developing healing techniques where these are available.

I. HEALING IN NEW TESTAMENT TIMES

There would appear to be three distinct lines of approach to healing in New Testament times:

1. The practice as established by the Lord Jesus Christ and continued by the Apostles though with reduced frequency;

2. The exercise of the 'gifts of healing' by individual church members as implied in 1 Corinthians 12:9, 28, 30 but not illustrated; and

3. The new procedure described and advocated in the Epistle of James.

Much modern-day faith-healing would appear to be based on, and to combine aspects of, each of these three patterns.

(i) The practice of Christ and the Apostles

We have seen that the practice of Christ and the Apostles was clearly the standard procedure during the period of the Gospels and Acts. Modern faith-healing claims the example and commission of Christ to his disciples as the basic justification and pattern of its practice. But this seems a doubtful claim since the modern practice of faith-healing, in so far as it can be generalised, bears little relationship to the fourteen characteristics of Jesus' healing which we noted at the end of chapter 2 (p. 24). Scarcely a single feature of Jesus' healing or that of the Apostles, is found in modern faith-healing. Its very purpose is different from his in that whereas his healing endeavours were intended to convince men of his glory and power, and thereby lead them to saving faith in him, the faith-healer's purpose is primarily, at least so far as the patient is concerned, to secure physical health and relief from the pain, distress or hopelessness of his physical or mental condition, with the bonus of some psychological or spiritual benefit added perchance.

But, as a general rule, the healing is not immediate or complete, often the necessity of convalescence is insisted upon, and frequently there is a relapse of the condition, sometimes with fatal results. Further visits to or by the healer and further treatments are common. Often the effects of the healing are not obvious to others, or even to the sufferer at least immediately. Rarely, if ever, can the sufferer be offered relief without his being in the presence of the healer at the time of the ministration of healing, except where 'prayer-cloths' or other devices are used. Failure to effect any immediate physical improvement in the sufferer's condition is frequently covered over, or compensated for, by the promise or expectation of psychological or spiritual benefit. The use of psychological or symbolic aids such as anointing or laying on of hands is common. Responsibility for success or failure is often pinned on the faith of the sufferer. And seldom, if ever, are physical organs, limbs, or faculties restored to their normal condition or function.

The word of divine authority by which immediate and permanent cures were effected in the New Testament times seems to be lacking. Exciting claims are made by some faith-healers, and while they often prove difficult to substantiate, or to refute, there is no doubt that in his sovereign purposes God does deign to manifest his divine power in miraculous ways from time to time, but it certainly cannot be said that the incidence of such eventualities is to be compared with the regular pattern of events in the time of Jesus and the Apostles. Clearly the pattern of healing as practised by the Lord and the Apostles changed with the end of the Apostolic era, and there is nothing in the Scriptures to warrant the claim or the expectation of its continuance. Its express purpose declined as the written Word of God became available to the church, and, in the opinion of many, ceased when the Scriptural witness and authentication of the church and its ministry made it no longer necessary.

In the New Testament healings 'faith' was not a decisive element. It is true that Jesus was greatly pleased to find evidence of faith on the part of some who sought or received healing, and commended it warmly even to the extent of crediting them with having contributed to the healing by such faith—'Thy faith hath made thee whole', or, 'I have not found so great faith, no, not in Israel'. But in no recorded case did the work of healing by Jesus or the Apostles depend on the faith of the sufferer, and certainly none ever failed to be healed because of the weakness or absence of faith. But in modern faith-healing the position is fundamentally different. The healer, in fact, in praying for the sick must do so 'in faith'. His prayer must be 'the prayer of faith'. And the sole ground on which he can offer healing to any is that of his own faith in the promises and the power of God. While most faith-healers deny that the effectiveness of healing rests upon the faith of the patient, nevertheless, sadly, the failure of healing is too often attributed to the failure of faith on the part of the patient. In the case of Christ and the Apostles the question of failure never arose, nor did the necessity of 'faith' on the part of the healer because he was the Son of God exercising the divine power, and the Apostles exercised the same power by his specific commission.

(ii) The exercise of 'gifts'
The exercise of the gifts of healing as implied in 1 Corinthians 12:9, 28, 30 presents many problems. To begin with, there is no other

Scriptural reference to these gifts as such. There is no example given of any who exercised them, nor is there any instance in the New Testament of their being exercised. Might we then conclude that Paul mentions them among the 'spiritual gifts' because he himself as an Apostle did heal in the name of Jesus, though only on five recorded occasions? Furthermore, while he himself exercised the gift, he never claimed to have received it, and he seems to have had very strong feelings regarding the relative importance of the gifts. He exhorts his readers, for example, to 'covet the best gifts', but then goes on to speak of 'a more excellent way' pointing to the primary importance of the gift of 'love' (1 Cor. 12:31; 13:1). And again, while urging his readers to 'desire spiritual gifts', he adds, 'but rather that ye may prophesy' (1 Cor. 14:1). It would appear that for Paul, next to love the most important gift was that of 'preaching'. Certainly it is beyond question that while Paul did set much store by the exercise of the 'gifts' in general, he was at pains to discourage the abuse of, or unsatisfactory indulgence in the use of, the more spectacular gifts like that of 'tongues' which only had their place when exercised under proper restraints. And the reason for this was obvious, since being spectacular their use would be specially open to undesirable curiosity or improper use.

How is the fact to be explained that there is nowhere recorded in the New Testament a case of healing effected through a member of the church claiming to possess or exercise the 'gift of healing', apart from the Apostles? There are two possibilities, one, that it simply did not happen; the other, that it was so common and normal that there was no need to mention it.

The first possibility, that healing effected through the exercise of the 'gift' of healing by members of the church did not happen, apart from the Apostles and a few others who are named, seems not unlikely. In the Corinthian Church, for example, there was so much controversy and division over many things including the exercise of the 'gift of tongues', that in such a volatile situation it seems incredible that the gift of healing could have been exercised without also becoming an occasion of comment one way or another by the Apostle. Or again, in Paul's correspondence with Timothy he has much to say about the responsibilities of ministers and elders. He speaks of the importance of sound teaching and preaching (1 Tim. 4:14–16), of faithful prayer and intercession (1 Tim. 2:1), of wise discipline (1 Tim. 3:15), of spiritual zeal (1 Tim. 6:11, 12), and summarises them in 2 Timothy 4:2. But there is not a word about healing—no command or exhortation to Timothy as the minister; no obligation upon the elders; no reference to the exercise of any gift by members of the congregation. The same is true of Paul's letter to Titus, and these two letters are generally regarded as being the touchstone of church administration as the era of the Apostles came to an end. Every aspect of the work of the minister, elders and members of the congregation is dealt with, but there is not a single mention of the subject of healing. As we noted already, the silence of Scripture does not in itself establish or preclude a doctrine or practice, but it cannot be unreasonable to deduce from these letters of Paul to Timothy and Titus, on which so much of our church discipline and practice is based, that healing was not regarded by the great Apostle as a primary or definitive aspect of the work of the ministry or such an essential element in the life of the congregation as the modern 'signs and wonders' concept would suggest. Indeed it was in one of these very letters that Paul advised Timothy to use medicine ('wine') for his chronic stomach complaint without the least reference to the possibility of 'miraculous' healing.

Moreover, there is no evidence in the New Testament that the 'gifts' of 1 Corinthians 12 would continue to operate beyond the time of the Apostles or those to whom they would commit them. There is no doctrine of 'Apostolic Succession' in the New Testament other than that of the succession of those who 'continued in the apostles' doctrine and fellowship, in the breaking of bread and of prayers' (Acts 2:46).

The second of these possibilities, that it was so common and normal that there was no need to mention it, seems remote for if the practice of faith-healing was of such considerable importance in the church as it appears to have been in the ministry of the Lord and the Apostles, it must surely have been taken notice of by the Apostles in their correspondence. For example, Paul writes with much enthusiasm of the 'work of faith, and labour of love, and patience of hope' of the Thessalonian Christians (1 Thes. 1:3), yet there is not a word about their prowess in faith-healing. The church in Philippi had a special place in the affections of Paul, and his letter to the Christians there is full of thanksgiving and appreciation of their practical faith and generosity, but again, not a word about faith-healing. Indeed, it is in this very letter that we learn of the almost fatal illness of Epaphroditus without any reference to the exercise of the healing gift even by the Apostle or anyone else (Phil. 2:27).

The Epistle of James is surely convincing evidence that by the time of its writing the gifts of healing were unknown through the *diaspora* to whom he writes, hence his instruction regarding a totally different means of healing.

We may summarise the features of the 'gifts of the Spirit' thus:

1. They are to be distinguished from 'natural' gifts or talents, charms, or the use of ritual or relics.

2. They are either supernatural capacities bestowed by the Holy Spirit or natural abilities enriched and empowered by the Holy Spirit

in particular circumstances or for specific purposes.

3. They are bestowed according to the sovereign purposes of God on particular individuals; not all the gifts are given to each or every believer.

4. There is no recorded instance of their use in the New Testament apart from the Apostles except Ananias and Philip.

5. Some were evidently intended to be permanent (*e.g.* apostles, prophets, evangelists, pastors and teachers) and others occasional in their use.

6. There is no declaration in Scripture regarding their withdrawal after the time of the Apostles and they appear to continue to be manifested in the edification and extension of the Body of Christ.

7. They are not marks of spiritual superiority but of increased capacity and responsibility for witness to Christ and service to others by those who possess them.

(iii) The procedure in James 5

Does James 5:14–18 establish the form of the ministry of healing for the church? The answer would appear to be in the affirmative and generally accepted as such by those who practise faith-healing. Indeed, as we have seen, the answer of faith-healers to the question 'On what do you base your healing ministry?' is almost universally and immediately, 'James 5' even though, as we have also seen, their practice is often not in keeping with the teaching and pattern of this passage. It is clear in this passage that the ministration of healing is to be done in private by the 'elders' (plural) of the local congregation at the request of the sufferer, the request presumably being made either by himself or someone on his behalf. There is no suggestion whatever of a 'Service of Divine Healing'. There is no suggestion that the procedure should involve any other than the elders of the local church.

This raises the problem of the validity of 'Healing Services'. John Richards, the Director of Renewal Servicing, an off-shoot of the Fountain Trust, and Anglican Representative on the Churches' Council for Health and Healing, has written extensively from his experience of the healing ministry. In his volume, *The Question of Healing Services*, he deals at length with the issue. He frankly sets out a number of problems relating to such services:

1. *There is no biblical equivalent.* There are twenty occasions of public group healings. But, as he says, 'spontaneous ministry to the gathered is not the same as planned ministry to the invited' (p. 51). Nevertheless, 'in the New Testament the church had no hesitation in risking pastoral dangers to meet pastoral *needs*. If it erred it was on the side of caring'.[1]

But in the New Testament there was *no* risk. Those who were ministered to were *always* healed! And besides, as he himself says, the circumstances were not those of a pre-arranged and advertised 'Healing Service' with all the 'hype' and pre-conditioning which is characteristic of many such services in modern times.

2. *Preparation is not possible.* This may be compensated for, he says, by making an appropriate introduction, and/or ensuring the ministry of the Word is appropriate. But here again we see the contrast with the New Testament experience where 'preparation' was neither provided nor required.

3. *Raising false hopes.* He makes a contrast between Christian healing and spiritualist healing by suggesting that the former is 'God-orientated' whereas the latter is 'sickness-orientated'. Hence he says,

Such ministry should take place in a context of worship.[2]

Since this will ensure that

Our hope rests on the loving faithfulness of our Father to whom all present come afresh as his children.[3]

Here again we note that healing seldom took place in the context of worship in the New Testament. And, alas, often many of those who attend such services are only 'sickness-orientated' and have little interest in spiritual encounter or renewal. Moreover, it is misleading to say, as Richards does, that hopes of healing cannot be false even if 'All our hope on God is founded', for he may deign not to heal.

4. *Over-emphasis of this ministry.* While he acknowledges that this ministry can be over-emphasised, he maintains that under-emphasis is as much a heresy. Moreover, he adds,

When healing is placed within the context of the Eucharist then its right position is assured.[4]

This may appear to some to be good ecclesiology but it has no basis in biblical theology. There is no instance anywhere in the New Testament of physical healing having been associated with, or administered as part of, the Lord's Supper. As we have seen, it is easy to over-emphasise the place of the ministry of healing in the pattern of the New Testament church life, and it certainly had no place in the observance of the Lord's Supper.

5. *The difficulty of after-care.* In the context of healing services open to all comers the difficulty of after-care is obvious. But the problem is greatly reduced in the context of the Christian fellowship or congregation.

Richards concludes,

The aim of a public healing service is that God would be glorified.... It is all too easy to glorify sickness, healers, ministers, the healed, and/or the church.[5]

Having dealt with these very real and relevant problems, Richards goes on to justify healing services on the following principles:

Firstly, they are right but only so if they are 'good', that is,
if they reflect the mind of the church in such matters as health,
medicine, faith and so on.[6]
Secondly, healing will bring joy to those who know and acknowledge
their need and receive it, but to those whose pride and self-esteem
prevent them from believing and yielding, it often only arouses anger
and opposition.
Thirdly, healing Services should be both 'one-church' and
'ecumenical'.
There are no universal rules. In some situations the natural
development will be within one local church, while in others the
next step forward will be an ecumenical venture.[7]
Fourthly, in healing the church must not become pre-occupied with
itself, it must be a part of the church's mission.
The place of a public healing service can only be assessed within
the total life of a parish. It will be quite clear whether the local
church offers merely an escape from society or a servicing point
for it.[8]
Fifthly, while he believes, as we have seen, there are many advantages
in healing taking place in a 'eucharistic setting', nevertheless he
acknowledges some serious problems and he himself favours its taking
place 'after communion'.[9]
Sixthly, whether Healing Services are held on a one-off or regular
basis depends upon the local situation. Again there are no rules.
We may summarise the general teaching of the James passage thus:
1. The passage is dealing with physical healing rather than spiritual,
though the two are not completely separable.[10]
2. There is no biblical warrant for the doctrine of 'Extreme Unction'
to be derived from this passage, nor indeed is there any reference to
sacramental healing being established.[11]
3. The healing offered in this passage is to be:
—administered once;
—administered privately not publicly;
—sought in the first instance by the patient.[12]
4. The 'elders' are not commissioned to exercise the gifts of healing
of 1 Corinthians 12 but to offer prayer and anoint with oil.[13]
5. The elders are not to act individually but as a body.[14]
6. The anointing with oil was symbolic either of medical healing or
of spiritual healing and consecration.[15]
7. If sin were involved directly or indirectly in relation to the
sickness then reconciliation and restitution were necessary.[16]
8. Mutual confession between Christians (not to a priest) and mutual
intercession will increase understanding and mutual support in trial.[17]
9. There is no reference to the 'laying on of hands'.[18]

10. There is no reference to the exorcism of demons.[19]

The contrast of the pattern of healing in this passage with that of the Lord and the Apostles is evident:

—there is no command to exercise a ministry of healing;
—healing is to be effected not by a word of authority but by prayer;
—the work of prayer is a work of faith (the 'prayer of faith');
—the use of oil is required.

The import of the James 5 passage is to provide the Christian believer with the challenge to seek the counsel, intercession and anointing of the spiritual oversight of the congregation to furnish healing for sickness of body or mind in accordance with the divine purpose, or to enable the sufferer to bear with faith and fortitude the trial or discipline to which he is being subjected, and to save him from doubt or despair in the assurance that 'the prayer of faith will save the sick'. This, in fact, is the usual consequence of the ministry of faith-healing, but it is often not what faith-healers claim or teach as the pattern or purpose of their ministry.

II. HEALING IN MODERN TIMES

The age of the Apostles was not long gone before the church began to put other constructions upon the principles and practices of healing contained in the Scriptures, and to build up its own systems and traditions many of which bore little relationship to the biblical patterns and purposes of healing, and brought the whole doctrine and practice into the realm of magic and superstition. As the influence of the 'Apostles' doctrine and fellowship' receded, and the ecclesiastical constitution and hierarchy of the church developed with its claim to a false 'Apostolic Succession' through the Bishop of Rome, the ministry of healing, including the exorcism of demons became sacramentalised as part of the liturgy. Anointing with oil, specified in James 5, became first 'healing unction' and then preparation for death in 'Extreme Unction'. And the power of God bestowed on the Apostles and believers through the 'gifts of the Spirit' gradually was transformed into a complex system of mystery and magic effected through manifestations of the Virgin Mary or the 'Saints', and dispensed by means of holy pictures, sacred shrines, holy relics, mysterious apparitions, and the paraphernalia of religious superstition and human credulity. The post-Apostolic age of 'signs and wonders' led farther and farther from the exercise of divine power to heal by the authority of the Word of God and the gift of the Holy Spirit to the chaos and confusion of the spirit world and the realms of the powers of darkness.

In abhorrence of, and reaction to, this unbiblical religion of fear and counterfeit miracle, the Reformation of the sixteenth century virtually 'threw out the baby with the bath water'. Repudiating the false 'Apostolic Succession' and the delegation of supernatural powers to the priesthood and the ritual, the 'saints' and the sacraments, of the church in the past ages, the Reformers took the view that the 'gifts of the Spirit' identified in the New Testament church with the Apostles and those to whom they ministered, were withdrawn or ceased to be operative. They had, of course, a very clear and lofty doctrine of the Holy Spirit as the third Person of the Godhead, and the work of the Holy Spirit as the Interpreter and Applicant of the Word of God to the believer. But they rejected both the fact and the necessity of further revelation of the power or purposes of God through miracle or supernatural gift, on the ground that all that is required for the saving knowledge of God is already given in the Word of God written (*i.e.* the Bible) and faithfully preached and effectually applied to the believer by the Holy Spirit. Thus during post-New Testament times, on the one hand, miracle-working by non-biblical means increased, while, on the other hand, the true 'gifts of the Spirit', especially those of supernatural effect, languished generally unsought and unused in the fellowship and witness of the church at large.

With the rise of Pentecostalism at the beginning of the twentieth century a new interest in, and pursuit of, spiritual gifts broke upon the Protestant Churches with a special emphasis on the gifts of 'tongues' and 'healing'. Inevitably there was a degree of fanaticism and excess, but the Pentecostal movement became firmly established in the many branches of Pentecostalism represented by the new Churches which repudiated the doctrine of the withdrawal or cessation of the New Testament 'gifts' at any time. A doctrine and practice of faith-healing based on the power and promise of 'signs and wonders', and exercised in accordance with James 5 became an important part of the 'normal' activity and experience of the life and witness of the church. For the first half of the 20th century the new Pentecostalism was largely confined to, and expressed in, the growth and spread of new Churches, especially in the 'Third World' where Pentecostalism is the overwhelming manifestation of evangelical Christianity, while the traditional Protestant Churches, Anglican, Lutheran, Methodist, Calvinist and Evangelical remained unaffected. Today the Pentecostal Churches are the largest and fastest growing Christian Churches across the world.

But by the beginning of the second half of the twentieth century a new wave of Pentecostalism, in the form of the Charismatic Movement, swept across the established Churches, Protestant and Roman Catholic, giving a new dimension and impetus to interest in the supernatural 'gifts of the Spirit' especially 'tongues' and 'healing'. Apart altogether from the ecumenical aspects of charismaticism which has brought together members of Churches Reformed and non-reformed, Western and Eastern, Orthodox and Evangelical, the charismatic emphasis has, on the one hand, fostered a new awareness of, and interest in the phenomenon of faith-healing, and on the other hand, has created a new need to take account of the nature and implications of the manifestation of the divine power of God in miracle and the supernatural working of the Holy Spirit in and through sanctified humanity. Thus, we have seen in modern healing ministries the same kinds of phenomena taking place in an Anglican Cathedral, a Roman Catholic Retreat, and a Vineyard 'Spiritual Warfare Conference', not to mention the individual healing ministries of both ordained and freelance healers. Throughout our review of modern healing principles and practices we have noted many of the areas of difference in belief or procedure from that of the New Testament scene. It remains therefore to attempt some assessment of the validity or relevance of the healing ministry to the life and witness of the church as set forth in the teaching and pattern of Scripture. Is it essential to the church's witness to the world? Does it edify the church? Is it a valid method of evangelism? Does it prove the spiritual maturity of the church or the believer? Does it produce spiritual fruit unto holiness in the healed? In the answers to such questions the significance and value of faith-healing may surely be discerned.

III. TWO ALTERNATIVES

(i) The 'gifts' withdrawn

There are two prevailing attitudes within the church to faith-healing. The first is that promulgated at the Reformation to the effect that with the passing of the Apostles and those to whom they conveyed spiritual gifts, the 'gifts of the Spirit', especially those involving miraculous or supernatural manifestations such as 'prophecy', 'tongues' or 'healing', were withdrawn and ceased to operate primarily because their original purpose—to authenticate the divine authority and power of Christ and the Apostles in the newly formed church—was no longer required since the Word of God had by divine inspiration become available in the Scriptures which were 'the only infallible rule of faith and practice and the supreme standard of the church'. As Calvin put it,

> The Lord, doubtless, is present with his people in all ages, and cures their sicknesses as often as there is need, not less than formerly; and yet he does not exert those manifest powers, nor dispense miracles by the hands of apostles, because the gift was temporary, and owing, in some measure, to the ingratitude of men, immediately ceased.[20]

Such a view did not call in question the sovereignty of God in all the affairs of men to 'overrule all things to his own glory' by means either natural or supernatural. But it did call in question the whole system of sacrament and superstition which down the preceding centuries had held men and women in thrall. Calvin saw the whole paraphernalia of healing by means of sacrament, saint or priesthood as fraud or even worse.

> Let no man now wonder that they have with so much confidence deluded souls, which they knew to be stupid and blind, because deprived of the word of God, that is, of his light and life, seeing they blush not to attempt to deceive the bodily perceptions of those who are alive, and have all their senses about them. They make themselves ridiculous, therefore, by pretending that they are endued with the gift of healing.[21]

Such an aversion to the unacceptable face of unreformed religion led evidently not to the rejection of the possibility of miracles of healing or of other kinds, but to the conclusion that miracles claimed to be effected through the sacraments or saints were in fact counterfeits by Satan of the works of the Lord and of the Apostles.

But with regard to the conclusion that the 'gifts of the Spirit' were withdrawn or ceased to operate after the close of the Apostolic period, there seems to be a problem as to why a distinction should have been made between some of the 'gifts' and others. The Reformers accepted that the gifts of prophecy (in the sense of 'preaching'), teaching, pastoring, evangelising, and most of those mentioned in 1 Corinthians 12 continued to be operative in the church in their own day, but they rejected the continuance of those gifts which manifested themselves in the supernatural (such as 'prophecy' in the sense of 'forecast', 'tongues' and 'healing') without furnishing the kind of biblical evidence for such a conclusion that they demanded for other aspects of doctrine and practice.

(ii) The 'gifts' continue

The second of the prevailing attitudes is that of those who believe that there is nothing in Scripture to indicate that the 'gifts of the Spirit' were not intended to be available to true believers in all ages or that any distinction is to be made between the 'miraculous' and 'non-miraculous' gifts. But having accepted that the gifts, and in particular the gift of healing, are, and always have been, available since New Testament times, there is considerable variety of opinion as to how they should be exercised.

As Table VIII shows, some believe that all Christians are commissioned to participate in the ministry of healing, while others insist that only certain individuals are entrusted with the capacity to effect healing. Some believe that anointing with oil is essential, while others insist on the necessity of the 'laying on of hands', and yet others are persuaded that healing can be effected without either of these procedures. Some believe that the exercise of healing is an essential and inseparable part of the ministry of the Word, while others see it as a specialised ministry to be exercised as required in response to the further gift of 'prophecy' (in the sense of 'insight' or 'foresight') or 'discernment'. Some believe that healing should be offered in the name of Christ to all who are sick and that they should expect, and be encouraged to expect, to be healed, while others insist that healing should be offered only to those who seek it and that not all who are ministered to will be, or should expect to be, healed. Some see healing as a valid method of evangelism, while others see it as related to the inner fellowship and edification of the church. Some believe all ministers of the Gospel should practice healing, while others believe only those specially called and 'gifted' should do so. Some believe healing is effected by the exercise of spiritual gifts, while others believe it is a ministry of prayer and is made effective through the 'prayer of faith'. Some believe healing is to be the work of individual healers, while others believe it is to be the work of a plurality of 'elders' or spiritual leaders within the local church fellowship. Some believe that healing is to be exercised in private, while others believe it is to be part of public Services of Worship. Practically all profess to believe that medical treatment is the normal God-given means of healing, while some believe that faith-healing should be sought after medical treatment has been exhausted, some believe that faith-healing should be sought in conjunction with medical treatment, and some believe that faith-healing should be sought as an alternative to medical treatment.

Not all of these positions are mutually exclusive, but it is clear that there is no simple or commonly-accepted pattern of doctrine or practice amongst Christian believers. One thing is obvious, that is, that while modern faith-healing practice in its various forms can be said to be derived from Scripture texts and concepts, *it cannot legitimately be said to be reproducing either the methods or the effects of the healing works of Christ and the Apostles.* Nor need it do so. The James passage set a new and different pattern from that of Christ and the Apostles, and apparently was intended to be the model for the church henceforth, just as the later Epistles of Paul and Peter are accepted as establishing the model of church government for succeeding ages.

IV. SUMMARY

We may therefore identify the following general principles:

1. God can and does heal both by the normal processes of treatment, medical and psychiatric, temporary remission, and spontaneous cure, and by divine intervention according to his sovereign purposes of love.

2. He may choose to do so either directly, without human agency or through the ministry of a person or persons acting under the guidance and power of the Holy Spirit.

3. He may do so in answer to the prayer of the sufferer or of one or more others interceding on his or her behalf. Such intercession on behalf of others is the privilege and duty of every individual Christian and of the church in fellowship.

4. He may withhold healing in accordance with his sovereign purposes of love.

5. He may and does use suffering for his own glory and for the good of those directly or indirectly concerned as a witness to his power and love, so that, like the Saviour himself, the sufferer may 'learn obedience by the things which he suffers' (Heb. 5:8) and thus be spiritually healed and enriched.

NOTES

1 J. Richards, *The Question of Healing Services,* Daybreak, London, 1989, pp. 51, 56.

2 *Ibid.,* p. 57.

3 *Ibid.,* p. 57.

4 *Ibid.,* p. 58.

5 *Ibid.,* p. 64.

6 *Ibid.,* p. 100.

7 *Ibid.,* p. 107.

8 *Ibid.,* p. 107.

9 *Ibid.,* p. 109.

10 *Ibid.,* pp. 93–99.

11 *Ibid.,* pp. 99–102.

12 *Ibid.,* pp. 102f.

13 *Ibid.,* p. 103.

14 *Ibid.,* p. 104.

15 *Ibid.,* p. 105.

16 *Ibid.,* p. 107.

17 *Ibid.,* p. 107.

18 *Ibid.,* p. 108.

19 *Ibid.,* p. 108.

20 J. Calvin, *Institutes of the Christian Religion,* James Clarke & Co., London, 1949, Bk. 4:19.19. p. 637.

21 *Ibid.,* p. 637.

21

PASTORAL PRACTICE

We have examined in some detail the biblical teaching and practice of faith-healing; the history and experience of the beliefs and practices of the church as exhibited in some of the main Reformed and unreformed traditions; and the most up-to-date developments of the phenomenon in contemporary faith-healing ministries. Now we must attempt to set out what we have learned in the context of the pastoral ministry of the church to the needs temporal and spiritual of those who are either already within its fellowship and wrestling with the challenge of demonstrating the faith that is, in all the vicissitudes of life in this present evil world, 'more than conqueror', or who, as yet strangers to the 'newness of life' that is in Christ Jesus, must be the concern and mission of those who having themselves obtained 'so great salvation' are commissioned to present Christ in the fulness of his Spirit and power to them.

I. PROPER PERSPECTIVES

When all the biblical material, especially that of the New Testament, is examined it is clear that healing, in the particular sense of faith-healing, had a significant but comparatively small place in the programme of God's revelation of himself through patriarchs, prophets and his Son, Christ Jesus. Designed primarily to authenticate, in the absence of any objective or written revelation, the authority and power of God manifested in and by his Son and his human servants, its importance and frequency receded with the growth and establishment of the church and the spread of the New Testament writings.

This is not to suggest that the 'gifts of the Spirit' were withdrawn or ceased to operate. In his sovereign graciousness God is free at any time, or in any circumstances, to manifest his power and purposes in accordance with the principles and means, natural and supernatural, revealed in the Scriptures. It is simply to assert what has been demonstrated again and again in the history of Christian work and witness, that the availability of the divine resources is specifically related to the needs and circumstances of the situation to which they are applied. The Lord did not feed every crowd with a handful of bread; he did not raise to life every corpse he met; he did not calm every storm on the lake. Peter did not heal everyone at the Beautiful Gate of the temple.

It is important to keep things in proper perspective. For example, when the paralytic man was brought to Jesus by his friends, the Lord made it clear to the patient himself and to all present that the healing of his physical affliction was only secondary to the healing of his spiritual malady through the forgiveness of his sin (Mark 2:10, 11). So, it would appear also to have been in the case of the paralytic healed at the Pool of Bethesda, for when Jesus found him later in the temple he counselled him with regard to his spiritual condition (John 5:14). It is clear that the healing effected by Jesus and the Apostles was directed toward the spiritual needs of the sufferer and those who may have been involved with him, though whether spiritual wholeness was effected is not always made plain.

It is true, by many accounts, that in the modern practice of faith-healing some who receive physical benefit do subsequently come to saving faith in Christ. But it must also be said that many of those who seek physical benefit from faith-healers have no concern about, or interest in, anything other than physical healing and bodily comfort. And it must also be said that the practice of many faith-healers, and especially that of public Healing Services, tends to foster such an attitude, especially when those who seek such help are pre-conditioned by more or less sensational publicity, or the sheer despair of having been diagnosed as suffering from an 'incurable' condition.

Moreover, the general increase of interest in, and charismatic obsession with, the practice of faith-healing has, for many, dangerously tilted the balance between the physical and the spiritual, the temporal and eternal values of life. In a sinful world where the material is increasingly crowding out the importance of the spiritual needs and destiny of so many in our modern society, it is all the more tragic when Christian perspectives too become 'conformed to this world'. Instead of the faith, courage, hope and confidence of Abraham, Moses, Job, the

Prophets and Apostles, and the host of those who down the centuries have endured and triumphed over physical and mental pain, weakness or trial 'as seeing him who is invisible', modern charismaticism would pander to earthbound fears and futilities rather than 'glory in the cross of our Lord Jesus Christ', or prove the sufficiency of that grace which from the very cauldron of personal trial could write, not in arrogance but in the power and contentment of the Holy Spirit, 'We are troubled on every side, yet not distressed; we are perplexed, but not in despair; persecuted, but not forsaken; cast down, but not destroyed; always bearing about in the body the dying of the Lord Jesus, that the life also of Jesus might be made manifest in our body' (2 Cor. 4:8–10).

What a pity that in the name of a more spectacular religion people should be diverted from the victory of that 'cloud of witnesses' who 'through faith subdued kingdoms, wrought righteousness, obtained promises, stopped the mouths of lions, quenched the violence of fire, escaped the edge of the sword, out of weakness were made strong, waxed valiant in fight, turned to flight the armies of the aliens...were tortured, not accepting deliverance; that they might obtain a better resurrection' (Heb. 11:33–35)! Here is real miracle, not the miracle of healing and deliverance which God sometimes works for his glory in the lives of his children, but the miracle of that divine support and sufficiency which triumphs not in escape from the assaults of the Evil One, but, as in the experience of the Lord himself when in the desert he was tempted of Satan, in the real victory of faith which proves that 'neither death, nor life, nor angels, nor principalities, nor powers, nor things present, nor things to come, nor...any other creature shall be able to separate us from the love of God which is in Christ Jesus' (Rom. 8:38, 39)!

Instead, in faith-healing people are being offered, not always but too often, not the immediate and total healing of body, mind and spirit effected by the word or touch of Christ and the Apostles, but little more than the counsel of the psychiatrist's couch, or the bromide of the doctor's consulting room, sanctified by prayer and the laying on of hands, and with similar temporary effect demonstrated by dependence on repeated or prolonged treatment by the faith-healer. All of which should rightly and effectively be, and often is, part of the normal pastoral ministry of ordained ministers, elders or Christian believers called and equipped by God to offer such healing by means of prayer and spiritual counsel either at the request of the sufferer, and in accordance with the pattern of James 5, or in the normal course of Christian concern and care for those in need in body, mind or spirit— but not as a pretence of simulating the miracle-working of Jesus and the Apostles, nor as a specialised ministry indicative of a superior spiritual charismaticism beyond that which was displayed in the

Churches of the New Testament period, and based upon the erroneous belief that Christians, as such, have the right to expect, in this world, exemption from the natural consequences of the fall, or the normal diseases and afflictions of the world, wrongly deduced from certain specific promises made in particular circumstances by God to ancient Israel, for example, Exodus 15:26; Deuteronomy 7:15 (*cf.* 2 Cor. 1:3–11; 12:5–7).

II. 'SIGNS AND WONDERS'

While Jesus and the Apostles manifested the divine power and authority of their work by effecting 'signs and wonders', it is clear that neither used that power or authority to deliver themselves from the afflictions or diseases of this world. In fact, in his personal encounter with Satan in the desert, Christ explicitly rejected the temptation to use 'signs and wonders' as the means of accomplishing his mission of redemption for mankind. He refused to turn the stones miraculously into bread when he was hungry; to cast himself down from the pinnacle of the temple presuming upon the divine power to save him from injury or death; to gain the kingdoms of the world by acknowledging the counterfeit power and authority of Satan (Matt. 4:1–11). Could the idea of a 'signs and wonders' ministry have been more decisively or convincingly rejected?

Moreover, it is clear that the Lord equally rejected 'signs and wonders' as an evangelistic method. While it is true that many people followed him and heard his preaching because of the miracles they witnessed or heard of, two things must be noted. Firstly, he often required those who were healed or witnessed his miraculous power not to tell others. Now whatever his particular reason may have been in any given instance, it is evident that it was not his intention to impress others as a mere wonder-worker, nor was his miracle-working intended by him to become an evangelistic method for attracting huge and curious audiences so that he might have the opportunity of preaching the 'good news of the Kingdom' to them. In fact, secondly, on occasions he actually rejected demands for a 'sign' (Matt. 12:38, 39; 16:4; Mark 8:11, 12; John 6:30), and even while accommodating the refusal of Thomas to be convinced of his resurrection by anything less than the opportunity to see and touch him in person, Jesus had words of special encouragement and commendation for those whose faith rose above dependence upon 'signs and wonders', 'Blessed are they that have not seen, and yet have believed' (John 20:29; 4:48).

The method of publicly convening a great crowd of people by the promise or expectation of seeing or benefiting from a display of his divine power for the purpose of inducing mass conversions or charismatic revival would appear to have been utterly rejected by the Lord. While, on occasions, many believed because of what they had heard, seen, or experienced (John 2:23; 7:31; 12:11), it is clear that this was not the immediate purpose for which he had performed the miracles in question. The fact, too, that the working of miracles steadily decreased in the ministry of the Apostles at the very time when the evangelistic mission of the church both to Jews and to Gentiles was at its peak, suggests that 'power-evangelism' had a place of declining, or at least receding, importance in the evangelistic strategy of the New Testament church.

It cannot be unimportant that the only ascription of the term 'signs and wonders' in the Gospels to any other than Christ is his own references to the advent and activity of 'false Christs' at the end of the age (Matt. 24:24; Mark 13:22). The term, with some variations, is used more frequently in the Acts of the Apostles (2:19, 22, 43; 4:30; 5:12; 7:36; 8:13; 14:3; 15:12), but always in reference to the sovereign activity of God himself (2:19; 7:36), of Christ (2:22), the Apostles (2:43; 5:12), Philip (8:13), Paul and Barnabas (14:3; 15:12). It is twice used by Paul with reference to himself (Rom. 15:19; 2 Cor. 12:12), and once in reference to the 'man of sin' who is to appear at the end of the age (2 Thes. 2:9) corresponding to the Lord's prediction (Matt. 24:24). It is used once with reference to God's messengers in the Old Testament times (Heb. 2:4). Apart therefore from the ministry of the Apostles who were specifically endowed and commissioned to exercise the divine power to work miracles through the enabling of the Holy Spirit, and the counterfeit miracles of Satan and the powers of evil, there is no indication whatever of 'signs and wonders' or 'power-evangelism' as a valid evangelistic method in the New Testament. On the contrary, it is 'through the foolishness of preaching' (1 Cor. 1:21) that Paul believes God is pleased 'to save them that believe', and he specifically sets the ministry of preaching over against the 'signs' and 'wisdom' which were particularly sought after by the Jews and Gentiles (1 Cor. 1:22, 23). Moreover, when Paul makes reference to the 'power' with which he preached to the Thessalonians, it was evidently not the power of miracle-working in himself (1 Cor. 2:4), but the power of 'miracle-living' in them by the Holy Spirit (1 Thes. 1:5, 9, 10).

Now the implication of all this is not for a moment to deny either the possibility or the fact of God's revelation of himself and his gracious purposes of love through the manifestation of 'signs and wonders' (particularly in faith-healing) either in the New Testament church or in the present time. On the contrary, we have repeatedly acknowledged the importance and effectiveness of the 'gifts of the Spirit' as catalogued in the New Testament, and their continuing demonstration by the Spirit of God in the life and witness of the church. It is neither possible, necessary nor desired to dispute the truth of the witness given by many of God's servants in the work of the Kingdom around the world that miracles do happen and are happening in the sovereign purposes of God's love, and the obedient reaping of his harvest-fields. But that is wholly different from asserting that the only true and effective method of evangelism and church-building is by a conscious and deliberate effort to cultivate and propagate 'signs and wonders' as evidence of obedience to the biblical pattern, or of the presence and blessing of God on the enterprise.

III. PATTERN FOR TODAY

What then is the place or pattern of the ministry of faith-healing for today?

1. When overtaken by some illness or affliction of body or mind, are we to seek medical or faith-healing? Although faith-healers themselves appear to pay lip-service to the value and importance of medical treatment, does depending on medical treatment indicate either a lack of faith in the power of God to heal, or a want of obedience to his Word? Certainly not. Christians believe that all medical knowledge and skill is God-given (though not always God-directed), and is to be used, as in Scripture, for the alleviation and cure of disease or affliction wherever it is available. With the blessing of God medical treatment is to be the normal procedure in the cure of physical or mental disorder, and to be received with trust and confidence both in God and in his agents of health and restoration. To regard medical skill and treatment as merely human or distinct from the working of his divine power, is to deny or disown the wisdom and love of the divine Physician who is pleased to use human brains, and hands which he has created, to do his work of compassion and healing often with effects that in relation to mere human wisdom and skill are nothing short of miraculous. Medical healing *is* faith-healing when seen in its proper perspective.

2. But what if medical skill or treatment is not available? For example, what is to be done in primitive societies where out of ignorance or superstition people are dependent upon the chicanery of the witch-doctor or the spiritist charmer; or in circumstances where because of accident, tragedy, or other cause beyond human control medical help or treatment is not available or cannot be obtained? We have seen (p. 225) God at work in 'missionary' situations, for example, with astonishing effect. And why not? Where he has not provided real medical skills or treatments, it is not in the least surprising that he should exert his divine power directly both to provide physical healing and to reveal his greater purposes of redemption for sin-sick souls.

3. And what if medical treatment has been sought but has proved unable to provide healing or hope? Should one then seek the ministry of faith-healing, and if so, how? There are a number of possibilities. For those who are believers the James 5 passage invites them, in the context of the general pastoral care of the local church, to call for the elders or spiritual leaders of the local congregation or fellowship to which they belong to come and pray for them anointing them with oil in the confidence that 'the prayer of faith will save the sick'. It is to be hoped that the nature and atmosphere of the local fellowship to which they belong is such that they could with confidence put the biblical injunction into effect. Failing that, as we have seen, there is no reason why any who are sick or in need of healing of any kind should not seek prayer on their behalf by a Christian believer or believers who may be known to them personally or known by them to carry on a ministry of prayer and intercession for and with the sick.

Or again, they may seek the Lord's help for themselves in fervent and believing prayer with confidence in God's promises to hear and answer. 'There is one mediator between God and men, the man Christ Jesus' (1 Tim. 2:5), but all who in repentance and faith have received his grace are 'brought nigh by the blood of Christ' (Eph. 2:13) and made 'kings and priests unto God' (Rev. 1:6) so that now without the need of priest or human mediator of any kind we have 'access by one Spirit unto the Father' (Eph. 2:18) and are every one invited to 'come boldly unto the throne of grace, that we may obtain mercy, and find grace to help in time of need' (Heb. 4:16). Another possibility is to seek healing or help by sharing in a 'Divine Healing Service'. Many have done so and have testified to the healing and help they have received. It is therefore difficult either to question the reality of the blessing that has been experienced, or to discourage others who may be in deep distress or need to seek help in this way, but, as we have seen, there is no biblical precedent for such services, nor is there any injunction in Scripture to seek public ministry of prayer or the exercise of healing gifts.

4. In taking any of these courses it must be accepted, of course, that the glory of God and the spiritual wellbeing of the sufferer must override all other considerations. This means that, in accordance with his gracious purposes God may respond (a) with immediate and total physical healing bringing with it a challenge to renewed dedication of body, mind and spirit to the service of Christ and to the witness of the Gospel and the work of the Kingdom of God, (b) with a greater or lesser degree of physical relief, but with increase of faith or grace with which to cope in peaceful and patient dependence upon himself in the sure confidence that 'all things work together for good to them that love God' (Rom. 8:28). It is clear both from the Scriptures and from

the experience of the most eminent servants of Christ that, in spite of its origin in the world, suffering can be and often is part of the divine purpose for his children and for the witness of his power and grace in the lives of those who know and love him best (Rom. 8:35–37). It is also to be remembered that for the Christian believer physical death is the ultimate enemy which has been conquered by Christ and so has been transformed into the very portal of 'life everlasting'. For 'to depart and be with Christ is far better' (Phil. 1:23) if indeed that is the will and way of God.

5. Prayer for healing is one facet of the whole mystery and wonder of prayer in its many forms and applications revealed in Scripture. In respect of healing it may be exercised by the individual sufferer on his own behalf; by the pastor of the local church in the normal course of his pastoral ministry to his 'flock'; by the spiritual oversight of the local church or fellowship at the request of the sufferer, as in James 5; by other believers individually or together in intercession on behalf of the sufferer either at his own request or other initiative. In recent times there appears to be an emphasis on the establishment of 'prayer-groups' or 'prayer-chains' specifically geared to obtaining healing or relief for the sick and afflicted. Each of these forms of prayer is illustrated in the New Testament. Paul prayed for himself three times with particular reference to release from his 'thorn' and the answer was 'No', but 'My grace is sufficient' (2 Cor. 12:8). In each of his letters, as in the writings of the other Apostles, Paul refers repeatedly to his intercession on behalf of the churches and their individual members as their 'pastor', and he calls on them to pray for him (Col. 1:9; 4:3). In the Acts of the Apostles we read of 'the church' gathered for prayer on behalf of individuals such as Peter and John (Acts 4:29, 30; 12:5).

The Bible speaks, for example, of 'believing' prayer (the 'prayer of faith') for, alas, prayer can so easily be offered without real confidence or expectation of being heard or granted; of 'fervent' prayer, that is, warm-hearted, motivated by love and affection both for God and for those who are being prayed for, as so easily it can become cold, mechanical, ritualistic; of 'persistent' prayer, for unlike Abraham or Elijah or Daniel or the early church members huddled in the 'upper room', it is so easy to give up in doubt or disappointment. The wonder of prayer lies in the realisation that in his own sovereign graciousness and loving ways God is pleased to hear and answer the pleas of his humble, penitent and obedient children. But he can not be manipulated, pressurised or cajoled into doing what we want by the numerical strength, the emotional passion, or the pious intention of those who pray.

This is the danger of such modern devices as 'soaking prayer' or 'telephone chain prayer' which, with the best of intention, may attempt to convince others, or even those who are engaged in the operation, that the sheer weight or strength of supplication must produce the desired effect. The gravity of such mistaken belief was surely poignantly demonstrated in the story of David Watson, who, in spite of repeated programmes of 'soaking prayer' for healing, was not healed. But, mercifully, the love and power of God are not diminished by our mistaken notions. We can be sure that when we 'take it to the Lord in prayer' with humble submission and loving dependence upon his divine wisdom and grace, 'The effectual, fervent prayer of a righteous man availeth much' (James 5:16).

IV. IN CONCLUSION

Healing, and especially faith-healing, cannot and must not be divorced from the cross of Christ and the redemption accomplished there for sinful and suffering mankind. We have seen already (p. 54) that the quotation in the Gospel of St. Matthew (8:17) from the prophecy of Isaiah (53:5) is not to be applied to the atoning work of Christ on Calvary, but was intended to refer to his earthly life and ministry. Moreover, it is clear that while the redemptive work of Christ will one day be brought to complete fulfilment in the restoration of the whole creation, saving faith in Christ promises and secures ultimate restoration of body and soul to the perfection of the eternal realm, but does not provide deliverance from the normal decay or afflictions of this fallen world. It is therefore essential to set the whole issue of healing in its proper context and perspective.

A faith-healing ministry which simply becomes another form of 'alternative medicine', or is regarded as such by those who seek to benefit from it, has no place in the biblical programme of the church. When Christ spoke of the coming of the Holy Spirit, he expressly declared the purpose of his coming to be 'He shall glorify me; for he shall receive of mine and shall show it unto you' (John 16:14). There can be no 'gifts' or activity of the Holy Spirit that do not relate to Christ and his work of redemption. In this sense, all healing whether of body, mind or soul, whether by medicine or by the power of the Holy Spirit, must relate to the glory of Christ and the eternal purposes of God for the sufferer. The human struggle with weakness, disease and the ravages of the fall whether physical, mental or spiritual, is the consequence of mankind's rebellion and estrangement from his Creator and can only be ultimately stilled and healed by the saving power of Christ. That struggle reached its climax when he 'who knew no sin (was) made to be sin for us, that we might be made the righteousness of God in him' (2 Cor. 5:21). And now 'the Sun of righteousness (is) risen) with healing in his wings' (Mal. 4:2).

Any healing which falls short of this divine dimension is only a temporary panacea which may make the journey of life in this world more comfortable, but must end in darkness and despair when the final 'examination' comes. But for the Christian there is real healing and hope, 'for our light affliction which is but for a moment, worketh for us a far more exceeding and eternal weight of glory, while we look not at the things which are seen, but at the things which are not seen; for the things which are seen are temporal, but the things which are not seen are eternal' (2 Cor. 4:17, 18). Here is the healing of faith!

APPENDIX—THE ECUMENICAL MOVEMENT

Nowadays any survey of church thought and activity would scarcely be regarded as adequate or complete which did not take some account of ecumenical considerations. And indeed, health is a subject that has received considerable attention in the consultations of the WCC.

I. THE 1990 CMC STUDY

> The Christian Medical Commission (CMC), a sub-unit of the Unit of Justice and Service of the World Council of Churches (WCC) has been engaged for the past twelve years in a study of health and healing from the Christian perspective.[1]

So begins the 1990 Report of a study by the CMC. The CMC, founded in 1968, arose out of two consultations in Tubingen, Germany, and organised jointly by the WCC and the Lutheran World Federation. The first in 1964 focused on medical missions in the Third World, and the second in 1968 dealt with the role of the church in healing. The WCC Assembly of 1975 in Nairobi mandated the CMC to

> serve as an enabling organisation to churches everywhere as they search for an understanding of health and healing which is distinctive to the Christian faith.[2]

From this one might have expected a serious interest in the rapid growth and experience of Pentecostalism and Charismaticism with their particular emphasis on faith-healing. Not surprisingly, however, the CMC enquiries quickly began to see health and healing as 'a justice issue', or 'a peace issue', or an environmental or political issue as well as a 'spiritual issue'. Even as a 'spiritual issue' healing is set largely in the context of 'community' and inter-personal relationships.

Health is a dynamic state of well-being of the individual and society; of physical, mental, spiritual, economic, political and social well-being; of being in harmony with each other, with the material environment, and with God.[3]

In fact the Report goes so far as to say,

He (Jesus) always related healing to the life of the community.... Jesus' concept of health, healing and wholeness is to set people free from all that stands in the way of life. But first he invites us to carry his yoke, to be burden-bearers, witnessing to and working for the kingdom of God.[4]

And by way of example the Report gives a peculiar twist to the story of the healing of the man at the Pool of Bethesda concluding

Jesus told him to 'Rise up, take up your mat and walk' rather than to wait for the commonly believed phenomenon of the 'whirling of the pool'[5]

thus suggesting that the healing of the man had more to do with the feelings of 'the community' than with the display of the power and love of God to heal. Or again, in the case of the woman who was healed by touching the clothes of Jesus from behind, the Report gives unwarranted significance to the breach of social custom rather than recognising the wonder of the power of faith:

To the 'unclean' woman who, despite the prohibition against touching a man, reached out and touched the hem of his garment, Jesus said: 'Daughter, your faith has made you whole'.[6]

Now of course it would be foolish and wrong not to recognise that personal 'wholeness' and social relationships are interrelated both in terms of cause and effect. But in Scripture, health in the sense of wholeness is first and foremost a matter of personal release from the power of sin and evil and their consequences in the life of the individual. In the New Testament when Jesus sent out his disciples to 'heal the sick and cast out demons' there is no indication whatever that he was referring to the resolution of the great social problems created by poverty, need, conflict or oppression in the society of his day, or to the establishment of local or national agencies of social welfare, but rather that he was commissioning them to deal with the physical and mental afflictions that are common to poor and rich alike. To say

He always related healing to the life of the community. He questioned existing laws, cultural values and practices that did not serve the interest of the poor[7]

is in many senses true. But to imply that his healing works were always related to a campaign for social justice, or always directed to the

benefit of the poor is contradicted by the fact that often he ministered
to those who were not 'poor' such as the centurion whose servant was
healed at his master's request or the Syrophoenician woman who
sought help for her daughter.

Making reference to 'Healing Practices' the Report says, 'Among
the practices which can aid in healing are scientific medicine,
traditional medicine' (presumably meaning the witch-doctor, spirits or
folklore), 'alternative forms of medicine, prayer, meditation and liturgy.
Each, especially when coupled with faith, can provide healing'.[8]

Whatever 'faith' is intended here to mean it cannot be the Christian
faith if it applies to each of the practices mentioned. But even this
account of 'Healing Practices' taken together with the added dimension
of 'church-related hospitals' and 'specialisation' in health care which,
the Report says, fails to deal with the patient as a whole person, is set
in social rather than spiritual perspectives:

> Each can also be used , intentionally or unintentionally, for evil.
> For example, the purpose may be to exploit or harm the
> individual. Or limited resources may be used to provide
> sophisticated treatment for a few while others are denied basic
> health care.[9]

The Report does acknowledge

> In many of the regional consultations, we learned of people who
> are actively engaged in healing through laying on of hands,
> prayer, anointing the sick with oil, caring for people by providing
> food and medicines, and visiting the sick at home or in hospitals
> and hospices.[10]

But again, we are warned,

> These activities are not to be set in opposition to other
> instruments through which God also acts to heal the human
> being. The Honduras Consultation said, 'We cannot exempt
> ourselves from the responsibility of using the resources of
> medical science or from political participation simply because we
> are praying for the sick!' Intercessory prayer creates a spiritual
> atmosphere that supports health workers.[11]

Well of course it does. It also supports surgeons, physicians,
psychiatrists and all who are engaged in the work of healing by God-
given and God-directed means. But, according to Scripture, it can also
provide direct, immediate and complete healing when conducted in
obedience to the Word of God and in commitment to the divine will
(Jas 5:15).

In chapter 4 the Report under the subtitle 'The congregation as a
healing place' acknowledges,

> Jesus sent the disciples out to preach, teach, and heal. Most
> churches today preach and teach but have abdicated healing to

medical professionals. Yet many ways in which churches are involved in healing were reported at the regional meetings: praying for the sick, confession and forgiveness, laying on of hands, anointing with oil, holy communion, using creative healing liturgies, supporting those who are committed to the healing task, training healers, using the charismatic gifts.[12] But there is no discussion of any of these and the Report goes on immediately to deal with 'The congregation as a caring community', as a 'Health teaching place' and as 'Advocate for justice, peace and integrity of creation'.

II. THE 1964 WCC CONSULTATION

The Report of the Tubingen Consultation in 1964 entitled 'The Healing Church' is equally dismissive of the biblical teaching and practice of faith-healing. It is true that the basic subject of the Consultation was the work of Christian medical missions. But it is of interest that while one of the 'preparatory papers' dealt specifically with the subject of 'Christian healing and the congregation', the 'Findings' of the Consultation took little cognisance of the substance of the paper. As Lesslie Newbigin, Director of the Division of World Mission and Evangelism says in the preface of the Report,

> The reader will note that the background papers really do not lead up to the statement ('Finding'), though they form its background. The gap between the two is an indication of the fact that something happened at Tubingen which went beyond the preparatory material.[13]

But whatever 'happened' no account was taken in the 'Finding' of the biblical phenomenon of faith-healing beyond this summary reference,

> In addition to practical acts of love and service the congregation is entrusted with sanctified means of healing by the ministry of the word, the sacraments and prayer with and for the sick. The manner in which these means are administered will vary according to the tradition of the individual church and the condition of the patient. They may include healing services, laying on of hands, anointing, etc. We do, however, disapprove of those healing services which disregard proper medical means, take place without preparation and follow-up and have a tendency to exploit the patient.[14]

The Finding goes on to discuss such matters as the need for training of theological students and members of the laity, but the purpose of the training is said to be

> to train chaplains to work as a member of a healing team, but also to train pastors to increase and deepen the care and cure of souls

as part of the healing ministry of the congregation.[15]
But the nature of the training envisaged is not directed towards the
exercise of spiritual gifts but rather apparently to the understanding and
experience of medical and psychological techniques.

Theological teaching staff should be encouraged along two lines.
Firstly, to develop courses in which the church's ministry of
healing is studied and practised. These courses should be based
in the seminary or college, but should include periodic hospital
and field visitation. Secondly to initiate courses in clinical
pastoring training where these do not exist, and to include these
in normal theological training.[16]

The remainder of the Report deals with the planning and development
of Christian medical work, so that, as in the CMC Report, while the
possibility of Christian healing apart from medical, psychiatric or
sociological means is formally acknowledged, it is not given serious
or systematic investigation or discussion.

III. THE 1970 LIMURU CONFERENCE

The Report of the Limuru Conference of 1970 sponsored by the
Protestant Churches Medical Association of Kenya and the Lutheran
Institute of Human Ecology, and involving the staff of the Christian
Medical Commission of the WCC, presents a similar approach to the
issue of 'Health and Wholeness'. Again the Conference 'Bible
Readings' actually dealt with such matters as 'The Bible view of
Healing' and 'The Biblical Practice of Healing', covering the meanings
of both the Old and New Testament terms and methods and including
discussion of the basic issues of 'faith', 'signs', 'gifts', *etc*. But the
Conference addresses concentrated on such matters as Christian
medical work, 'The meaning of human ecology', community aspects
of health and healing, and 'the practice of community medicine', but
there was no discussion or consideration of the phenomenon of faith-
healing. And 'the future pattern of the church's ministry of healing' is
set out under six features which relate to medical, social and
environmental issues.

The ecumenical approach to the nature of the church as a healing
community is discussed at some length by Karin Granberg-Michaelson
in the WCC publication *Healing Community* in which she draws on the
twelve-year study by the WCC's Christian Medical Commission of
health, healing and wholeness. In it she says,

The early church described in Acts had a very clear vision of its
purpose. It understood its primary function to be that of witness
and proclamation of the good news of Jesus Christ. Members

enacted their commitment through a radical sharing of their economic resources with one another and the poor. They also devoted much time to prayer, fasting, preaching, healing and corporate acts of worship.[17]
She notes the place and importance attached to 'spiritual gifts' in the church's life both in the choice of leadership and in its vision and witness.

> Spiritual gifts are those gifts or graces that have been entrusted to a person for the benefit of the whole community of the church.... Those gifts include the commonly understood and publicly recognised services associated with churches such as preaching, teaching, administration and music.... And further there are the controversial and often misunderstood gifts like prophecy, speaking in tongues, and healing.... 1 Corinthians 12 makes it clear that everyone has a gift to offer the body...and in 2 Corinthians 14:1 we are advised to earnestly desire the spiritual gifts.[18]

But beyond listing many 'gifts' outside as well as within the categories of 1 Corinthians 12, there is no further theological examination or explanation of them or their use. Mrs. Granberg-Michaelson concludes her book with a report of a seminar on Christian Perspectives on Health, Healing, Wholeness and Suffering which was held at the Bossey Conference Centre of the WCC in May 1990, but again it dealt with these matters in terms of healing through the mutual loving and caring of the members of Christian congregations and communities without reference to the ministry of faith-healing.

IV. THE 1980 BOSSEY CONSULTATION

The report of the 1980 Bossey Consultation entitled 'The Church is Charismatic' and edited by Arnold Bittlinger runs to over two hundred and forty pages. It deals with many aspects of the Charismatic Renewal which began at the beginning of the 1960s, and which, the Report says, was due primarily to a longing on the part of Christians for, amongst other things,

> strength in reaction against a Christianity which denied or explained away the miracles and mighty works attested in the New Testament.[19]

One might therefore have expected the Report at least at some point to deal with the implications of 'the miracles and mighty works attested in the New Testament'. But we are to be disappointed. There is widespread reference to the 'gifts' of the Spirit. For example, in a 'Survey of the Worldwide Charismatic Movement', we read,

> While few churches have adopted an explicitly dispensationalist

position of maintaining that the endowments of power in the New
Testament were intended only for the period of the church's
foundation, most Christians assume this to have been the case.
Charismatic Renewal challenges this mentality, affirming that
what the Holy Spirit did in the first century, he can and does in
the twentieth.[20]
And there are frequent references to the various gifts listed in the New
Testament. For example, it is said,

> *Gifts of healing* are given to members of the body of Christ so
> that human diseases and disabilities of every kind, organic and
> non-organic, psychological as well as physical, can be healed
> through the direct action of Jesus Christ and the ministry of the
> Christian.[21]

Moreover, the 'holistic' view of man is expressed in a number of ways
including healing

> which expresses a more integral understanding of the relationship
> between sin and sickness, health and salvation.[22]

In his paper on 'Church reactions to the Charismatic Renewal' Kilian
McDonnell refutes the suggestion that in some way Paul sets the gift
of 'love' over against, or as superior to, the other gifts.

> It is a perversion of Paul's meaning if one makes it appear that
> one has to choose between charity and the gifts. One chooses
> them both. Charity is the absolutely essential context in which
> the gifts are exercised, without the presence of charity there are
> no charisms.[23]

Thus healing, in the sense of faith-healing, is clearly set within the
evidence of spiritual renewal. But sadly there is no theological
treatment of the ministry of faith-healing within the church. Even in
his 'Models of Christian Community in the New Testament', J. D. G.
Dunn insists,

> The ongoing life of the (local) community is charismatic in
> character. As the shared experience of the Spirit is the beginning
> of community, so it is the continuing manifestations of the Spirit
> or gifts of the Spirit which constitute the life and growth of the
> community of the body of Christ. The 'functions' of the body are
> precisely the *charismata* of the Spirit (Rom. 12:4)—*charisma* for
> Paul denoting *any* word or act which embodies or manifests
> grace (*charis*), which is a *means of grace* to another...without
> them the body is dead. Christian community exists only in the
> living interplay of charismatic ministry, in the actual being and
> doing for others in word and deed.[24]

Now of course all these matters which have been the substance of
ecumenical consultation and report are valid and important aspects of
healing in general terms, but, it would appear that faith-healing, as

such, while it is fully and frequently acknowledged as being an essential aspect of the church's ministry, has not, as yet, been made the subject of specific examination or comment.

NOTES

1 *Healing and Wholeness, the Churches' Role in Health,* Christian Medical Commission, WCC, Geneva, 1990 p. 1.

2 *Ibid.,* p. 1.

3 *Ibid.,* p. 6.

4 *Ibid.,* pp. 6, 7.

5 *Ibid.,* p. 6.

6 *Ibid.,* p. 6

7 *Ibid.,* p. 6.

8 *Ibid.,* p. 9.

9 *Ibid.,* pp. 9, 10.

10 *Ibid.,* p. 13.

11 *Ibid.,* p. 14.

12 *Ibid.,* p. 31.

13 *The Healing Church,* World Council Studies No. 3, WCC, Geneva, 1965, p. 6.

14 *Ibid.,* p. 37.

15 *Ibid.,* p. 38.

16 *Ibid.,* p. 38.

17 *Healing Community,* Risk Book Series, WCC, Geneva, 1991, p. 30.

18 *Ibid.,* p. 74.

19 *The Church is Charismatic,* WCC, Geneva, 1981, p. 9.

20 *Ibid.,* p. 127.

21 *Ibid.,* p. 128.

22 *Ibid.,* p. 131.

23 *Ibid.,* p. 149.

24 *Ibid.,* pp. 104f.

Table I—Individual Healings of Jesus

No.	HEALINGS BY JESUS	Mark	Matthew	Luke	John	Physical	Exorcism of Demons	Raising of dead	Compassion	Response to Request	Response to Faith	Glory of Christ	Spoken Word	Touch	Word and Touch	Use of Saliva	At a Distance	Jesus	Patient	Friend of Patient	Enemies of Jesus	Faith Discerned	Faith Demanded	Faith Expressed	Faith Unmentioned
1	Peter's Mother-in-Law	1:30-31	8:14-15	4:35-39		●								●						●					●
2	Man with Leprosy	1:40-45	8:1-4	5:12-15		●			●						●				●					●	
3	Synagogue Demoniac	1:21-28		4:31-37			●						●					●							●
4	Paralysed Man	2:1-12	9:1-8	5:18-26		●					●		●							●		●			
5	Man with Withered Hand	3:1-6	12:10-13	6:6-11		●							●					●							●
6	Gadarene Demoniac	5:1-20	8:28-34	8:26-39			●						●						●						●
7	Jairus' Daughter	5:22-43	9:18-26	8:41-56				●		●					●					●			●		
8	Woman with Haemorrhage	5:25-34	9:20-22	8:43-48		●					●			●					●					●	
9	Syrophoenician Girl	7:24-30	15:22-28				●				●						●			●				●	
10	Deaf Mute	7:31-37				●										●				●					●
11	Blind Man of Bethsaida	8:22-26				●										●				●					●
12	Epileptic Boy	9:14-29	17:14-21	9:37-43			●			●					●					●			●		
13	Blind Bartimaeus	10:46-52	20:29-34	18:35-43		●					●		●						●					●	
14	Two Blind Men		9:27-31			●					●			●					●				●		
15	Centurion's Servant		8:5-13	7:1-10		●					●						●			●		●			
16	Dumb Demoniac		9:32-34				●						●							●					●
17	Blind and Dumb Demoniac		12:22-24	11:14-16			●						●								●				●
18	Woman bent over			13:11-17		●			●						●			●				●			
19	Man with Dropsy			14:1-6		●								●				●							●
20	Man with Leprosy			17:11-19		●				●			●						●					●	
21	Malchus' Ear			22:50-51		●								●							●				●
22	Widow of Nain's Son			7:11-18				●	●						●			●							●
23	Nobleman's Son				4:46-54	●					●						●			●		●			
24	Impotent Man				5:1-16	●						●	●					●							●
25	Man born Blind				9:1-41	●						●				●		●							●
26	Lazarus				11:1-46			●				●	●					●							●

Table II—Summary of Table I

GOSPEL REFERENCES	Mark	13
	Matthew	14
	Luke	17
	John	4
NATURE OF HEALING	Physical	17
	Exorcism	6
	Raising of Dead	3
REASON FOR HEALING	Compassion	3
	Response to Request	5
	Response to Faith	6
	Glory of Christ	3
METHOD OF HEALING	Spoken Word	12
	Touch	4
	Word and Touch	8
	Use of Saliva	3
	At a Distance	3
WHOSE INITIATIVE	Jesus	4
	Patient	7
	Friend of Patient	13
	Enemies of Jesus	2
FAITH FACTOR	Faith Discerned	5
	Faith Demanded	5
	Faith Expressed	9
	Faith Unmentioned	14

Table III—Multiple Healings of Jesus

#	INCIDENT	GOSPEL REFERENCES	Physical	Exorcism	Unspecified	All	Many	Some	Scripture Fulfilled	Compassion
	GENERAL HEALINGS									
1	Capernaum	Matt. 8:16–17	•	•		•			•	
		Mark 1:32–34	•	•			•			
		Luke 4:40–41	•	•		•				
2	Galilee	Matt. 4:23–25	•	•		•				
		Mark 1:39		•						
		Luke —								
3	Seaside	Matt. 12:15–16			•	•				
		Mark 3:10–12	•	•		•				
		Luke 6:17–19	•	•		•				
4	Nazareth	Matt. 13:58			•			•		
		Mark 6:5	•					•		
		Luke —								
5	Villages	Matt. 9:35	•				•			
		Mark —								
		Luke —								
6	After Murder of John the Baptist	Matt. 14:14	•			•				•
		Mark —								
		Luke 9:11			•		•			
7	Gennesaret	Matt. 14:35–36			•		•			
		Mark 6:54–56	•				•			
		Luke —								
8	Hillside in Galilee	Matt. 15:30–31	•			•				
		Mark —								
		Luke —								
9	Judea	Matt. 19:2			•		•			
		Mark —								
		Luke —								
10	At time of John's Enquiry	Matt. —								
		Mark —								
		Luke 7:19–23	•	•			•			
11	The Temple	Matt. 21:12–14	•					•		
		Mark —								
		Luke —								
12	Galilee	Matt. —								
		Mark —								
		Luke 5:15			•		•			

Table IV—Healings of the Apostles

INCIDENT	BIBLICAL REFERENCE	HEALING BY WHOM	Physical	Exorcism of Demons	Raising of dead	Unspecified	The Healer	The Patient	Friends of Patient	Response to Request	Compassion	Response to Faith	Witness to Gospel	Spoken Word	Touch	Word and Touch	Other Means	Faith Discerned	Faith Demanded	Faith Expressed	Faith Unmentioned
INDIVIDUAL HEALINGS																					
1 At the Temple Gate	Acts 3:1–10	Peter (and John)	•				•						•			•					•
2 Paul's Sight	Acts 9:17–19	Ananias	•				•						•		•						•
3 Aeneas Healed	Acts 9:32–35	Peter	•				•						•	•							•
4 Dorcas	Acts 9:36–41	Peter			•				•	•				•							•
5 Cripple at Lystra	Acts 14:8–11	Paul	•				•					•		•				•			
6 Girl at Philippi	Acts 16:16–18	Paul		•			•				•			•							•
7 Eutychus	Acts 20:9–12	Paul			•		•				•						•				•
8 Father of Publius	Acts 28:8	Paul	•				•				•					•					•
GENERAL HEALINGS																					
1 In Jerusalem	Acts 2:43	The Apostles				•							•								•
2 In Jerusalem	Acts 5:12	The Apostles				•							•								•
3 In Jerusalem	Acts 5:15–16	Peter				•	•						•								•
4 In Jerusalem	Acts 6:8	Stephen				•							•								•
5 In Samaria	Acts 8:6–7	Philip		•			•						•								•
6 In Iconium	Acts 14:3	Paul and Barnabas				•							•								•
7 In Ephesus	Acts 19:11–12	Paul	•	•			•						•				•				•
8 In Malta	Acts 28:9	Paul	•				•						•								•

Table V—Old Testament Healings

No.	Biblical Reference	Whom Concerned	Physical	Mental	Raising Dead	Cure of Childlessness	Relief of Judgement	Reward of Faithfullness	Response to Request	Patient	Other	God Alone	Moses (Aaron)	Elijah	Elisha	Isaiah	Healing Refused	Illness Prevented
1	Genesis 18:14	Sarah	●			●						●						
2	Genesis 20:17–18	Women of Abimelech	●			●			●		●							
3	Genesis 25:21	Rebekah	●			●			●		●							
4	Genesis 30:22–24	Rachel	●			●						●						
5	Numbers 12:14	Miriam's Leprosy	●				●		●		●		●					
6	Numbers 16:47–48	Plague on Israel	●				●						●					
7	Numbers 21:9	Brazen Serpent	●				●						●					
8	1 Kings 13:1–6	Jeroboam's Hand	●				●		●	●								
9	Daniel 4:33–36	Nebuchadnezzar		●			●					●						
10	1 Kings 17:21–22	Widow's son	●		●				●		●			●				
11	2 Kings 4:33–35	Shunamite boy	●		●			●	●		●				●			
12	2 Kings 5:14	Naaman	●						●	●					●			
13	2 Kings 20:1–11	Hezekiah	●					●	●	●						●		
14	Job 42:10	Job	●					●	●	●		●						
15	1 Kings 14:12	Jeroboam's son	●														●	
16	2 Kings 1:4, 17	Amaziah	●														●	
17	2 Kings 5:27	Gehazi	●														●	
18	2 Kings 13:21	Corpse in Tomb	●		●							●			●			
19	Exodus 15:23–25	Poisoned Water	●										●					●
20	2 Kings 2:21–22	Poisoned Spring	●												●			●
21	2 Kings 4:38–41	Poisoned Food	●												●			●

Column groupings: **NATURE OF HEALING** (Physical, Mental, Raising Dead, Cure of Childlessness); **REASON FOR HEALING** (Relief of Judgement, Reward of Faithfullness, Response to Request); **WHOSE REQUEST** (Patient, Other); **AGENT OF HEALING** (God Alone, Moses (Aaron), Elijah, Elisha, Isaiah); **OTHER** (Healing Refused, Illness Prevented).

Table VI—Spiritual Gifts

		Romans 12:6–9	1 Corinthians 12:8–10	1 Corinthians 12:28	1 Corinthians 12:29–30	Ephesians 4:11	1 Peter 4:10–11	TOTAL
1	Prophecy/Prophets	•		•	•	•	•	5
2	Ministry	•					•	2
3	Teaching/Teachers	•		•	•	•		4
4	Exhortation	•						1
5	Giving	•						1
6	Ruling/Governments	•		•				2
7	Showing Mercy	•						1
8	Love	•						1
9	Wisdom		•					1
10	Knowledge		•					1
11	Faith		•					1
12	Healing(s)		•	•	•			3
13	Miracles		•		•			2
14	Discerning of Spirits		•					1
15	Tongues		•		•			2
16	Interpretation of Tongues		•		•			2
17	Apostles			•	•	•		3
18	Helps			•				1
19	Evangelists					•		1
20	Pastors					•		1

Table VII—Comparison of the answers of the five 'Healers' to the questionnaire

		A	B	C	D	E
1	Why did you take up the ministry of healing?	Convinced by Pentecostal teaching	—	Healing received: challenged by other's need	Challenged by a sufferer to heal	Healing received
2	Do you see yourself as:					
	(a) Doing as Christ and the Apostles did?	Yes	Yes	Yes	Yes	Yes
	(b) Exercising a 'gift' of healing?	Yes, but gift in church not healer	Yes, seven gifts	Yes. Also tongues	No	Yes
	(c) Fulfilling the pattern of James 5?	Yes	Yes, but not with 'Elders'	Yes. But rarely anointing	Yes	Yes, but not anointing
	(d) Praying for the sick with fruitful results?	No	No	No	No	No
3	In your ministry does healing:					
	(a) Take place immediately?	Seldom	Not always	Usually not	Occasionally	Have never seen it
	(b) Require repeated treatment?	Yes. Four or five or more times	Yes, usually three	Sometimes	Sometimes	Sometimes. Helped by prayerful atmosphere
	(c) Suffer relapse?	Yes	Yes	Yes	Sometimes	
	(d) Fail completely?	Yes it can	Never	Yes	Yes	Yes
4	In your work:					
	(a) What is the nature of faith?	(a) The faith is in the healer, not the healed	(a) The faith is for healing, not saving faith	(a) Not saving faith	—	—
	(b) What part does faith play?	(b) It is necessary	(b) It is important	(b) Not required in healed, may be in others	(b) Essential in healer. Desirable in healed	(b) Little or no faith in patient
5	How do you explain failure in a particular case?	The sovereignty of God	The disease too far advanced	Could be due to faulty ministry	No explanation. Could be test of healer	Sovereignty of God or only apparent
6	(a) Do you expect miracles to happen?	Yes	Yes	Yes	Yes 'as a blessing'	Yes
	(b) Do you encourage patients to expect such?	Yes	Yes	Yes	Yes 'as a blessing'	Yes as indicating positive faith
7	How far do you use psychology or psychiatry?	Not at all	When necessary	To some extent	Yes but not as a psychiatrist	Not consciously
8	How important in your work is:					
	(a) Anointing with oil?	Used on request	Not used at all	Rarely	Rarely	Not at all
	(b) Laying on of hands?	It is essential	Always	Usually	Central and very important	Necessary as symbol of concern and love
9	Do you share in or encourage Healing Services?	Yes and No	Not any longer	Yes	Yes	Yes
10	Should all ministers exercise healing?	In a limited way	No, only those with gifts	Yes if open to the gift of the Spirit	No. The ideal is a healing group	Yes but the Spirit is required

Table VIII—Comparison of attitudes to Healing

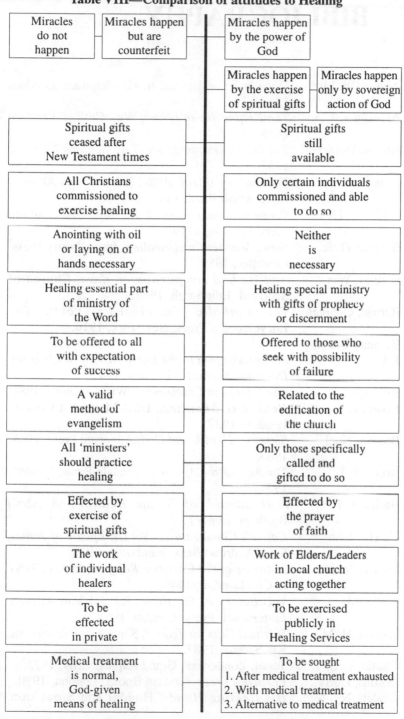

Miracles do not happen	Miracles happen but are counterfeit		Miracles happen by the power of God	
			Miracles happen by the exercise of spiritual gifts	Miracles happen only by sovereign action of God

Spiritual gifts ceased after New Testament times	Spiritual gifts still available
All Christians commissioned to exercise healing	Only certain individuals commissioned and able to do so
Anointing with oil or laying on of hands necessary	Neither is necessary
Healing essential part of ministry of the Word	Healing special ministry with gifts of prophecy or discernment
To be offered to all with expectation of success	Offered to those who seek with possibility of failure
A valid method of evangelism	Related to the edification of the church
All 'ministers' should practice healing	Only those specifically called and gifted to do so
Effected by exercise of spiritual gifts	Effected by the prayer of faith
The work of individual healers	Work of Elders/Leaders in local church acting together
To be effected in private	To be exercised publicly in Healing Services
Medical treatment is normal, God-given means of healing	To be sought 1. After medical treatment exhausted 2. With medical treatment 3. Alternative to medical treatment

BIBLIOGRAPHY

Abbott, W. M.   *Documents of Vatican II*, G. Chapman, London, 1967.

Alexander, J. A.   *The Prophecies of Isaiah*, Wm. Collins, London, 1848.

Alford, Dean H.   *The Greek Testament Vol.II*, Rivingtons, London, 1857.

Amsler, S.   *Vocabulary of the Bible*, Ed. J-J Von Allmen, Lutterworth Press, London, 1958.

Andrews, H. T.   *Peake's Commentary on the Bible*, Nelson and Sons, London, 1919.

Barclay, O. R.   *Signs, Wonders and Healing*, Inter-Varsity Press, Leicester, 1989.

Barclay, Wm.   *And He had compassion on them*, Church of Scotland, Edinburgh, 1966.

Bertrin, Georges   *The Catholic Encyclopedia* Vol.9, The Encyclopedia Press, New York, 1910.

Bethune-Baker,
J. F.   *An Introduction to the Early History of Christian Doctrine*, Methuen, London, 1949.

Bittlinger, A.   *The Church is Charismatic*, WCC, Geneva, 1981.

Booth, H.   *Healing is Wholeness*, DSR Methodist Church, London, 1987.

Brooks, Noel   *Sickness, Health and God*, Advocate Press, USA, 1965.

Bruce, F. F.   *The Acts of the Apostles*, Tyndale Press, London, 1951.

Butlin, J. T.   *A Handbook of Divine Healing*, Marshall Brothers, London.

Calvin, John   *Calvin's Commentaries Vol.III, Epistle of James*, Saint Andrew Press, Edinburgh, 1972.

Calvin, John   *Institutes of the Christian Religion*, James Clarke & Co., London, 1949.

Carez, M.   *Vocabulary of the Bible*, Ed. J-J Von Allmen, Lutterworth Press, London, 1958.

Carson, H. M.   *Spiritual Gifts for Today?*, Kingsway Publications, Eastbourne, 1987.

Chafer, L. S.   *Satan*, Zondervan, Grand Rapids, USA, 1973.

Collins, Doris   *Positive Forces*, Grafton Books, London, 1990.

Coslett, N.   *His Healing Hands*, Hodder and Stoughton,

	London, 1985.
Creed, J. M.	*The Gospel according to St. Luke*, Macmillan, London, 1950.
Cressey, M. H.	*New Bible Dictionary*, IVF, London, 1962.
Dale, David	*Health and Healing* No.1, CCHH, London, 1989.
Dearmer, Percy	*Body and Soul*, Dutton, New York, 1923.
Duncan, Denis	*Health and Healing*, Saint Andrew Press, Edinburgh, 1988.
Edmunds, V. &	
Scorer, C. G.	*Some Thoughts on Faith Healing*, Tyndale Press, London, 1956.
Edwards, T. C.	*Commentary on First Corinthians*, 1885.
Foakes-Jackson,	
F. J.	*Peake's Commentary on the Bible*, Nelson and Sons, London, 1919.
Gardner, R.	*Healing Miracles*, Darton, Longman and Todd, London, 1988.
Glennon, J.	*Your Healing is Within You*, Hodder & Stoughton, London, 1969.
Gray, M.	*New Bible Dictionary*, IVF, London, 1962.
Gunstone, J.	*Signs and Wonders*, Darton, Longman and Todd, London, 1989.
Granberg-	
Michaelson, K.	*Healing Community*, Risk Book Series, WCC, Geneva, 1991.
Gwatkin, H. M.	*Selections from Early Christian Writers*, Macmillan & Co., London, 1929.
Hodge, A. A.	*Commentary on the Westminster Confession of Faith*, T. Nelson and Sons, London, 1870.
Holifield, E. B.	*Health and Medicine in the Methodist Tradition*, Crossroad, New York, 1986.
Hoskyns & Davey	*The Fourth Gospel*, Faber & Faber, London, 1948.
Inglis, B.	*Fringe Medicine*, Faber and Faber, London, 1964.
Irenaeus	*Adv. Haer. II*, cited by B. B. Warfield.
Jamieson,	
Fausset & Brown	*Commentary on the Whole Bible*, Oliphants, USA, 1966.
Jeffreys, G.	*The Miraculous Foursquare Gospel-Doctrinal*, Elim Publishing Co., London, 1929.
Jeffreys, G.	*The Miraculous Foursquare Gospel-Supernatural*, Elim Publishing Co., London, 1930.
Jeffreys, G.	*Pentecostal Rays*, Elim Publishing Co., London, 1933.
Jensen, P. and	

Payne, T.   *John Wimber, Friend or Foe?*, St. Matthias Press, London, 1990.

Kaye, Bishop J.   *The Ecclesiastical History of the Second and Third Centuries*, 1845, cited by B. B. Warfield.

Kirby, G. W.   *The Question of healing*, Victory Press, London, 1967.

Koch, K.   *Demonology Past and Present*, Kregel Publications, Grand Rapids, USA, 1981.

Lambourne, R. A.   *Community, Church and Healing*, Darton, Longman and Todd, London, 1963.

Lewis, C. S.   *Miracles*, Fontana Books, London, 1947.

Lightfoot, J. B.   *Commentary on Philippians*, Macmillan and Co., London, 1881.

Maddocks, M.   *The Christian Healing Ministry*, SPCK, London, 1981.

Marsh, Thomas   'A Theology of the Anointing of the Sick', *The Furrow*, Gill and Son, Dublin, 1978.

Marshall, N.   (cited by B. B. Warfield).

Martin, Bernard   *Healing for You*, Lutterworth Press, London, 1965.

Martin, R. P.   *Commentary on Philippians*, Tyndale Press, London, 1960.

Martyr, Justin   *Second Apology*, cited by P. Dearmer.

Mayor, J. B.   *The Epistle of St. James*, Macmillan and Co., London, 1910.

Morris, L. L.   *New Bible Dictionary*, IVF, London, 1962.

Morris, L. L.   *Commentary on I Corinthians*, Tyndale Press, London, 1958.

Macgregor,
G. H. C.   *The Gospel of John*, Hodder and Stoughton, London, 1928.

MacNutt, F.   *Healing*, Ave Maria Press, Indiana, 1975.

MacNutt, F.   *The Power to Heal*, Ave Maria Press, Indiana, 1977.

McNeile, A. H.   *The Gospel according to St. Matthew*, Macmillan, London, 1949.

Northridge, W. L.   *Psychology and Pastoral Practice*, Epworth Press, London, 1947.

Origen   *Con. Celsius, Bks I, III*, cited by P. Dearmer.

Orr, James   *The Christian View of God and the World*, Andrew Elliott, Edinburgh, 1902.

Osborne, T. L.   *Healing the Sick and Casting out Devils*, Voice of Faith Ministry, Inc., Tulsa, USA, 1953.

Parker, P. G.   *Divine Healing*, Victory Press, London, 1931.

Peake, A. S.   *Commentary on the Bible*, Nelson and Sons,

Peake, A. S.   London, 1919.
The Problem of Suffering in the Old Testament.

Peck, M. S.   *People of the Lie*, Rider, London, 1983.

Peddie, J. C.   *The Forgotten Talent*, Fontana Books, London, 1966.

Plummer, A.   *An Exegetical Commentary on the Gospel according to St. Matthew*, Robert Scott, London, 1928.

Plummer, A.   *Expositor's Bible St. James and St. Jude*, Hodder and Stoughton, London, 1891.

Pope, R. M.   *Hastings Dictionary of the Apostolic Church.*

Putman, W. G.   *New Bible Dictionary*, IVF, London, 1962.

Pytches, D.   *Some Said it Thundered*, Hodder and Stoughton, London, 1990.

Quadratus   c.126 cited by P. Dearmer.

Rackham, R. B.   *The Acts of the Apostles*, Methuen, London, 1947.

Rawlinson, A. E. J.   *The Gospel according to St. Mark*, Methuen, London, 1947.

Richards, J.   *The Question of Healing Services*, Daybreak, London, 1989.

Robertson, A. T.   *Word Pictures in the New Testament VI*, Broadman Press, Tennessee, 1933.

Robinson, H. W.   *Religious Ideas of the Old Testament*, Duckworth, London, 1947.

Ropes, J. H.   *ICC Commentary Epistle of James*, T. and T. Clark, Edinburgh, 1948.

Roux, H.   *Vocabulary of the Bible*, Ed. J-J Von Allmen, Lutterworth Press, London, 1958.

Salmond, S. D. F.   *Christian Doctrine of Immortality*, T. and T. Clark, Edinburgh, 1895.

Sanders, J. O.   *The Holy Spirit and His Gifts*, Marshall, Morgan and Scott, London, 1970.

Seventh-Day Adventism   *Questions on Doctrine*, Review and Herald Publishing Co., Washington D.C., 1957.

Simpson, A. B.   *The Gospel of Healing*, Morgan and Scott, London, 1915.

Springer, K.   *Riding the Third Wave*, Marshall Pickering, Basingstoke, 1987.

Stott, J. R. W.   *Baptism and Fullness*, IVP, Leicester, 1977.

Tasker, R. V. G.   *Tyndale NT Commentaries, Epistle of James*, Tyndale Press, London, 1957.

Tasker, R. V. G.   *Commentary on II Corinthians*, Tyndale Press,

London, 1958.
Taylor, J. V.   *The Go Between God*, SCM Press, London, 1972.
Taylor, W. M.   *The Miracles of our Saviour*, Hodder and
                    Stoughton, London, 1906.
Temple, Wm.   *Readings in St. John's Gospel*, Macmillan,
                    London, 1945.
Thurston, Herbert   *Encyclopedia of Religion and Ethics*, Vol.8.
Ulhorn, Gerhard   *The Conflict of Christianity with Heathenism.*
Wade, G. W.   *Peake's Commentary on the Bible*, Nelson and
                    Sons, London, 1919.
Warfield, B. B.   *Counterfeit Miracles*, Banner of Truth Trust,
                    London, 1972.
Watson, David   *Fear no Evil*, Hodder and Stoughton, Sevenoaks,
                    1984.
Weatherhead,
L. D.   *Psychology, Religion and Healing*, Hodder and
                    Stoughton, London, 1951.
Wilkinson, J.   *Health and Healing*, Handsel Press, Edinburgh,
                    1980.
Wilson, M.   *The Church is Healing*, SCM Press, London,
                    1966.
Wimber, J.   *Power Evangelism*, Hodder and Stoughton,
                    London, 1985.
Wimber, J.   *Power Healing*, Hodder and Stoughton, London,
                    1986.
Wimber, J.   *Practical Healing*, Hodder and Stoughton,
                    London, 1987.
Wiseman, D. J.   *New Bible Dictionary*, IVF, London, 1962.
Witherow, T.   *The Form of the Christian Temple*, T. and T. Clark,
                    Edinburgh, 1889.
Woodward, C.   *A Doctor heals by Faith*, Hodder and Stoughton,
                    London, 1964.
Wright, J. S.   *New Bible Dictionary*, IVF, London, 1962.
Wyman, F. L.   *The Dead are Raised Up*, Ken-Pax Publishing Co.,
                    Minehead, 1954.

Council of Trent Sess. 14, De Extrema Unctione.
Constitution and Government of the Presbyterian Church in Ireland,
        Belfast, 1980.
Pastoral Care of the Sick and Dying, Study Text 2, United States
        Catholic Conference, Washington, 1984.
Presbyterian Church in Ireland, General Assembly Reports, Belfast,
        1959.

Presbyterian Church in Ireland, General Assembly Belfast, 1982.
Shorter Catechism of Westminster Assembly of Divines, J. G. Eccles, Inverness, 1981.
Westminster Confession of Faith, J. G. Eccles, Inverness, 1981.
The Ministry of Healing—Report of Lambeth Conference on Healing 1920, SPCK, London, 1924.
The Healing Church, World Council Studies No.3, WCC, Geneva, 1965.
Healing and Wholeness—The Churches' Role in Health—Christian Medical Commission, WCC, Geneva, 1990.
The Church and the Ministry of Healing—A Methodist Statement, 1977.
Health and Healing Bulletin Issue 21, The Methodist Church, London, 1991.

SCRIPTURE INDEX

1:50	39	2:22	300
2:11	18, 98, 198	2:43	300
2:23	300	2:43, 44	65
3:14	45	2:46	286
4:48	18, 107, 299	2:47	68
4:52, 53	11, 15	3:1–10	32
4:54	18, 198	3:1ff	195, 200
5:1–9	82, 103, 214	3:8	240
5:1–9, 14	82	3:21	118
5:1–16	10	4:16	38
5:3	10	4:27	88
5:7, 8	16	4:29, 30	38, 303
5:14	200, 297	4:30	98, 300
5:20	39	5:12	300
5:28, 29	118	5:15	33, 35, 36, 39
6:14	107	5:16	99
7:31	300	5:41	109, 195, 241
9	195	7:22	52
9:2	48, 198	7:36	300
9:3	43	7:49	12
9:6	16, 200	8:4–8	195
9:7	10	8:6, 7	99
10:10	49	8:9	275
11:4	18	8:9, 11	99
11:40	18	8:9, 23	63
11:44	15	8:11	63
14:2, 3	120	8:13	300
14:11	19, 38	8:13–24	29
14:12	38, 249	9	120
14:13	40	9:17	32
14:16–18	39	9:32–43	200
16:13	35	10:38	88
16:14	304	10:42	31
16:23f	39	11:30	86
20:22, 23	195	12:5	303
20:30, 31	17	13:2, 3	30
21:15–19	195	13:6	61, 63
21:25	5	13:8–11	63
		13:36	118
Acts		14:3	300
1:8	31, 39, 41, 195	14:8, 9	195
1:21, 22	73	14:23	30, 215
1:25	118	15:2	86
2:19	300	15:12	300

SUBJECT INDEX